Consultations in Liver Disease

Editor

STEVEN L. FLAMM

CLINICS IN
LIVER DISEASE

www.liver.theclinics.com

Consulting Editor
NORMAN GITLIN

August 2020 • Volume 24 • Number 3

ELSEVIER

1600 John F. Kennedy Boulevard • Suite 1800 • Philadelphia, Pennsylvania, 19103-2899

http://www.theclinics.com

CLINICS IN LIVER DISEASE Volume 24, Number 3
August 2020 ISSN 1089-3261, ISBN-13: 978-0-323-71068-8

Editor: Kerry Holland
Developmental Editor: Donald Mumford

Clinics in Liver Disease (ISSN 1089-3261) is published quarterly by Elsevier Inc., 360 Park Avenue South, New York, NY 10010-1710. Months of issue are February, May, August, and November. Business and Editorial Offices: 1600 John F. Kennedy Blvd., Ste. 1800, Philadelphia, PA 19103-2899. Customer Service Office: 3251 Riverport Lane, Maryland Heights, MO 63043. Periodicals postage paid at New York, NY and additional mailing offices. Subscription prices are $313.00 per year (U.S. individuals), $100.00 per year (U.S. student/resident), $572.00 per year (U.S. institutions), $409.00 per year (international individuals), $200.00 per year (international student/resident), $709.00 per year (international instiiutions), $343.00 per year (Canadian individuals), $100.00 per year (Canadian student/resident), and $709.00 per year (Canadian institutions). Foreign air speed delivery is included in all *Clinics* subscription prices. All prices are subject to change without notice. **POSTMASTER:** Send address changes to *Clinics in Liver Disease*, Elsevier Health Sciences Division, Subscription Customer Service, 3251 Riverport Lane, Maryland Heights, MO 63043. **Customer Service: Telephone: 1-800-654-2452 (U.S. and Canada); 314-447-8871 (outside U.S. and Canada). Fax: 314-447-8029. E-mail: journalscustomer service-usa@elsevier.com (for print support); journalsonlinesupport-usa@elsevier.com (for online support).**

Reprints. For copies of 100 or more of articles in this publication, please contact the Commercial Reprints Department, Elsevier Inc., 360 Park Avenue South, New York, NY 10010-1710. Tel.: 212-633-3874; Fax: 212-633-3820; E-mail: reprints@elsevier.com.

Clinics in Liver Disease is covered in *MEDLINE/PubMed (Index Medicus)*, Science Citation Index Expanded, Journal Citation Reports/Science Edition, and Current Contents/Clinical Medicine.

Contributors

CONSULTING EDITOR

NORMAN GITLIN, MD, FRCP (LONDON), FRCPE (EDINBURGH), FAASLD, FACP, FACG
Head of Hepatology, Southern California Liver Centers, San Clemente, California, USA

EDITOR

STEVEN L. FLAMM, MD
Chief, Hepatology Program, Professor, Department of Medicine, Division of Gastroenterology and Hepatology, Northwestern University Feinberg School of Medicine, Chicago, Illinois, USA

AUTHORS

ARIEL ADAY, MD
Assistant Professor and Associate Program Director for GI Fellowship, The University of Texas Southwestern Medical Center, Dallas, Texas, USA

JOSEPH AHN, MD
Professor of Medicine, Division of Gastroenterology and Hepatology, Oregon Health & Science University, Portland, Oregon, USA

JASMOHAN S. BAJAJ, MD, MS
Division of Gastroenterology, Hepatology and Nutrition, Virginia Commonwealth University, McGuire VA Medical Center, Richmond, Virginia, USA

JUSTIN R. BOIKE, MD, MPH
Assistant Professor, Department of Medicine, Northwestern University Feinberg School of Medicine, Chicago, Illinois, USA

ROBERT S. BROWN JR, MD, MPH
Gladys and Roland Harriman Professor of Medicine, Division of Gastroenterology and Hepatology, NewYork-Presbyterian/Weill Cornell Medical College, New York, New York, USA

ADAM P. BUCKHOLZ, MD
Gastroenterology Fellow, Division of Gastroenterology and Hepatology, NewYork-Presbyterian/Weill Cornell Medical College, New York, New York, USA

AMANDA CHEUNG, MD
Clinical Assistant Professor of Medicine, Division of Gastroenterology and Hepatology, Stanford University School of Medicine, Palo Alto, California, USA

AUDREY DEEKEN-DRAISEY, MD
Department of Pathology, Northwestern University Feinberg School of Medicine, Northwestern Memorial Hospital, Chicago, Illinois, USA

SIRINA EKPANYAPONG, MD
Department of Medicine, Division of Gastroenterology and Hepatology, Vejthani Hospital, Bangkok, Thailand

STEVEN L. FLAMM, MD
Chief, Hepatology Program, Professor, Department of Medicine, Division of Gastroenterology and Hepatology, Northwestern University Feinberg School of Medicine, Chicago, Illinois, USA

GUADALUPE GARCIA-TSAO, MD
Professor of Medicine, Section of Digestive Diseases, Yale School of Medicine, New Haven, Connecticut, USA; Chief, Section of Digestive Diseases, VA Connecticut Healthcare System, West Haven, Connecticut, USA

KENNETH B. GORDON, MD
Professor and Chair, Department of Dermatology, Medical College of Wisconsin, Milwaukee, Wisconsin, USA

LAMIA Y.K. HAQUE, MD, MPH
Fellow, Section of Digestive Diseases, Yale School of Medicine, New Haven, Connecticut, USA

SOFIA SIMONA JAKAB, MD
Associate Professor of Medicine, Section of Digestive Diseases, Yale School of Medicine, New Haven, Connecticut, USA; Section of Digestive Diseases, VA Connecticut Healthcare System, West Haven, Connecticut, USA

KIMBERLY KATZ, MD
Department of Dermatology, Medical College of Wisconsin, Milwaukee, Wisconsin, USA

KRIS V. KOWDLEY, MD, AGAF, FAASLD, FACG, FACP
Seattle, Washington, USA

PAUL KWO, MD
Professor of Medicine, Division of Gastroenterology and Hepatology, Stanford University School of Medicine, Palo Alto, California, USA

JOSEPH K. LIM, MD
Professor of Medicine, Yale Liver Center, Section of Digestive Diseases, Yale School of Medicine, New Haven, Connecticut, USA

VIGNAN MANNE, MD
Sunrise Health Consortium GME, Las Vegas, Nevada, USA

LAUREN MYERS, PA-C
Instructor of Medicine, Division of Gastroenterology and Hepatology, Oregon Health & Science University, Portland, Oregon, USA

KATHY M. NILLES, MD
Division of Gastroenterology and Hepatology, MedStar Georgetown Transplant Institute, Georgetown University School of Medicine, Washington, DC, USA

JACQUELINE G. O'LEARY, MD, MPH
Associate Professor of Medicine, The University of Texas Southwestern Medical Center, Chief of Hepatology, Dallas Veterans Affairs Medical Center, Dallas, Texas, USA

ASHAKI D. PATEL, MD
Department of Dermatology, Medical College of Wisconsin, Milwaukee, Wisconsin, USA

SAMBASIVA M. RAO, MD
Department of Pathology, Northwestern University Feinberg School of Medicine, Northwestern Memorial Hospital, Chicago, Illinois, USA

K. RAJENDER REDDY, MD
Department of Medicine, Division of Gastroenterology and Hepatology, Ruimy Family President's Distinguished Professor of Medicine, University of Pennsylvania, Philadelphia, Pennsylvania, USA

BRADLEY REUTER, MD
Division of Gastroenterology, Hepatology and Nutrition, Virginia Commonwealth University, McGuire VA Medical Center, Richmond, Virginia, USA

GUANG-YU YANG, MD, PhD
Department of Pathology, Northwestern University Feinberg School of Medicine, Northwestern Memorial Hospital, Chicago, Illinois, USA

Contents

Hepatitis B virus (HBV) reactivation, in the background of cleared and overt chronic HBV infection, can be seen in patients receiving immunosuppressive agents. Risk of reactivation is variably associated with HBV serologic status and types of immunosuppressive therapy. Prevention of HBV reactivation by antiviral prophylaxis is an effective strategy to reduce morbidity and mortality in those with immunocompromised states. This article defines HBV reactivation, discusses risk stratification and common medications that can induce HBV reactivation as well as guideline recommendations for prevention of HBV reactivation, and describes the prognosis and management of patients who experience HBV reactivation.

Variceal bleeding is a complication of cirrhosis that defines decompensation. Important advances in the management of gastroesophageal varices have led to a significant decrease in the morbidity and mortality. Achieving these results in clinical practice is contingent on clinicians applying the best practice strategies and appropriate referral to a tertiary center. Several quality metrics were developed by the American Association for the Study of Liver Diseases. This article aims to update outpatient and inpatient strategies to include the latest recommendations on variceal screening and surveillance, primary and secondary prophylaxis of variceal bleeding, and therapy for patients with acute variceal bleeding.

Given the visibility of cutaneous findings, skin manifestations are often a presenting symptom of underlying systemic disease, including chronic liver disease. Many cutaneous signs and symptoms that correlate with chronic liver disease are common physical examination findings in patients with no history of liver disease. It is nonetheless important to be aware that these cutaneous findings may be an indication of underlying liver disease and often occur in the setting of such hepatic dysfunction. This article covers general cutaneous signs that may correlate with various liver diseases and describes specific cutaneous signs as they relate to more specific liver diseases.

Liver biopsy and histologic examination are the mainstay for diagnosing liver diseases, despite advances in imaging and molecular procedures. Liver biopsy can provide useful information regarding the structural integrity and type and degree of injury, disease activity, response to treatment, progression of disease and degree/staging of fibrosis. Liver biopsies evaluate acute and chronic liver diseases, and mass-forming lesions. The role of the pathologist is to integrate clinical, serologic, and biochemical data with morphologic changes and provide a comprehensive diagnosis. This review focuses on basic principles necessary for proper interpretation of liver biopsy specimens in patients with chronic liver disease.

Transjugular intrahepatic portosystemic shunts is an established treatment for portal hypertensive complications. Advancements in technology and technique have led to novel indications, including treatment of chronic portal vein thrombosis and use before abdominal surgery to alleviate portal hypertensive complications. Use of TIPS can facilitate the embolization of large portal-systemic shunts to alleviate refractory hepatic encephalopathy owing to excessive portal shunting. Despite these advances, transjugular intrahepatic portosystemic shunts is an invasive procedure with risk for complications and should be performed at a center with expertise to ensure a successful patient outcome.

Focal nodular hyperplasia and hepatocellular adenoma are benign liver lesions that occur most frequently in women and may be found as incidental findings on imaging. Hepatocellular adenomas may be infrequently associated with malignant progression or risk of rupture and as such, require surveillance or definitive treatments based on their size threshold. It is important clinically to differentiate these lesions, and utilizing imaging modalities such as contrast enhanced ultrasound or magnetic resonance imaging can be helpful in diagnosis. Further molecular subtyping of hepatocellular adenoma lesions may be beneficial to describe risk factors and potential future clinical complications.

Viral hepatitis can cause a wide spectrum of clinical presentations from a benign form with minimal or no symptoms to acute liver failure or death. Hepatitis D coinfection and superinfection have distinct clinical courses, with the latter more likely leading to chronic infection. Management of chronic hepatitis D virus is individualized because of the paucity of treatment options and significant side effect profile of currently available treatments. Sporadic cases of hepatitis E caused by contaminated meats are becoming increasingly prevalent in immunocompromised hosts. Human herpesviruses are an important cause of disease also in immunocompromised individuals.

Cholangiocarcinoma: Diagnosis and Management

Adam P. Buckholz and Robert S. Brown Jr.

Cholangiocarcinoma is a highly lethal biliary epithelial tumor that is rare in the general population but has increased rates in patients with primary sclerosing cholangitis (PSC). It is heterogenous, and management varies by location. No effective prevention exists, and screening is likely only feasible in PSC. Patients often present in an advanced state with jaundice, weight loss, and cholestatic liver enzymes. Diagnosis requires imaging with magnetic resonance cholangiopancreatography, laboratory testing, and endoscopic retrograde cholangiopancreatography. Potentially curative options include resection and liver transplant with neoadjuvant or adjuvant chemoradiation. Chemotherapy, radiation, and locoregional therapy provide some survival benefit in unresectable disease.

Thrombocytopenia in Chronic Liver Disease: New Management Strategies

Kathy M. Nilles and Steven L. Flamm

Thrombocytopenia is common in advanced liver disease, and such patients frequently need invasive procedures. Numerous mechanisms for thrombocytopenia exist, including splenic sequestration and reduction of levels of the platelet growth factor thrombopoietin. Traditionally, platelet transfusions have been used to increase platelet counts before elective procedures, usually to a threshold of greater than or equal to 50,000/μL, but levels vary by provider, procedure, and specific patient. Recently, the thrombopoietin receptor agonists avatrombopag and lusutrombopag were studied and found efficacious for increasing platelet count in the outpatient setting for select patients with advanced liver disease who need a procedure.

Budd-Chiari Syndrome: An Uncommon Cause of Chronic Liver Disease that Cannot Be Missed

Lamia Y.K. Haque and Joseph K. Lim

Budd-Chiari syndrome (BCS), or hepatic venous outflow obstruction, is a rare cause of liver disease that should not be missed. Variable clinical presentation among patients with BCS necessitates a high index of suspicion to avoid missing this life-threatening diagnosis. BCS is characterized as primary or secondary, depending on etiology of venous obstruction. Most patients with primary BCS have several contributing risk factors leading to a prothrombotic state. A multidisciplinary stepwise approach is integral in treating BCS. Lifelong anticoagulation is recommended. Long-term monitoring of patients for development of cirrhosis, complications of portal hypertension, hepatocellular carcinoma, and progression of underlying diseases is important.

Alpha1-antitrypsin deficiency (A1ATD) is an inherited cause of chronic liver disease. It is inherited in an autosomal codominant pattern with each inherited allele expressed in the formation of the final protein, which is primarily produced in hepatocytes. The disease usually occurs in pediatric and elderly populations. The disease occurs with the accumulation of abnormal protein polymers within hepatocytes that can induce liver injury and fibrosis. It is a commonly under-recognized and underdiagnosed condition. Patients diagnosed with the disease should be regularly monitored for the development of liver disease. Liver transplant is of proven benefit in A1ATD liver disease.

The gut microbiome is an exciting new area of research in chronic liver disease. It has shown promise in expanding our understanding of these complicated disease processes and has opened up new treatment modalities. The aim of this review is to increase understanding of the microbiome and explain the collection and analysis process in the context of liver disease. It also looks at our current understanding of the role of the microbiome in the wide spectrum of chronic liver diseases and how it is being used in current therapies and treatments.

Acute on chronic liver failure (ACLF) is an inflammation-based disorder that occurs in patients with underlying liver disease and is characterized by hepatic and extrahepatic organ failure. Morbidity and mortality are high in patients with ACLF, and therefore prevention and early identification are critical to improve outcome. The purpose of this article is to define ACLF, describe ways to identify the expected outcome of ACLF after development, and illustrate interventions to prevent it and when it is not preventable reduce associated morbidity and mortality.

CLINICS IN LIVER DISEASE

FORTHCOMING ISSUES

November 2020
**Hepatocellular Carcinoma: Moving
Into the 21st Century**
Catherine Frenette, *Editor*

February 2021
Liver Transplantation
David Goldberg, *Editor*

May 2021
Complications of Cirrhosis
Andres Cardenas and Thomas Reiberger,
Editors

RECENT ISSUES

May 2020
Hepatic Encephalopathy
Vinod K. Rustgi, *Editor*

February 2020
Drug Hepatotoxicity
Pierre M. Gholam, *Editor*

November 2019
Portal Hypertension
Sammy Saab, *Editor*

THE CLINICS ARE AVAILABLE ONLINE!
Access your subscription at:
www.theclinics.com

Preface

Consultations in Liver Disease

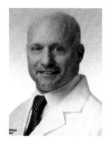

Steven L. Flamm, MD
Editor

Community practitioners in the field of Gastroenterology are frequently consulted to evaluate inpatients and outpatients with acute and chronic liver issues. Many of the medical problems are complex, and recent advances in the field may be difficult to follow for busy providers. This issue of *Clinics in Liver Disease* on Consultations in Liver Disease is the fourth in a series dedicated to supporting community providers with pertinent clinical information about consultations that are commonly encountered in community practice. The first issue, "Approaches to Consultation for Patients with Liver Disease," was published in May 2012, and the second and third, each entitled "Consultations in Liver Disease," were published in February 2015 and November 2017, respectively. These issues present concise, clinically oriented reviews of complicated topics with an emphasis on diagnosis and management. In this issue, additional topics have been selected to help practitioners care for patients with liver-related problems.

Reactivation of chronic hepatitis B virus infection has been increasingly recognized as a problem with potentially severe consequences and has been observed more frequently in the age of immunotherapy for various disease states. Drs Ekpanyapong and Reddy discuss the contemporary approach to evaluation and management of patients in this setting.

Bleeding from esophagogastric varices continues to be a frightening complication of cirrhosis. Management of patients with varices is guided by recommendations that are routinely updated. Drs Jakab and Garcia-Tsao detail the current practice strategies.

Many patients with liver disease have dermatologic manifestations. Drs Patel, Katz, and Gordon discuss commonly encountered dermatologic problems observed in such patients. In addition, one of the central modalities in the diagnosis of the cause of liver disease is histologic evaluation. Common pathologic terms and presentations are reviewed by Drs Deeken-Draisey, Rao, and Yang.

Clin Liver Dis 24 (2020) xiii–xiv
https://doi.org/10.1016/j.cld.2020.05.001
1089-3261/20/© 2020 Published by Elsevier Inc.

liver.theclinics.com

Transjugular transhepatic portosystemic shunts have been used for more than 20 years in patients with certain complications of end-stage liver disease. There are emerging data on newer uses for the procedure, and they are reviewed by Dr Boike and me.

Benign liver lesions are frequently identified on abdominal imaging. Distinguishing between focal nodular hyperplasia and hepatic adenoma is an important but difficult distinction because the management is different. Ms Myers and Dr Ahn discuss the approach to evaluation of such benign liver lesions.

Patients with elevated liver enzymes are commonly encountered in practice. Viral hepatitis is always a consideration. The common hepatitis virus infections (A, B, and C) are generally easy to diagnose. However, viral hepatitis from other viruses is not uncommon and yet is difficult for the community practitioner. Drs Cheung and Kwo review the causes of non-A, -B, and -C viral hepatitis.

Cholangiocarcinoma (intrahepatic and extrahepatic) is a grave diagnosis. Drs Buckholz and Brown review the approach to evaluation and management of this condition.

Severe thrombocytopenia is frequently observed in the setting of advanced liver disease. There have been recent advances in the management of severe thrombocytopenia in patients with cirrhosis who are undergoing elective procedures. These advances are discussed by Dr Nilles and me.

Budd-Chiari and alpha-1 antitrypsin deficiency are uncommon problems seen in patients with liver disease. However, it is important not to miss either diagnosis. Drs Haque and Lim detail the approach to evaluation and management of Budd-Chiari, and Drs Manne and Kowdley discuss alpha-1 antitrypsin deficiency.

An evolving area of investigation in the field of hepatology is the understanding of the effects of the microbiome on patients with chronic liver disease. It is expected that the therapeutic landscape in patients with chronic liver disease will eventually involve the microbiome. Drs Reuter and Bajaj discuss this important topic.

Finally, acute on chronic liver failure is a relatively new concept for which there have been increasing data. Inpatient consultation for providers who care for patients with liver disease is not uncommon for this entity. Drs Aday and O'Leary elaborate on this topic.

This issue of *Clinics in Liver Disease* complements the previous issues by introducing additional important clinical topics that help the community practitioner evaluate and manage common problems observed in the inpatient and outpatient setting.

Once again, I would like to thank Dr Norman Gitlin for offering me the opportunity to serve as the editor for this issue of *Clinics in Liver Disease*. Furthermore, I would like to thank Kerry Holland and Donald Mumford for their enthusiastic support in preparing the articles for publication.

Steven L. Flamm, MD
Division of Gastroenterology and Hepatology
Northwestern University
Feinberg School of Medicine
676 North St Clair, 19th Floor
Chicago, IL 60611, USA

E-mail address:
s-flamm@northwestern.edu

Hepatitis B Virus Reactivation

What Is the Issue, and How Should It Be Managed?

Sirina Ekpanyapong, MD[a], K. Rajender Reddy, MD[b],*

KEYWORDS

- Hepatitis B virus • Reactivation • Immunosuppression • Hepatitis flare
- Antiviral prophylaxis

KEY POINTS

- Hepatitis B virus (HBV) reactivation is not uncommon in patients receiving immunosuppressive therapy, which can then lead to serious complication such as hepatitis flare, hepatic decompensation, and hepatic failure.
- Prevention of HBV reactivation by antiviral prophylaxis in patients who are planned to receive immunosuppressive agents is an effective strategy to reduce morbidity and mortality caused by HBV reactivation.
- Risk of HBV reactivation can be classified into low- (<1%), moderate- (1%–10%), and high-risk (>10%) groups according to HBV serologic status and types of immunosuppressive therapy.
- All patients who are candidates for chemotherapy or immunosuppressive therapy should be screened for HBV serologic status before initiating treatment. Patients with moderate-to-high risk for HBV reactivation should be considered for antiviral prophylaxis.
- Every immunosuppressed patient who develops HBV reactivation (with or without hepatitis flare) should be treated with a high barrier to resistance antiviral agent as early as possible. However, despite initiation of antiviral treatment, some patients may still develop hepatic decompensation or hepatic failure.

INTRODUCTION

Hepatitis B virus (HBV) reactivation can be precipitated following the use of immunosuppressive agents and chemotherapy and can be a serious manifestation. HBV

[a] Department of Medicine, Division of Gastroenterology and Hepatology, Vejthani Hospital, 1 Soi Lat Phrao 111, Khlong Chan, Bang Kapi District, Bangkok 10240, Thailand; [b] Department of Medicine, Division of Gastroenterology and Hepatology, University of Pennsylvania, 3400 Spruce Street, 2 Dulles HUP, Philadelphia, PA 19104, USA
* Corresponding author.
E-mail address: ReddyR@pennmedicine.upenn.edu

Clin Liver Dis 24 (2020) 317–333
https://doi.org/10.1016/j.cld.2020.04.002
1089-3261/20/© 2020 Elsevier Inc. All rights reserved.

liver.theclinics.com

reactivation commonly occurs in hepatitis B surface antigen (HBsAg)-positive patients, but also can be encountered in those with a positive antibody to hepatitis B core antigen (anti-HBc) while they are HBsAg-negative.[1] Although there is lack of consistency on the definition of HBV reactivation, it can be defined as virologic, biochemical, or clinical, although most often there is an overlap of various features. Reactivation initially is characterized by a sudden rise of HBV DNA, which can be followed by a hepatitis flare (defined by an elevation of alanine transaminase [ALT] levels ± bilirubin) several weeks after.[2] Therapeutic interventions that can induce HBV reactivation have increased over the past few years, while B cell-depleting agents, such as rituximab, remain the cornerstone for their frequent association with HBV reactivation. Corticosteroid is another drug that is commonly used in combination with immunosuppressive regimens, although the dosage and duration of corticosteroid treatments may affect the risk of HBV reactivation. In addition, a non-cancer drug class such as tumor necrosis factor (TNF) inhibitors can also induce HBV reactivation, a concern among physicians when treating inflammatory bowel disease or rheumatologic diseases.[3] As a consequence of HBV reactivation, there is associated severe morbidity and high mortality because of hepatic decompensation and hepatic failure.[4] Prevention of HBV reactivation is necessary in order to reduce the risk of morbidity and mortality in patients who are targeted to receive immunosuppressive agents. This article discusses the heterogeneous definitions, the risk of reactivation with a spectrum of immunosuppressive and cancer chemotherapeutic agents, the risk with targeted biologics, guideline recommendations for the prevention of HBV reactivation, and the prognosis and management of HBV reactivation.

DEFINITION OF HEPATITIS B VIRUS REACTIVATION

The updated American Association for the Study of Liver Diseases (AASLD) guideline recommendation on prevention, diagnosis, and treatment of chronic hepatitis B 2018 defined HBV reactivation in HBsAg-positive, anti-HBc positive patients as any of the following[2]: (1) at least 2 log (or 100-fold) increase in HBV DNA compared with the baseline level, (2) HBV DNA at least 3 log (or 1000) IU/mL in a patient with previously undetectable HBV DNA, or (3) HBV DNA at least 4 log (or 10,000) IU/mL if the baseline level is not available.

For HBsAg-negative, anti-HBc positive patients, HBV reactivation is defined as[2] detectable HBV DNA or reverse HBsAg seroconversion or reappearance of HBsAg. A clinical hepatitis flare is defined as an ALT rising to at least 3 times the baseline level and greater than 100 U/L.

Some individuals with HBV reactivation are asymptomatic with a normal hepatic biochemical profile, while some can have a flare of HBV infection with increased aminotransferase levels. However, a hepatitis flare can be with or without clinical signs and symptoms (such as nausea and vomiting), but severe flare can be associated with hepatic decompensation, jaundice, and poor outcome, especially in patients with underlying cirrhosis.[5]

NATURAL HISTORY OF HEPATITIS B VIRUS REACTIVATION

Hepatitis B virus (HBV) can infect individuals and lead to acute infection or chronic infection and the latter especially when exposed to the virus in infancy and childhood. HBV virus enters the hepatocytes via the sodium-taurocholate cotransporter (NTCP) receptor.[6] After viral entry, it releases double-stranded viral genomes that are then transported into the nucleus. In the nucleus, viral genomes are repaired by polymerase enzymes into covalently closed circular DNA (cccDNA). The cccDNA is stabilized in

HBV-infected hepatocytes that can then persist as a latent state and serve as a reservoir for HBV reactivation despite evidence for recovery as denoted by the development of anti-HBs.[7] Treatment with nucleoside/nucleotide analogue (NA) can suppress HBV DNA, but cccDNA still remains after several years of treatment.[1,8]

Specific CD4+ and CD8+ T cells target HBV infected cells for viral elimination via cytopathic mechanisms and suppress viral replication via noncytopathic cytokine-mediated pathways.[9] The activated B cells produce neutralizing antibodies that contribute to viral clearance. Although these immune responses can control active HBV replication, they are not potent enough to eliminate cccDNA. Thus, these infected cells serve as a reservoir for HBV reactivation when the immune mechanisms are suppressed.[1] The various types of chemotherapies and immunosuppressive agents may variably be associated with potential risks of reactivation differently.

The evolution of HBV reactivation can be classified into stages[1]:

- Viral replication: After immunosuppression, HBV DNA may increase and patient may still be asymptomatic and without aspartate transaminase (AST) or alanine transaminase (ALT) elevation.
- HBV-reactivation related hepatitis (hepatitis flare): A few days to weeks after viral replication, AST and ALT levels start rising up to 5 to 10 times from baseline levels. Patients may experience constitutional symptom and jaundice; however, some may remain asymptomatic.
- Resolution: Some patients can have spontaneous improvement after hepatitis flare after cessation of immunosuppressive agents. However, if HBV reactivation is recognized, starting antiviral therapy can also lead to decline in HBV DNA levels, amelioration of immune-mediated injury of HBV infected hepatocytes, and subsequent resolution of hepatitis flare.
- Liver failure: A minority of patients may have progressive decline in hepatic function and end up with hepatic decompensation or liver failure despite initiation of antiviral agents. These clinical manifestations may lead to significant morbidity and mortality. Unfortunately, liver transplantation, although it would be considered the logical rescue strategy, might present a contraindication because of the uncertain course and prognosis of the underlying conditions of lymphoma or other malignancy, which are the basis for immunosuppressive treatment that has led to HBV reactivation (**Fig. 1**).

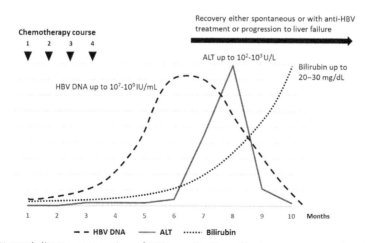

Fig. 1. Natural disease progression of HBV reactivation after immunosuppressive therapy.

A recent retrospective multicenter study (n = 156) from the Acute Liver Failure Study Group (ALFSG) noted that 18% of HBV-associated acute liver failure (ALF) occurred after receiving immunosuppressive therapy. Survival beyond 21 days in patients with HBV-associated ALF after immunosuppression was significantly lower than in nonimmunosuppression HBV-associated ALF.[10] Another systematic review and meta-analysis in patients with solid tumors receiving chemotherapy had demonstrated that without prophylaxis, there was a 23% (range 2%–60%) risk of HBV-related hepatitis and chemotherapy interruption, a 2% (range 1%–20%) risk of HBV-related acute liver failure, and a 2.3% (range 0.4%–20%) mortality risk.[11]

RISK STRATIFICATION OF HEPATITIS B VIRUS REACTIVATION
Status of Hepatitis B Serology

HBsAg-positive
Patients who are HBsAg positive are at higher risk for HBV reactivation than those with HBsAg-negative and anti-HBc positive serologic status. HBsAg-positive patients with HBeAg-positive and/or high baseline HBV DNA levels may have highest risk of hepatitis B virus reactivation, with the highest risk being in those with an HBV DNA of greater than 10^5 copies/mL (approximately 10^4 IU/mL).[12]

HBsAg-negative with anti-HBc positive
These are patients with resolved HBV infection who may also present a risk for reactivation when receiving immunosuppressive therapy, especially including a regimen containing an anti-CD20 (eg, rituximab)[13] or from hematopoietic stem cell transplantation with high predictors of HBV reactivation that include age of at least 50 years (P=.004, hazard ratio[HR] = 8.2) and chronic graft-versus-host disease (P=.010, HR = 5.3).[14]

Of note, based on available data, it is unclear if anti-HBs is protective against HBV reactivation.[15] However, it does appear that patients with detectable anti-HBs have a lower risk of reactivation.[15,16] A prospective study from Taiwan on chemotherapy-induced HBV reactivation in lymphoma patients with resolved HBV infection had noted that HBV reactivation occurred in 9 of 116 (7.8%) patients with positive anti-HBs, and in 8 of 34 (23.5%) patients with negative anti-HBs.[15] Another prospective study from Taiwan also found that quantification of anti-HBc and anti-HBs may help predict HBV reactivation risk in patients with lymphoma; patients with both high anti-HBc ($\geq$6.41 IU/mL) and low anti-HBs (<56.48 mIU/mL) at baseline had higher risk of reactivation (HR = 17.29; P < .001).[16]

Types of Immunosuppressive Therapy

Anti-CD20 agents (eg, rituximab and ofatumumab)
Anti-CD20 agents (eg, rituximab and ofatumumab) are B cell-depleting agents used to treat hematologic malignancies. Rituximab is a CD20-directed cytolytic monoclonal antibody indicated for the treatment of various conditions, including non-Hodgkin's lymphoma (NHL), chronic lymphocytic leukemia (CLL), and rheumatoid arthritis (RA) in combination with methotrexate in adult patients with moderately to severely active RA who have inadequate response to one or more TNF antagonist therapies, and granulomatosis with polyangiitis (GPA) (Wegener granulomatosis) and microscopic polyangiitis (MPA), in adult patients in combination with glucocorticoids.[17] Ofatumumab is indicated in combination with chlorambucil, for the treatment of previously untreated patients with CLL for whom fludarabine-based therapy is considered inappropriate, recurrent or progressive CLL, or patients with CLL refractory to fludarabine.[18] According to an US Food and Drug Administration (US-FDA) warning,

rituximab and ofatumumab are associated with increased risk of HBV reactivation in patients with HBsAg-positive and/or anti-HBc positive serologic status. The incidence of HBV reactivation following rituximab use has ranged from 3% to 55%.[19] Risk factors that are associated with high probability of HBV reactivation include HBsAg-positivity with active HBV replication (positive HBV DNA), male sex, HBeAg positivity, lack of anti-HBs, anthracycline/steroid use, younger age, and pre-existing hepatic biochemical test abnormalities.[19–21] The overall mortality rate from reactivation is reported to be as high as 30% to 60%.[20,22] A recent study from Japan in HBsAg-negative, anti-HBc positive patients receiving obinutuzumab or rituximab-containing immunochemotherapy (n = 326) (phase 3 GOYA and GALLIUM studies) noted HBV reactivation in around 8.2% of cases, occurring at a median of 125 days (IQR 85-331) after the first dose.[23] In 232 patients without prophylactic NA, 10.8% had HBV reactivation, while in 94 patients with prophylactic NA use, 2.1% had HBV reactivation. Prophylactic NA was significantly associated with a reduced risk of HBV reactivation (adjusted HR = 0.09; 95% confidence interval [CI] 0.02-0.41; P=.0018).[23]

Anthracyclines (eg, doxorubicin and epirubicin)

Anthracycline-containing chemotherapy regimens are commonly used in treatment for breast cancer, ovarian cancer, lymphoma, and Kaposi sarcoma.[24] This drug class has been associated with a significant risk of HBV reactivation in chronic hepatitis B.[3] The mechanism is believed to be associated with regulatory factor X box 1 gene (RFX1) expression[25] and the activation of ataxia-telangiectasia mutated (ATM), ATM-, and RAD3-related (ATR) transcription.[26] An increasing trend for surveillance and HBV prophylaxis started after Yeo W and colleagues demonstrated HBV reactivation risk in HBsAg-positive breast cancer patients (n = 41) receiving cytotoxic chemotherapy (anthracycline-containing regimens were also included).[27] Forty-one percent developed HBV reactivation, and 71% of the patients who developed reactivation encountered premature termination of chemotherapy.[27] Lamivudine prophylaxis in HBV carrier breast cancer patients receiving adjuvant chemotherapy (n = 165) (80% anthracycline-containing regimens) was associated with significantly lower incidence of hepatotoxicity than in those who were not on prophylaxis (2.7 vs 14.1%, P=.011) and with fewer premature terminations of planned adjuvant chemotherapy (0 vs 10.9%, P=.004).[28] Accordingly, the American Gastroenterological Association (AGA) guideline recommends antiviral prophylaxis for chronic hepatitis B patients treated with anthracycline derivatives as they are deemed to be at high risk for HBV reactivation.[3,29]

Glucocorticoids

Corticosteroids enhance HBV replication by 2 mechanisms: depressed cytotoxic T-cell function and direct stimulation of HBV genomic sequence.[3] Once glucocorticoids are administered, HBV replication tends to increase, while serum aminotransferase tends to decline.[30] Subsequently when glucocorticoids are withdrawn, HBV replication declines (presumably because of immune system rebound), while serum aminotransferase increases (often peaking at around 4 to 6 weeks after withdrawal).[30,31] In HBsAg-positive individuals receiving corticosteroids, there is evidence of HBV reactivation in both moderate-to-high dose and rapidly tapered-to-prolonged regimens, but reactivation occurs less in patients receiving low-dose regimens (prednisone < 10 mg/d) even after prolonged use.[3,29] As such, short periods of corticosteroid use of less than 1 week regardless of dosage were believed to present a low risk for HBV reactivation; however, a recent study from Hong Kong to evaluate an impact of dose and duration of corticosteroid on the risk of hepatitis flare in patients with chronic hepatitis B (5254 chronic hepatitis B patients)[32] had shown that peak daily dose of greater than 40 mg compared with less than 20 mg prednisolone equivalents (adjusted HR = 1.64, P<.001) was an independent risk factor of hepatitis flare. Risk of hepatitis flare started to increase in those receiving corticosteroid of peak daily dose greater than 40 mg prednisolone equivalents even for less than 7 days (adjusted HR = 1.55, P=.026); the risk further increased with increasing duration of use for 7 to 28 days and greater than 28 days (adjusted HR = 1.90 and 1.64, P<.001). Thus, short courses of high-dose corticosteroid may also increase the risk of HBV flare in chronic hepatitis B patients, and thus, starting antiviral prophylaxis in this patient would be a consideration, although one would have to take into consideration the cost/benefit ratio of such an intervention.[32] A more recent study from the same group (n = 12,997) also reported that HBsAg-negative/anti-HBc positive individuals who received high peak daily doses of corticosteroids had an increased risk of hepatitis flare, but not HBsAg seroreversion (patients with anti-HBc positive only had 1-year incidence risk of HBsAg seroreversion of 1.8%), and liver failure rate was low, with no deaths identified.[33] Thus, HBV prophylaxis in this group would not appear to be cost -effective.

Tumor necrosis factor-α inhibitors (eg, infliximab, etanercept, adalimumab, certolizumab, and golimumab)

TNF-α inhibitors are also associated with HBV reactivation when used in patients with Crohn disease, RA, and psoriasis.[34–36] Patients who are HBsAg-positive may have risk of reactivation of around 1% to 10%. However, reactivation risk is less common in HBsAg-negative, anti-HBc positive patients (1%).[3] Recent systematic review and meta-analysis to assess the incidence of HBV reactivation among patients treated with anti-TNF-α estimated a pooled incidence of HBV reactivation of 4.2% (95% CI 1.4%–8.2%). The pooled incidence of reactivation was 3.0% (95% CI 0.6%–7.2%) for patients with occult infection compared to 15.4% (95%CI 1.2%–41.2%) in those with overt infection. The incidence of reactivation was 3.9% for etanercept and 4.6% for adalimumab.[37] In contrast, in patients with rheumatologic conditions with previously resolved HBV infection (HBsAg-negative, anti-HBc positive), long-term biologic therapy (n = 146/179 patients with anti-TNF-α) was not associated with HBV reactivation, suggesting that prophylaxis is not indicated in those on anti-TNFs when the patients are anti-HBc alone positive.[38] A large retrospective study (n = 8887) in patients on long-term treatment with TNF antagonists for autoimmune diseases found HBV reactivation in 39% of patients who were HBsAg-positive before therapy, but not in any patients who were HBsAg-negative/anti-HBc positive before therapy, indicating that HBsAg-positive patients should receive prophylactic antiviral therapy, but not HBsAg-negative/anti-HBc positive patients.[39] Another study in resolved HBV infection (HBsAg-negative, anti-HBc positive, HBV DNA negative) with RA (n = 152) treated with biological disease-modifying antirheumatic drugs (bDMARDs) found reactivation rate around 4.6% and that the absence of anti-HBs may be a risk factor for HBV reactivation in resolved HBV patients.[40] It is important to appreciate that in the net aggregate, the risk of reactivation in those who are HBsAg-negative/anti-HBc positive while on anti-TNFs is negligibly low to none, and thus HBV prophylaxis is not indicated in such patients while they are monitored for hepatic biochemical flare on therapy.

Cytokine inhibitors, monoclonal antibodies, and integrin inhibitors (eg, abatacept, ustekinumab, mogamulizumab, natalizumab, and vedolizumab)

Abatacept is a drug indicated for the treatment of moderate-to-severe RA. It is a fusion receptor protein that is fused to the extracellular domain of CTLA-4 and prevents T cell activation by binding to CD80 and CD86 molecules.[41] HBV reactivation was reported in a patient with RA and with HBsAg-negative and anti-HBc positive state and treated with abatacept. After 2 years of treatment, HBV DNA levels became detectable and with abnormal hepatic biochemical tests, at which time the drug was stopped and lamivudine treatment was introduced. After 1 month of lamivudine, HBV DNA became undetectable and with normalized hepatic biochemical profile.[42]

Belatacept, an example of another fusion protein indicated for the prevention of acute rejection after kidney transplant (KT) in adult patients, has also been reported to cause HBV reactivation in a HBsAg-negative/anti-HBc positive/anti-HBs positive patient who underwent KT for HIV-associated nephropathy (HIVAN) and after 2 years of belatacept treatment. However, after entecavir initiation, HBV DNA became undetectable, and there was a favorable outcome.[43]

Ustekinumab is a human interleukin-12 and -23 antagonist indicated for the treatment of adult patients with moderate-to-severe plaque psoriasis, active psoriatic arthritis, and moderate-to-severe active Crohn disease who have failed or were intolerant to treatment with immunomodulators or corticosteroids, or intolerant to treatment with 1 or more TNF blockers.[44] A study from Taiwan using ustekinumab in the treatment of patients with psoriasis and concurrent hepatitis B (14 patients) found few cases of HBV reactivation in HBsAg-positive patients. Among HBsAg-positive patients, 2 of 7 patients (29%) who did not receive HBV prophylaxis experienced reactivation (one was an inactive carrier, the other had chronic hepatitis B and was HBeAg-negative). No reactivation was found in HBsAg-negative/anti-HBc positive patients. No significant increase in aminotransferase levels were observed in those with reactivation.[45] Another prospective study from Taiwan included 93 psoriasis patients receiving ustekinumab (54 inactive HBV carriers, resolved HBV infection, or isolated anti-HBc positivity); only 3 patients experienced HBV reactivation, and none had liver failure.[46] Although there is paucity of data, it is estimated that ustekinumab-associated risk of reactivation, at most, is at the lower end of moderate-risk category (1%–10%).[3]

A case report from Japan noted fatal HBV reactivation in a HBsAg-positive patient with detectable HBV DNA and adult T-cell leukemia-lymphoma (ATL) receiving the anti-CC chemokine receptor 4 (CCR4) monoclonal antibody, mogamulizumab. Despite concomitant entecavir treatment with mogamulizumab, HBV reactivation occurred and progressed into liver failure.[47]

Experience in HBV-infected patients has thus far not been reported with natalizumab and vedolizumab.[3]

Tyrosine kinase inhibitors (eg, imatinib, sunitinib, gefitinib, erlotinib)

Tyrosine kinase inhibitors (TKIs) are commonly used in the treatment of chronic myeloid leukemia (CML) and gastrointestinal stromal tumor (GIST). Imatinib and nilotinib are reportedly associated with moderate risk for HBV reactivation in chronic hepatitis B patients.[48,49] A large single-center retrospective study evaluating the incidence of HBV reactivation in CML patients who were HBsAg-positive and treated with TKIs (n = 1817, HBsAg-positive 4.2%) found a reactivation rate of 26% in patients without antiviral prophylaxis. This would strongly support routine screening for HBV serologic status prior to initiation of TKI therapy and following with antiviral prophylaxis in HBsAg-positive patients receiving TKIs.[50] Another multicenter retrospective study to evaluate HBV reactivation in CML patients receiving TKIs (n = 702, HBsAg-positive 6.1%) found an HBV reactivation rate of 34.9% in HBsAg-positive patients without antiviral prophylaxis. Median time to HBV reactivation was 9.3 months (range 2.3–

68.8 months). Nonuse of prophylactic strategy and HBV DNA levels at diagnosis were significantly associated with HBV reactivation (*P*=.011 and *P*=.036, respectively). This study also suggested the importance of antiviral prophylaxis to prevent HBV reactivation during TKI treatment.[51]

Immune checkpoint inhibitors
Immune checkpoint inhibitors target key regulators of immune system. Programmed cell death 1 (PD-1) is a transmembrane protein expressed on T-cells, B-cells, and NK cells. PD-1 is an inhibitory molecule that binds to programmed death-ligand 1 or 2 (PD-L1 or PD-L2); PD-L1 is usually expressed on many tumor cells. The binding between PD-1 and PD-L1/2 on the tumor cells can inhibit apoptosis of the tumor cells that the tumors use as an escape mechanism. PD-1 and PD-L1 inhibitors are immunotherapies that were developed in order to prevent this escape mechanism of tumor cells and facilitate restoration of T-cells' immune function. Cytotoxic T-lymphocyte antigen-4 (CTLA-4) is implicated as a negative regulator of T-cell activation, and inhibition of CTLA-4 can lead to T-cells activation and immune surveillance of cancers. Stimulating immune systems may lead to immune-related adverse events, including flare of viral hepatitis. There are few case reports on HBV reactivation related to immune checkpoint inhibitors (**Table 1**).

Programmed cell death protein-1 inhibitors
Nivolumab There is a case report on HBV reactivation after nivolumab treatment in a patient with known human immunodeficiency virus (HIV) infection who was HBsAg-negative, anti-HBc positive, and HBV DNA negative. He was on antiretroviral therapy with dolutegravir and abacavir and with undetectable HIV viral load. He experienced HBV reactivation (HBsAg-positive seroreversion with high HBV DNA) while on nivolumab treatment for stage IIIa poorly differentiated carcinoma of the lung. The patient was then switched from abacavir to tenofovir disoproxil fumarate (TDF), and finally HBV DNA decreased while hepatic biochemical profile returned to normal.[52] A pilot study using nivolumab in virally suppressed chronic HBV patients evaluating the hypothesis that increasing T-cell activity may provide durable control of HBV infection found that in HBeAg-negative patients who were virally suppressed by prior antiviral agents, adding nivolumab was well-tolerated and led to HBsAg decline in most patients.[53]

Table 1
Immunotherapeutic agents with reported cases of hepatitis B virus reactivation

Immune Checkpoint Inhibitors	HBsAg Positive/Anti-HBc Positive	HBsAg Negative/Anti-HBc Positive
PD-1 inhibitors		
• Nivolumab	✓[55]	✓[52]
• Pembrolizumab	A report with unknown baseline HBV status[54]	A report with unknown baseline HBV status[54]
PD-1 inhibitors		
• Atezolizumab, Avelumab, Durvalumab	Not available	Not available
CTLA-4 inhibitors		
• Ipilimumab	✓[55]	Not available

Pembrolizumab There is a case report of a patient with stage IV poorly differentiated adenocarcinoma of the lung (no hepatitis panel at baseline) who started on pembrolizumab; subsequently there was HBV reactivation attributed to the drug (newly elevated transaminases and HBV DNA, negative autoimmune profile). After the initiation of TDF, transaminases returned to normal range within 10 weeks, and HBV DNA became undetectable. Therefore, immunotherapy may possibly lead to HBV reactivation, and screening for chronic hepatitis B before initiating therapy is a justified strategy.[54]

Programmed death-ligand 1 inhibitors: atezolizumab, avelumab, and durvalumab Atezolizumab is the first drug in this class that received initial FDA approval for metastatic urothelial carcinoma and has since been approved for metastatic nonsmall cell lung cancer (NSCLC). Avelumab is approved for Merkel cell carcinoma, while durvalumab is approved for urothelial carcinoma and stage III NSCLC. Currently there are no reported cases of HBV reactivation from these agents. Of note is that clinical trials using these immunotherapeutic agents have usually excluded patients with chronic hepatitis B infection (HBsAg-positive). More data are needed, particularly in those with anti-HBc alone positive status, before any conclusions on the risk of HBV reactivation from this drug class.

Cytotoxic T-lymphocyte antigen-4 inhibitors

Ipilimumab A patient with malignant melanoma and HBsAg-positive state (normal ALT, no baseline HBV DNA) was treated with ipilimumab and was then switched to nivolumab and was believed to have HBV reactivation after treatment (ALT elevation, anti-HBc IgM positive, increased HBV DNA with the negativity of all autoimmune markers). The patient started treatment with TDF, and also remained on nivolumab treatment. Eventually, HBV DNA levels significantly decreased after 2 months of TDF.[55] A retrospective study from China to determine the safety of immune checkpoint inhibitors in melanoma patients receiving ipilimumab or pembrolizumab (n = 23) noted hepatic biochemical test abnormalities from immune-related adverse events in 22%; most toxicities were mild and easily managed. No toxicity was observed in 11 patients with previous HBV infection (antiviral drug was started in patients who were HBsAg-positive with or without detectable HBV DNA before receiving ipilimumab or pembrolizumab).[56]

Traditional immunosuppression

There is no convincing evidence of HBV reactivation from azathioprine or 6-mercaptopurine (active metabolite of azathioprine) when used as single agents. The AGA guideline assessment is that this is a low-risk group for reactivation (<1% risk) in both HBsAg-positive and HBsAg-negative, anti-HBc positive patients.[3]

Data from a prospective study from Japan evaluated reactivation of HBV in patients with RA who received immunosuppressive therapy (n = 50). HBV reactivation occurred in 2 out of 5 patients who were HBsAg-positive and in 1 out of 45 patients without HBsAg. Screening for HBV reactivation and prophylactic therapy with entecavir were effective in preventing HBV-associated hepatic failure in patients who were HBsAg-positive and in those who were anti-HBc positive in the background of receiving immunosuppression.[57] On the contrary, in a cross-sectional study evaluating long-term use of methotrexate in RA patients (n=173; 1 patient [0.58%] who was HBsAg-positive, 65 patients [37.6%] had anti-HBc immunoglobulin G [IgG] alone positive serology), none had HBV reactivation during 9.9 years of methotrexate treatment.[58] Because there are small numbers of case reports of HBV reactivation from methotrexate monotherapy (predominantly in HBsAg-positive patients), the AGA

Guideline assessed methotrexate use to present a low-risk group (<1% risk) for reactivation.[3]

Of note, apart from HBV reactivation, the differential diagnosis of patients receiving immunosuppressive therapy with increased aminotransferase levels should include drug-induced hepatotoxicity, infection by other viruses, and other causes of liver disease. Patients who are suspected to have drug-induced hepatotoxicity would have ALT elevation without an elevation of HBV DNA levels. Other viral-induced hepatitis (such as hepatitis A, C, D, E, cytomegalovirus, and herpes viruses) should be considered, and investigations should be sent, particularly in those who are immunocompromised. Further, other causes of liver disease such as ischemic hepatitis, hepatic veno-occlusive disease, and tumor infiltration should also be considered in the differential diagnosis.

Direct-acting antivirals

DAAs are not considered as immunosuppressive agents; however, there are some reports of HBV reactivation in HCV-infected patients treated with DAAs. The FDA reported 29 cases of HBV reactivation in patients receiving DAAs from 2013 to 2016, and this raised concern, particularly in patients with HBV-HCV coinfection treated with DAAs.[59] A report from a clinical trial of ledipasvir-sofosbuvir treatment in HCV-infected patients in Taiwan and Korea (103 of 173 patients [60%] with previous HBV infection [anti-HBc positive]) noted that none had evidence of HBV reactivation.[60] Recent systematic review and meta-analysis of HBV reactivation in HBV-HCV coinfected patients treated with antiviral agents demonstrated that among HCV patients with overt HBV (HBsAg-positive) (n = 779), the pooled HBV reactivation rate was 14.1%; HBV reactivation was reported to occur much earlier in those treated with DAAs (4–12 weeks during treatment) than in those treated with interferon (most at the end of treatment and some during follow-up).[61] However, HBV reactivation occurred less frequently in HCV patients with occult HBV infection (HBsAg-negative with positive HBV DNA), and sustained virologic response (SVR) was not affected by HBV reactivation.[61] An interesting study to evaluate potential risk of HBV reactivation in patients with resolved HBV infection (HBsAg-negative, undetectable HBV DNA, anti-HBc positive) undergoing DAA for HCV treatment found that anti-HBs titer was significantly decreased early on after DAA treatment, and patients with negative anti-HBs or very low titer of anti-HBs at baseline were at risk of transient detectable HBV DNA during HCV treatment.[62] As such, EASL Guideline recommends that patients who are HBsAg-positive and undergo DAA therapy be considered for concomitant NA prophylaxis until 12 weeks after DAA, and patients with HBsAg-negative/anti-HBc positive serology and undergoing DAA be monitored for HBV reactivation.[5]

Risk Categorization

HBV reactivation risk is categorized into high risk (>10% reactivation risk), moderate risk (1%–10% reactivation risk), and low risk (<1% reactivation risk) (**Table 2**).[3,29] Recommended HBV prophylaxis and treatment algorithm for chemotherapy candidates are described in (**Fig. 2**).

TREATMENT AND PROGNOSIS OF HEPATITIS B VIRUS REACTIVATION

Immunosuppressed patients who develops HBV reactivation (with or without hepatitis flare) should be treated with nucleoside/nucleotide analogue (NA) as early as possible regardless of ALT levels. Severe hepatitis and hepatic failure can develop in 25% to 50% of patients with HBV reactivation.[63] Tenofovir or entecavir should be the

Table 2
Hepatitis B virus reactivation risk according to Hepatitis B virus status and immunosuppressive agents and guideline recommendation for prevention of Hepatitis B virus reactivation

Risk Group	HBsAg-Positive/Anti-HBc Positive (% Risk)	HBsAg-Negative/Anti-HBc Positive (% Risk)
High risk (>10%)	• B cell-depleting agents such as rituximab and ofatumumab (30%–60%) • Anthracycline derivatives such as doxorubicin and epirubicin (15%–30%) • Corticosteroid therapy for ≥ 4 weeks (moderate-high dose[a]) (>10%)	• B cell-depleting agents such as rituximab and ofatumumab (>10%)
Recommendation	Antiviral prophylaxis regardless of HBV DNA levels and anti-HBs status, and prophylaxis should be continued to at least 18 months in B cell-depleting agents until after cessation of immunosuppression.	
Moderate risk (1%–10%)	• TNF-α inhibitors: etanercept, adalimumab, certolizumab, infliximab (1%–10%) • Other cytokine inhibitors and integrin inhibitors: abatacept, ustekinumab, natalizumab, vedolizumab (1%–10%) • Tyrosine kinase inhibitors: imatinib, nilotinib (1%–10%) • Corticosteroid therapy for ≥ 4 weeks (low dose) (1%–10%)	• TNF-α inhibitors: etanercept, adalimumab, certolizumab, infliximab (1%) • Other cytokine inhibitors and integrin inhibitors: abatacept, ustekinumab, natalizumab, vedolizumab (1%) • Tyrosine kinase inhibitors: imatinib, nilotinib (1%) • Corticosteroid therapy for ≥ 4 weeks (moderate-high dose) (1%–10%) • Anthracycline derivatives: doxorubicin and epirubicin (1%–10%)
Recommendation	Antiviral prophylaxis regardless of HBV DNA levels.	Monitoring of HBsAg, HBV DNA and ALT 3 months. Pre-emptive therapy when HBsAg seroreversion or detectable HBV DNA noted, regardless of ALT levels.
Low risk (<1%)	• Traditional immunosuppressive agents: azathioprine, 6-mercaptopurine, methotrexate • Intra-articular corticosteroids • Corticosteroid therapy for ≤ 1 week	• Traditional immunosuppressive agents: azathioprine, 6-mercaptopurine, methotrexate • Intra-articular corticosteroids • Corticosteroid therapy for ≤ 1 week • Corticosteroid therapy for ≥ 4 weeks (low dose)

(continued on next page)

Table 2
(continued)

Risk Group	HBsAg-Positive/Anti-HBc Positive (% Risk)	HBsAg-Negative/Anti-HBc Positive (% Risk)
Recommendation	In HBsAg-positive/anti-HBc positive patients, monitor HBV DNA levels and ALT every 3–6 months as routine practice. Viral suppressive therapy is recommended at baseline or during follow-up as per guidelines based on HBV DNA and ALT levels. In HBsAg-negative/anti-HBc positive patients, if biochemical flare noted, work-up for HBV reactivation is to be initiated, and treatment is indicated if HBsAg seroreversion or elevated HBV DNA noted.	

Abbreviations: ALT, alanine transaminase; DNA, deoxyribonucleic acid; HBV, hepatitis B virus; TNF, tumor necrosis factor.
[a] Corticosteroid: prednisone (or equivalent); low dose (<10 mg), moderate dose (10–20 mg), high dose (>20 mg).
Data from Refs.[2,3,5,29]

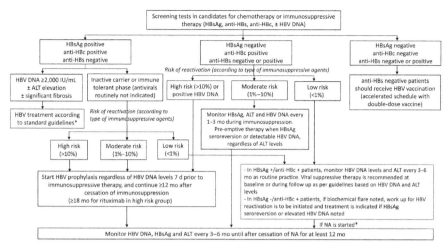

Fig. 2. Recommended HBV prophylaxis, follow up, and treatment algorithm (authors' modifications) for chemotherapy candidates. * High resistant barrier NA (e.g. entecavir, TDF, TAF) should be preferred over low-barrier NA (e.g. lamivudine). HBV, Hepatitis B virus; DNA, Deoxyribonucleic acid; ALT, Alanine transaminase; NA, Nucleoside/nucleotide analogue; TDF, Tenofovir disoproxil fumarate; TAF, Tenofovir alafenamide. (*Data from* Refs.[2,5,66])

treatment of choice once diagnosed with HBV reactivation, because lamivudine (LAM) may be associated with greater risk of drug resistance. Tenofovir is preferred rather than entecavir in patients who have history of prior LAM therapy. Data on efficacy of antiviral agents in reducing morbidity and mortality in patients with HBV reactivation are insufficient, and there are no trials that allow direct comparison of the effectiveness between third-generation antiviral drugs and earlier-generation therapies in patients with HBV reactivation during immunosuppressive therapy.[29] However, there is indirect evidence from randomized controlled trials (RCTs) noting lower drug failure rates and lower viral resistance from third-generation drugs compared with LAM in nonimmunosuppressed patients. Accordingly, the AGA Guideline recommends antiviral drugs with a high barrier to resistance over LAM in patients with HBV reactivation during immunosuppressive therapy.[29]

There are case reports demonstrating clinical improvement after antiviral treatment in patients with HBV flare, especially when early treatment was initiated.[64,65] However, some patients may develop severe flare despite antiviral therapy, which then leads to unnecessary interruption of chemotherapy for the patient's underlying condition, and some may progress to liver failure and with high mortality.[15,64] Thus, initiation of antiviral therapy is essential as early as possible in the HBV reactivation phase and before a clinical flare occurs.

SUMMARY

HBV reactivation in patients with immunosuppressive therapy can result in severe morbidity and mortality. Therefore, testing for HBV serology is suggested in all patients who are candidates for immunosuppressive therapy. High-risk patients for reactivation should be started with antiviral prophylaxis before initiating immunosuppressive regimen. To date, there are many newer agents used in autoimmune and oncologic patients such as biologics and immunotherapies that have been variably reported to lead to HBV reactivation; however, more data are needed in order to estimate their risk for

HBV reactivation and the role on antiviral prophylaxis. Further, when HBV reactivation is recognized during immunosuppressive therapy, prompt initiation of antiviral treatment is essential. While monitoring for resolution during reactivation, some patients may encounter hepatic decompensation, which leads to high morbidity and mortality.

DISCLOSURE

S. Ekpanyapong has nothing to disclose. K.R. Reddy is on the Advisory Board of Gilead, Merck and received grant support from Gilead, BMS, Merck.

REFERENCES

1. Loomba R, Liang TJ. Hepatitis B reactivation associated with immune suppressive and biological modifier therapies: current concepts, management strategies, and future directions. Gastroenterology 2017;152(6):1297–309.
2. Terrault NA, Lok ASF, McMahon BJ, et al. Update on prevention, diagnosis, and treatment of chronic hepatitis B: AASLD 2018 hepatitis B guidance. Hepatology 2018;67(4):1560–99.
3. Perrillo RP, Gish R, Falck-Ytter YT. American Gastroenterological Association Institute technical review on prevention and treatment of hepatitis B virus reactivation during immunosuppressive drug therapy. Gastroenterology 2015;148(1): 221–44.e3.
4. Hoofnagle JH. Reactivation of hepatitis B. Hepatology 2009;49(5 Suppl): S156–65.
5. EASL 2017 Clinical Practice Guidelines on the management of hepatitis B virus infection. J Hepatol 2017;67(2):370–98.
6. Yan H, Zhong G, Xu G, et al. Sodium taurocholate cotransporting polypeptide is a functional receptor for human hepatitis B and D virus. eLife 2012;1:e00049.
7. Rehermann B, Ferrari C, Pasquinelli C, et al. The hepatitis B virus persists for decades after patients' recovery from acute viral hepatitis despite active maintenance of a cytotoxic T-lymphocyte response. Nat Med 1996;2(10):1104–8.
8. Werle-Lapostolle B, Bowden S, Locarnini S, et al. Persistence of cccDNA during the natural history of chronic hepatitis B and decline during adefovir dipivoxil therapy. Gastroenterology 2004;126(7):1750–8.
9. Guidotti LG, Chisari FV. Immunobiology and pathogenesis of viral hepatitis. Annu Rev Pathol 2006;1:23–61.
10. Karvellas CJ, Cardoso FS, Gottfried M, et al. HBV-associated acute liver failure after immunosuppression and risk of death. Clin Gastroenterol Hepatol 2017; 15(1):113–22.
11. Paul S, Saxena A, Terrin N, et al. Hepatitis B virus reactivation and prophylaxis during solid tumor chemotherapy: a systematic review and meta-analysis. Ann Intern Med 2016;164(1):30–40.
12. Lau GK, Leung YH, Fong DY, et al. High hepatitis B virus (HBV) DNA viral load as the most important risk factor for HBV reactivation in patients positive for HBV surface antigen undergoing autologous hematopoietic cell transplantation. Blood 2002;99(7):2324–30.
13. Seto WK, Chan TS, Hwang YY, et al. Hepatitis B reactivation in patients with previous hepatitis B virus exposure undergoing rituximab-containing chemotherapy for lymphoma: a prospective study. J Clin Oncol 2014;32(33):3736–43.
14. Seto WK, Chan TS, Hwang YY, et al. Hepatitis B reactivation in occult viral carriers undergoing hematopoietic stem cell transplantation: a prospective study. Hepatology 2017;65(5):1451–61.

15. Hsu C, Tsou HH, Lin SJ, et al. Chemotherapy-induced hepatitis B reactivation in lymphoma patients with resolved HBV infection: a prospective study. Hepatology 2014;59(6):2092–100.

16. Yang HC, Tsou HH, Pei SN, et al. Quantification of HBV core antibodies may help predict HBV reactivation in patients with lymphoma and resolved HBV infection. J Hepatol 2018;69(2):286–92.

17. FDA. RITUXAN (rituximab) prescribing information. 1997. Available at: https://www.accessdata.fda.gov/drugsatfda_docs/label/2012/103705s5367s5388lbl.pdf. Accessed May 15th, 2019.

18. FDA. ARZERRA® (ofatumumab) prescribing information. 2009. Available at: https://www.accessdata.fda.gov/drugsatfda_docs/label/2016/125326s062lbl.pdf. Accessed May 15th, 2019.

19. Tsutsumi Y, Yamamoto Y, Ito S, et al. Hepatitis B virus reactivation with a rituximab-containing regimen. World J Hepatol 2015;7(21):2344–51.

20. Villadolid J, Laplant KD, Markham MJ, et al. Hepatitis B reactivation and rituximab in the oncology practice. Oncologist 2010;15(10):1113–21.

21. Chen YM, Chen HH, Huang WN, et al. Reactivation of hepatitis B virus infection following rituximab treatment in HBsAg-negative, HBcAb-positive rheumatoid arthritis patients: a long-term, real-world observation. Int J Rheum Dis 2019; 22(6):1145–51.

22. Markovic S, Drozina G, Vovk M, et al. Reactivation of hepatitis B but not hepatitis C in patients with malignant lymphoma and immunosuppressive therapy. A prospective study in 305 patients. Hepatogastroenterology 1999;46(29):2925–30.

23. Kusumoto S, Arcaini L, Hong X, et al. Risk of HBV reactivation in patients with B-cell lymphomas receiving obinutuzumab or rituximab immunochemotherapy. Blood 2019;133(2):137–46.

24. FDA. ADRIAMYCIN (Doxorubicin HCl) injection prescribing information. 2010. Available at: https://www.accessdata.fda.gov/drugsatfda_docs/label/2010/050467s070lbl.pdf. Accessed February 24th, 2020.

25. Wang J, Jia J, Chen R, et al. RFX1 participates in doxorubicin-induced hepatitis B virus reactivation. Cancer Med 2018;7(5):2021–33.

26. Kostyusheva A, Brezgin S, Bayurova E, et al. ATM and ATR expression potentiates HBV replication and contributes to reactivation of HBV infection upon DNA damage. Viruses 2019;11(11) [pii:E997].

27. Yeo W, Chan PK, Hui P, et al. Hepatitis B virus reactivation in breast cancer patients receiving cytotoxic chemotherapy: a prospective study. J Med Virol 2003; 70(4):553–61.

28. Lee HJ, Kim DY, Keam B, et al. Lamivudine prophylaxis for hepatitis B virus carrier patients with breast cancer during adjuvant chemotherapy. Breast Cancer 2014;21(4):387–93.

29. Reddy KR, Beavers KL, Hammond SP, et al. American Gastroenterological Association Institute guideline on the prevention and treatment of hepatitis B virus reactivation during immunosuppressive drug therapy. Gastroenterology 2015; 148(1):215–9 [quiz: e216–7].

30. Scullard GH, Smith CI, Merigan TC, et al. Effects of immunosuppressive therapy on viral markers in chronic active hepatitis B. Gastroenterology 1981;81(6):987–91.

31. Sheen IS, Liaw YF, Lin SM, et al. Severe clinical rebound upon withdrawal of corticosteroid before interferon therapy: incidence and risk factors. J Gastroenterol Hepatol 1996;11(2):143–7.

32. Wong GL, Yuen BW, Chan HL, et al. Impact of dose and duration of corticosteroid on the risk of hepatitis flare in patients with chronic hepatitis B. Liver Int 2019; 39(2):271–9.

33. Wong GL, Wong VW, Yuen BW, et al. Risk of hepatitis B surface antigen seroreversion after corticosteroid treatment in patients with previous hepatitis B virus exposure. J Hepatol 2020;72(1):57–66.

34. Esteve M, Saro C, Gonzalez-Huix F, et al. Chronic hepatitis B reactivation following infliximab therapy in Crohn's disease patients: need for primary prophylaxis. Gut 2004;53(9):1363–5.

35. Lee YH, Bae SC, Song GG. Hepatitis B virus (HBV) reactivation in rheumatic patients with hepatitis core antigen (HBV occult carriers) undergoing anti-tumor necrosis factor therapy. Clin Exp Rheumatol 2013;31(1):118–21.

36. Lee YH, Bae SC, Song GG. Hepatitis B virus reactivation in HBsAg-positive patients with rheumatic diseases undergoing anti-tumor necrosis factor therapy or DMARDs. Int J Rheum Dis 2013;16(5):527–31.

37. Cantini F, Boccia S, Goletti D, et al. HBV reactivation in patients treated with anti-tumor necrosis factor-alpha (TNF-alpha) agents for rheumatic and dermatologic conditions: a systematic review and meta-analysis. Int J Rheumatol 2014;2014: 926836.

38. Barone M, Notarnicola A, Lopalco G, et al. Safety of long-term biologic therapy in rheumatologic patients with a previously resolved hepatitis B viral infection. Hepatology 2015;62(1):40–6.

39. Pauly MP, Tucker LY, Szpakowski JL, et al. Incidence of hepatitis B virus reactivation and hepatotoxicity in patients receiving long-term treatment with tumor necrosis factor antagonists. Clin Gastroenterol Hepatol 2018;16(12):1964–73.e1.

40. Watanabe T, Fukae J, Fukaya S, et al. Incidence and risk factors for reactivation from resolved hepatitis B virus in rheumatoid arthritis patients treated with biological disease-modifying antirheumatic drugs. Int J Rheum Dis 2019;22(4):574–82.

41. Dubois EA, Cohen AF. Abatacept. Br J Clin Pharmacol 2009;68(4):480–1.

42. Talotta R, Atzeni F, Sarzi Puttini P. Reactivation of occult hepatitis B virus infection under treatment with abatacept: a case report. BMC Pharmacol Toxicol 2016;17:17.

43. Cambier ML, Canestri A, Lependeven C, et al. Hepatitis B virus reactivation during belatacept treatment after kidney transplantation. Transpl Infect Dis 2019;21: e13170.

44. FDA. STELARA® (ustekinumab) prescribing information. 2009. Available at: https://www.accessdata.fda.gov/drugsatfda_docs/label/2016/761044lbl.pdf. Accessed May 16th, 2019.

45. Chiu HY, Chen CH, Wu MS, et al. The safety profile of ustekinumab in the treatment of patients with psoriasis and concurrent hepatitis B or C. Br J Dermatol 2013;169(6):1295–303.

46. Ting SW, Chen YC, Huang YH. Risk of Hepatitis B reactivation in patients with psoriasis on ustekinumab. Clin Drug Invest 2018;38(9):873–80.

47. Ifuku H, Kusumoto S, Tanaka Y, et al. Fatal reactivation of hepatitis B virus infection in a patient with adult T-cell leukemia-lymphoma receiving the anti-CC chemokine receptor 4 antibody mogamulizumab. Hepatol Res 2015;45(13):1363–7.

48. Lai GM, Yan SL, Chang CS, et al. Hepatitis B reactivation in chronic myeloid leukemia patients receiving tyrosine kinase inhibitor. World J Gastroenterol 2013; 19(8):1318–21.

49. Ikeda K, Shiga Y, Takahashi A, et al. Fatal hepatitis B virus reactivation in a chronic myeloid leukemia patient during imatinib mesylate treatment. Leuk Lymphoma 2006;47(1):155–7.

50. Uhm J, Kim S-H, Oh S, et al. High incidence of Hepatitis B viral reactivation in chronic myeloid leukemia patients treated with tyrosine kinase inhibitors. Blood 2018;132(Suppl 1):3010.
51. Kim S-H, Kim HJ, Kwak J-Y, et al. Hepatitis B virus reactivation in chronic myeloid leukemia treated with various tyrosine kinase inhibitors: multicenter, retrospective study. Blood 2012;120(21):3738.
52. Lake AC. Hepatitis B reactivation in a long-term nonprogressor due to nivolumab therapy. AIDS 2017;31(15):2115–8.
53. Gane E, Verdon DJ, Brooks AE, et al. Anti-PD-1 blockade with nivolumab with and without therapeutic vaccination for virally suppressed chronic hepatitis B: a pilot study. J Hepatol 2019;71(5):900–7.
54. Pandey A, Ezemenari S, Liaukovich M, et al. A rare case of pembrolizumab-induced reactivation of Hepatitis B. Case Rep Oncol Med 2018;2018:5985131.
55. Koksal AS, Toka B, Eminler AT, et al. HBV-related acute hepatitis due to immune checkpoint inhibitors in a patient with malignant melanoma. Ann Oncol 2017; 28(12):3103–4.
56. Wen X, Wang Y, Ding Y, et al. Safety of immune checkpoint inhibitors in Chinese patients with melanoma. Melanoma Res 2016;26(3):284–9.
57. Tamori A, Koike T, Goto H, et al. Prospective study of reactivation of hepatitis B virus in patients with rheumatoid arthritis who received immunosuppressive therapy: evaluation of both HBsAg-positive and HBsAg-negative cohorts. J Gastroenterol 2011;46(4):556–64.
58. Laohapand C, Arromdee E, Tanwandee T. Long-term use of methotrexate does not result in hepatitis B reactivation in rheumatologic patients. Hepatol Int 2015; 9(2):202–8.
59. Bersoff-Matcha SJ, Cao K, Jason M, et al. Hepatitis B virus reactivation associated with direct-acting antiviral therapy for chronic Hepatitis C virus: a review of cases reported to the U.S. Food and Drug Administration adverse event reporting system. Ann Intern Med 2017;166(11):792–8.
60. Sulkowski MS, Chuang WL, Kao JH, et al. No evidence of reactivation of Hepatitis B virus among patients treated with ledipasvir-sofosbuvir for Hepatitis C virus infection. Clin Infect Dis 2016;63(9):1202–4.
61. Chen G, Wang C, Chen J, et al. Hepatitis B reactivation in hepatitis B and C co-infected patients treated with antiviral agents: a systematic review and meta-analysis. Hepatology 2017;66(1):13–26.
62. Ogawa E, Furusyo N, Murata M, et al. Potential risk of HBV reactivation in patients with resolved HBV infection undergoing direct-acting antiviral treatment for HCV. Liver Int 2018;38(1):76–83.
63. Shih CA, Chen WC, Yu HC, et al. Risk of severe acute exacerbation of chronic HBV infection cancer patients who underwent chemotherapy and did not receive anti-viral prophylaxis. PLoS One 2015;10(8):e0132426.
64. Liao CA, Lee CM, Wu HC, et al. Lamivudine for the treatment of hepatitis B virus reactivation following chemotherapy for non-Hodgkin's lymphoma. Br J Haematol 2002;116(1):166–9.
65. Clark FL, Drummond MW, Chambers S, et al. Successful treatment with lamivudine for fulminant reactivated hepatitis B infection following intensive therapy for high-grade non-Hodgkin's lymphoma. Ann Oncol 1998;9(4):385–7.
66. Arora A, Anand AC, Kumar A, et al. INASL guidelines on management of Hepatitis B virus infection in patients receiving chemotherapy, biologicals, immunosuppressants, or corticosteroids. J Clin Exp Hepatol 2018;8(4):403–31.

Evaluation and Management of Esophageal and Gastric Varices in Patients with Cirrhosis

Sofia Simona Jakab, MD[a,b,*], Guadalupe Garcia-Tsao, MD[a,b]

KEYWORDS

- Esophageal varices • Gastric varices • Nonselective beta-blocker
- Endoscopic variceal ligation • Variceal bleeding • Portal hypertension • Cirrhosis
- Decompensated cirrhosis

KEY POINTS

- Gastroesophageal varices can be seen endoscopically in patients with cirrhosis in the compensated and the decompensated stages but are more common in decompensated patients.
- In patients with compensated cirrhosis, the presence of gastroesophageal varices on endoscopy is indicative of the presence of clinically significant portal hypertension, the main predictor of decompensation.
- In patients with varices that have never ruptured, the use of nonselective beta-blockers is preferred, as they will not only prevent the first episode of variceal hemorrhage, but will also prevent the development of other decompensating events.
- Acute variceal bleeding is a life-threatening complication of cirrhosis, but the mortality associated with it has decreased with current management based on careful blood transfusion, vasoactive medications, antibiotics, and endoscopic and pre-emptive transjugular intrahepatic portosystemic shunts.
- Prevention of recurrent variceal hemorrhage is based on the combination of nonselective beta-blockers and endoscopic variceal ligation.

TYPES OF GASTROESOPHAGEAL VARICES

Esophageal varices are the most common type of gastroesophageal varices, with a prevalence of 50% to 60% among patients with cirrhosis, and up to 85% in patients with decompensated cirrhosis. Gastric varices are present in about 20% of patients with cirrhosis, and they can be of different types.[1] Sarin classification[2] is the most commonly classification used to define the type of gastric varices (**Fig. 1**). GOV type

---

[a] Section of Digestive Diseases, Yale University School of Medicine, PO Box 208056, 333 Cedar Street, New Haven, CT 06520-8056, USA; [b] Section of Digestive Diseases, VA Connecticut Healthcare System, West Haven, CT, USA
* Corresponding author. 40 Temple Street, Suite 1A, New Haven, CT 06510.
E-mail address: simona.jakab@yale.edu

Clin Liver Dis 24 (2020) 335–350
https://doi.org/10.1016/j.cld.2020.04.011
1089-3261/20/© 2020 Elsevier Inc. All rights reserved.

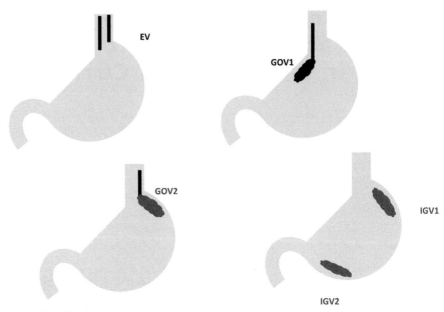

Fig. 1. Classification of gastroesophageal varices.

1 (GOV1) are esophageal varices extending below the cardia into the lesser curvature and are the most common (75% of gastric varices). GOV type 2 (GOV2) are esophageal varices extending into the fundus. Isolated GV type 1 (IGV1) are located in the fundus (IGV1). Isolated GV type 2 (IGV2) are located elsewhere in the stomach but are rare.

Esophageal varices and GOV1 will be considered together as gastroesophageal varices (GEV), because their management is the same. GOV2 and IGV1 will be referred to as fundal varices, and their specific therapeutic approach will be discussed separate from GEV.

In order to make an impact on the natural history of varices and improve clinical outcomes, specific interventions are recommended and will be discussed throughout this article. Variceal screening, surveillance, and prophylaxis of variceal bleeding are usually addressed in an outpatient setting, while acute variceal bleeding requires inpatient care and sometimes transfer to a tertiary center. Among the cirrhosis quality metrics developed by the American Association for the Study of Liver Diseases (AASLD),[3] 7 measures are applicable to the management of varices (**Table 1**). These measures aim to prevent variceal bleeding, but based on emerging data, the paradigm may change, with a focus on treating clinically significant portal hypertension rather than high-risk varices, and preventing any decompensations (eg, variceal bleeding, ascites, or hepatic encephalopathy) rather than just variceal bleeding (**Fig. 2**).

This new paradigm is based on a large randomized controlled trial (PREDESCI trial)[4] showing that nonselective beta-blockers (NSBBs) prevent decompensation (not only variceal hemorrhage, but mainly ascites) in patients with compensated cirrhosis and clinically significant portal hypertension (CSPH). In this trial, CSPH was diagnosed using invasive measures: hepatic venous pressure gradient (HVPG) of 10 mm Hg or higher. However, CSPH can be diagnosed noninvasively by liver stiffness measurement/platelet count, presence of gastroesophageal varices (any size) and/or presence of large collaterals on cross-sectional imaging. Therefore, in patients with compensated

Table 1
American Association for the Study of Liver Diseases cirrhosis quality metrics regarding gastroesophageal varices

Variceal screening	• Patients with cirrhosis, with platelet count < 150,000/mm³ or liver stiffness measurement > 20 kPa, and no documentation of previous gastrointestinal (GI) bleeding, should have EGD to screen for varices within 12 months of cirrhosis diagnosis. • Patients with decompensated cirrhosis and no documented history of previous GI bleeding should have EGD to screen for varices within 3 mo of cirrhosis diagnosis.
Primary prophylaxis of variceal bleeding	• Patients with cirrhosis, no documented history of previous GI bleeding, and medium/large varices on endoscopy should receive either NSBBs or EVL within 1 mo of varices diagnosis.
Variceal bleeding	• Patients who are admitted with or develop GI bleeding should receive antibiotics within 24 h of admission or presentation. Antibiotics should be continued for at least 5 d. • Patients with cirrhosis who present with upper GI bleeding should have EGD within 12 h of presentation. • Patients with cirrhosis who are found to have bleeding esophageal varices should receive EVL or sclerotherapy at the time of index endoscopy.
Secondary prophylaxis of variceal bleeding	• Patients with cirrhosis who survive an episode of acute variceal hemorrhage should receive a combination of EVL and NSBBs.

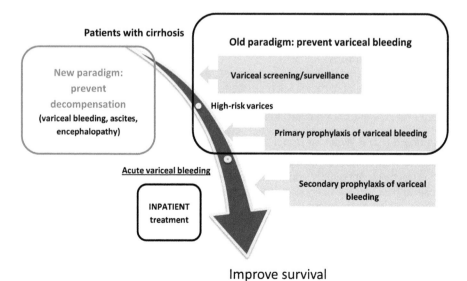

Fig. 2. Management of varices and points of intervention.

cirrhosis and varices, NSBBs would be preferred over endoscopic variceal ligation (EVL). In a patient who has obvious collaterals on imaging, esophagogastroduoendoscopy (EGD) may not even be necessary.

OUTPATIENT MANAGEMENT OF GASTROESOPHAGEAL VARICES

The most common scenario in an outpatient setting requiring gastroenterologists to think about GEV is when a patient presents for management of cirrhosis. A practical 3-pronged approach includes: establishing the stage of cirrhosis, deciding if or when to proceed with upper endoscopy, and determining if treatment is needed or what what type of treatment is necessary.

Establishing the Stage of Cirrhosis

The first step in the assessment of GEV is establishing the stage of cirrhosis: compensated or decompensated. Patients can transition from one stage to another, and the stage of cirrhosis is essential when deciding the management of GEV. When using Child–Turcotte–Pugh (CTP) classification, patients in CTP-A class are compensated, and patients in CTP-B/C class are mostly decompensated.

Compensated cirrhosis
Compensated cirrhosis is asymptomatic, and its diagnosis is based on:

- Clinical findings (eg, firm and/or enlarged left liver lobe, splenomegaly, spider angioma, or palmar erythema)
- Laboratory data (eg, thrombocytopenia, liver synthetic dysfunction with abnormal albumin, international normalized ratio [INR], bilirubin)
- Imaging (eg, nodular liver, with or without portal hypertension suggested by recanalized umbilical vein, portosystemic collaterals, splenomegaly)
- Liver elastography, if available (based on Baveno VI consensus,[5] patients with 2 separate liver stiffness measurements [LSM] > 15 kPa on transient elastography [TE] have severe fibrosis or compensated cirrhosis and are at risk to develop GEV)
- Liver biopsy, when data are discordant

Decompensated cirrhosis
Decompensated cirrhosis is easier to diagnose, as it is defined by the presence of any overt complications of cirrhosis such as ascites, hepatic encephalopathy, and/or variceal hemorrhage. In addition to the suggestive history and physical examination, laboratory and imaging data confirm the diagnosis, and liver biopsy is rarely needed.

Determining If and When an Upper Endoscopy Is Indicated

In patients with compensated cirrhosis, the severity of portal hypertension correlates with the development of GEV and risk of variceal bleeding.[6] Patients with compensated cirrhosis and without clinically significant portal hypertension (CSPH) are at a low risk of having or developing varices in the next 5 years. GEV usually occur once patients develop CSPH, and patients with CSPH not only have a higher risk of developing varices but also have a higher risk of decompensation.[7] The presence or absence of CSPH is determined by measuring the hepatic venous pressure gradient through transjugular hepatic vein catheterization, and is useful in research but impractical in routine clinical care. Noninvasive tests such as imaging showing portosystemic collaterals or recanalized umbilical vein or reversal of portal flow, liver stiffness measurement, platelet count, and spleen diameter can help identify patients with a high risk of CSPH across cohorts of patients with different etiology of cirrhosis or posthepatitis C eradication.[8–16]

Compensated cirrhosis
In the case of no EGD in patients with LSM greater than 20 to 25 kPa by TE or recanalized umbilical vein/portosystemic collaterals on imaging, it should be noted that these patients are likely to have CSPH. They benefit from NSBBs, with the goal of preventing decompensation (based on PREDESCI trial,[4] they should receive carvedilol or propranolol).

If there is EGD in patients with compensated cirrhosis with likely CSPH but who cannot tolerate or have contraindications to NSBBs, patients should be monitored for development of large varices that would benefit from EVL.

Decompensated cirrhosis
Screening EGD in patients with decompensated cirrhosis is still recommended to be performed at the time of diagnosis of cirrhosis decompensation, followed by annual surveillance EGD if no varices were seen on prior EGD.

Given the presence of decompensation, all these patients have CSPH. Turco and colleagues[17] showed in a meta-analysis including patients with and without ascites that those who respond to treatment with NSBBs (based on reduction of HVPG) have a reduced risk of events, death, or liver transplantation. These data suggest that patients with decompensated cirrhosis have additional benefits from NSBBs regardless of presence of varices at high risk of bleeding, and EGD may not be required in the future to initiate NSBB.

Of note, for patients already on NSBBs, either for primary prophylaxis of variceal bleeding or for other indications, as long as their heart rate is 55 to 60 beats per minute (on nadolol or propranolol) or carvedilol is dosed at least 12.5 mg/d regardless of heart rate, screening or surveillance EGD is no longer required, as it will not change their current regimen based on EGD findings. For patients in whom endoscopic variceal ligation is used for primary prophylaxis for variceal bleeding, EGD interval is discussed. If TIPS (transjugular intrahepatic portosystemic shunt) was inserted for ascites, having obtained a portosystemic gradient less than 12 mm Hg, and TIPS has remained patent, EGD for screening or surveillance of varices is not necessary, as the pressure reduction achieved by TIPS is sufficient to make variceal bleed unlikely or even to make varices disappear. Importantly, TIPS should not be placed with the purpose of preventing first variceal hemorrhage, as this portosystemic shunting has been associated with a higher mortality in this setting.

Are Nonselective Beta-Blocker and Endoscopic Variceal Ligation Indicated?

In patients without prior variceal bleeding, the current recommendations address solely the prevention of the first variceal bleeding in patients with high-risk varices (HRV) considered to have a high risk of bleeding (>15% per year): patients with medium or large varices (which constitute the largest group), patients with small varices with red wale marks, or CTP-class C patients with any size varices. Studies on primary prophylaxis of variceal bleeding, spanning almost 3 decades, have reported on the benefits of NSBBs such as propranolol, nadolol, and more recently carvedilol.[18–24] The other therapy with a proven beneficial effect in preventing first variceal bleeding in patients with HRV is EVL. Either one or the other should be used (**Table 2**), as combination therapy has no advantages and can increase adverse effects. Shared decision making considering patients' preference when choosing between NSBB and EVL should be strongly considered, to ensure patients' adherence.

Table 2
For patients with cirrhosis and no prior variceal bleeding: nonselective beta-blocker or endoscopic variceal ligation (also see Fig. 3)

Therapy	No Ascites	Ascites	Goal
Propranolol	20–160 mg twice daily	20–80 mg twice daily	Titrate to HR 55–60 or SBP <90
Nadolol	20–160 mg daily	20–80 mg daily	Titrate to HR 55–60 or SBP <90
Carvedilol	3.125–12.5 mg daily	Avoid	Titrate to *12.5–25* mg/d or SBP<90
EVL	EGD every 2–8 wks until EV eradication → repeat EGD at 3–6 mo → EGD every 6-12 mo if no large varices		Variceal eradication; if recurrent large varices → resume banding every 2-8 wks

In the PREDESCI trial, patients with compensated cirrhosis and CSPH but without HRV treated with propranolol (titrated to 160 mg twice daily or maximum dose tolerated) or carvedilol (titrated to 25 mg/d or maximum dose tolerated) had an increased decompensation-free survival, especially a delayed development of ascites.[4] Of note, this effect was seen after 2 years of follow-up, and most patients had untreated chronic hepatitis C. Based on PREDESCI trial, the new paradigm will aim to prevent any decompensation in patients with CSPH, not just the first variceal bleeding in patients with HRV. As such, in patients with compensated cirrhosis, NSBB will be initiated earlier without the requirement of finding HRV on EGD, as the decision will be based on noninvasive testing suggestive of CSPH. In patients with decompensated cirrhosis, recommendations may change as well to favor initiation of NSBBs without EGD, given the high prevalence of small varices in these patients, the difficulty to perform EVL for small varices, and possible additional benefits from NSBBs.[17] EGD may be reserved for patients who cannot tolerate NSBBs, with the goal to perform EVL if large varices are detected.

After initiating NSBBs, patients need to be carefully monitored for adverse effects while titrating the dose to goal (see **Table 2**) or to the maximally tolerated dose. For propranolol and nadolol, the treatment goal is to achieve a resting heart rate of 55 to 60 beats per minute, in the absence of hypotension or adverse effects. For carvedilol, a dose of 12.5 mg/d was found to prevent first variceal bleed, without a specific heart rate goal.[25,26] NSBBs have the advantage of decreasing portal pressure and therefore have the potential of reducing not only variceal hemorrhage, but other complications of cirrhosis.

Safety concerns have been raised regarding the use of NSBBs in patients with decompensated cirrhosis, particularly in patients with refractory ascites or after an episode of spontaneous bacterial peritonitis.[27,28] These earlier reports finding increased kidney dysfunction and mortality secondary to NSBBs have been challenged by subsequent studies.[29,30] It seems that the harmful effect is dose-dependent and related to a low mean arterial pressure.[31] Therefore, NSBBs are not contraindicated in patients with ascites, but they require careful use or interruption in the event of severe circulatory dysfunction (eg, hypotension, hyponatremia, or hepatorenal syndrome). Avoid high doses (not to exceed 80 mg propranolol orally twice a day or 80 mg nadolol orally daily); avoid carvedilol given its additional vasodilating effect and therefore higher likelihood to decrease blood pressure. Titrate NSBBs to avoid systolic blood pressure of less than 90 mm Hg, and temporarily discontinue NSBBs in the setting of bleeding, infection, or kidney dysfunction.[1]

EVL is a local therapy without an effect on portal pressure and carries the risk of bleeding from ligation-induced ulcers.[32,33] Additionally, EVL is not recommended in patients with high-risk small varices, because small varices are difficult to ligate. Importantly, if NSBBs are chosen as primary prophylactic therapy, there is no need for surveillance endoscopies. If EVL is chosen, endoscopy is done every 2 to 8 weeks if varices are large enough for band ligation; once variceal eradication is achieved, repeat endoscopy for surveillance is indicated at 3 to 6 months, followed by EGD every 6 to 12 months until large varices are detected, and band ligation is required again.[1]

SPECIAL CONSIDERATIONS REGARDING PRIMARY PROPHYLAXIS OF BLEEDING FROM FUNDAL VARICES

There is no specific approach regarding primary prophylaxis of variceal bleeding from fundal varices, given limited data in these patients.[1] The use of NSBBs or endoscopic obliteration with cyanoacrylate glue was evaluated in patients with large fundal varices (GOV2 or IGV1) and no prior bleeding.[34] There was a lower bleeding rate observed with endoscopic obliteration, but the small number of patients could support a firm recommendation. AASLD guidance suggests that NSBBs can be used for primary prophylaxis of bleeding from GOV2/IGV1, as this is the least invasive treatment, and it could also prevent decompensation of cirrhosis.[1] As discussed for esophageal varices, the issues regarding preventing decompensation in patients with compensated cirrhosis with fundal varices would favor the use of NSBBs.

SECONDARY PROPHYLAXIS OF VARICEAL BLEEDING: NONSELECTIVE BETA-BLOCKERS OR ENDOSCOPIC VARICEAL LIGATION

In patients who have bled from varices, the 1-year risk of recurrent variceal bleeding can be as high as 60% in the absence of secondary prophylaxis. The recommended treatment to prevent recurrent hemorrhage consists of combination therapy NSBB plus EVL.

Nonselective Beta-Blockers Used for Secondary Prophylaxis of Variceal Bleeding Are Nadolol or Propranolol

In this setting (dose and goals as per **Table 2**), there are not enough data to recommend carvedilol, as there are no randomized controlled trials, and patients may have more severe liver disease and are more prone to be more vasodilated. NSBBs should be started during hospitalization, once octreotide is discontinued, to allow monitoring of blood pressure, heart rate, and occurrence of any clinical adverse effects prior to discharge.

Endoscopic Variceal Ligation

In this setting, EVL is done every 2 to 8 weeks until varices are eradicated, followed by surveillance endoscopy at 3 to 6 months after variceal eradication, and every 6 to 12 months indefinitely. When large varices recur, EVL is resumed every 2 to 8 weeks until variceal eradication.

The key element of combination therapy is NSBBs, particularly in CTP-B/C class patients in whom a higher mortality has been shown when patients are on EVL alone compared with combination therapy NSBBs plus EVL.[35]

Patients who have had TIPS placed during the episode of acute variceal bleeding should not receive NSBB or EVL, as the shunt resolves portal hypertension and varices. However, they will require Doppler ultrasound of the TIPS every 6 months (at the time of HCC surveillance) to assess TIPS patency.

SPECIAL CONSIDERATIONS REGARDING SECONDARY PROPHYLAXIS OF BLEEDING FROM FUNDAL VARICES

If the initial bleeding resolved or it was controlled with cyanoacrylate glue obliteration, strategies to decrease the risk of rebleeding from fundal varices include repeat cyanoacrylate glue, TIPS, or intravascular obliteration with sclerosant (balloon-occluded retrograde transvenous obliteration or BRTO).[36–39] To allow retrograde access to the fundal varices, BRTO requires the presence of a spontaneous gastrorenal or splenorenal shunt, which actually occurs in 60% to 80% of patients with fundal varices. Because it does not divert the portal blood flow from the liver but actually increases it, BRTO does not cause hepatic encephalopathy, but it may cause worsening ascites or bleeding from esophageal varices. TIPS and BRTO are recommended by AASLD as first-line treatments to prevent rebleeding, reserving the use of cyanoacrylate glue injections for situations when TIPS and BRTO are not feasible.[1]

Fig. 3 presents a stepwise approach for the outpatient management of patients with cirrhosis to appropriately use NSBBs, EVL, and other interventions targeting gastroesophageal varices.

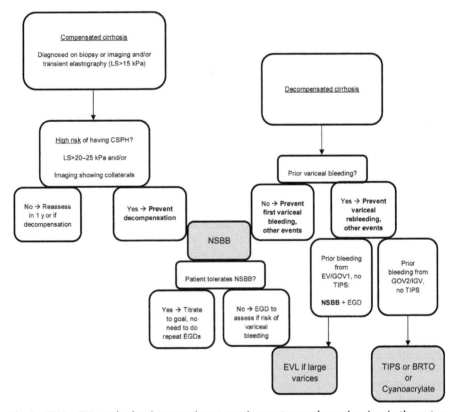

Fig. 3. NSBBs, EVL, and other interventions targeting gastroesophageal varices in the outpatient management of patients with cirrhosis.

INPATIENT MANAGEMENT OF GASTROESOPHAGEAL VARICES

Treatment of acute variceal bleeding is the most important aspect of inpatient management of GEV, but it is important to note that most hospital admissions for patients with cirrhosis are complications not related to variceal bleeding. These hospitalizations are opportunities to ensure patients receive appropriate management of GEV.

ACUTE VARICEAL BLEEDING

Advances in the management of acute variceal bleeding are associated with improved survival, but the 6-week mortality rate remains high, up to 20%.[40,41] Several therapies, including vasoactive medications, antibiotics, endoscopic methods (eg, EBL or sclerotherapy, glue injection, balloon tamponade, esophageal stent, and hemostatic powder), and interventional radiology treatments (TIPS, coil embolization, balloon-occluded retrograde transvenous obliteration) are currently used to treat acute variceal bleeding. **Fig. 4** summarizes the inpatient management of GEV, including interventions recommended by AASLD as quality metrics in cirrhosis care.

General management should focus on

- Resuscitation (intravenous access: airway/breathing/circulation) and orotracheal intubation, especially in patients with massive hematemesis or mental status changes
- Restrictive transfusion of packed red blood cells - transfuse when hemoglobin is less than 7 g/dL, with the goal of 7 to 9 g/dL[42]

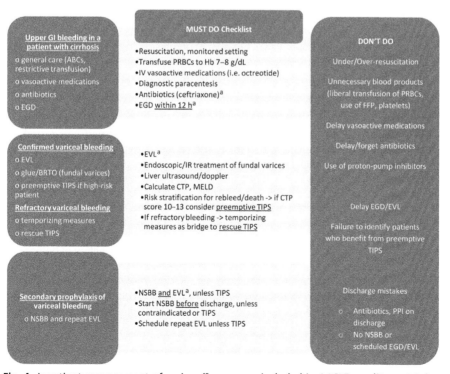

Fig. 4. Inpatient management of varices ([a] measures included in AASLD quality metrics).

- Avoid unnecessary correction of coagulopathy, as there is no evidence that correcting platelet count or INR are of benefit in variceal hemorrhage[1]
- Discontinue outpatient medications (diuretics, NSBBs) if low blood pressure in the setting of bleeding; of note, NSBBs could blunt the sympathetic response to hemorrhage

Specific pharmacologic therapy for acute variceal hemorrhage should be initiated as soon as diagnosis is suspected and while planning for an urgent upper endoscopy. This includes

- Vasoactive therapy causes splanchnic vasoconstriction and reduction in portal pressure - octreotide, terlipressin or somatostatin, with similar efficacy,[43] or vasopressin, which is less commonly used
  - Octreotide: intravenous bolus of 50 μg followed by a continuous infusion of 50 μg/h (2–5 days)
  - Terlipressin: 2 mg intravenously every 4 hours (initial 48 hours), followed by 1 mg intravenously every 4 hours (2–5 days)
  - Somatostatin: intravenous bolus of 250 μg followed by a continuous infusion of 250 to 500 μg/h (2–5 days)
- Antibiotic prophylaxis to decrease the variceal rebleeding rate and mortality by decreasing the risk of bacterial infection (in particular spontaneous bacterial peritonitis)[44]
  - Intravenous ceftriaxone 1 g/24 h, 5 to 7 days (stop once off vasoactive therapy, or at the time of discharge)

Proton pump inhibitors (PPIs) have no effect on variceal bleeding. While it is reasonable to start intravenous PPIs while awaiting EGD, they should be discontinued once variceal bleeding is confirmed. If used briefly to help with postbanding ulcer, although the evidence is limited, PPIs should not be continued after discharge.

EGD needs to be performed within 12 hours of admission, with EVL if a diagnosis of variceal hemorrhage is established based on several criteria[1]:

- Active bleeding from a varix
- Stigmata of recent hemorrhage are observed on a varix (clot, white nipple)
- Only nonbleeding varices are seen and there is no other source of bleeding

For patients in whom bleeding is brisk and banding cannot be performed, or if refractory bleeding not controlled with medical and endoscopic therapy, several temporizing measures may help. Balloon tamponade involves using a tube with an esophageal and a gastric balloon. It requires training and following a specific protocol, to avoid complications. It is effective in controlling bleeding temporarily, as a bridge to TIPS or, less likely, liver transplantation. It can cause lethal complications such as aspiration, esophageal ulceration, and perforation. Recently, self-expandable esophageal stents were found to have greater efficacy and less complications than balloon tamponade in the control of EVH in treatment failures.[45] Early application of hemostatic powder was also evaluated for acute variceal bleeding,[46] but it requires follow-up EGD for EVL after 24 hours, and more data are needed to establish its role. Balloon tamponade and esophageal stents are temporary bridge therapies, as ultimately, patients with refractory bleeding require TIPS placement (rescue TIPS). Because patients who rebled despite standard therapy and require rescue TIPS are mostly Child C patients, the mortality after rescue TIPS is high.

Pre-emptive (early) TIPS (pTIPS) placement is a strategy that anticipates treatment failure and death by pre-emptively placing TIPS soon after therapeutic EVL in patients at high risk of failing standard therapy. In a randomized trial including patients with a CTP score of 10 to 13 (excluding those with score 14 or 15) and CTB-B patients with active bleeding at endoscopy, pTIPS was associated with a 25% absolute risk reduction in mortality.[47] Subsequent studies have confirmed lower mortality with pTIPS in CTB-C (10–13 points),[48–50] despite which pTIPS is placed in only a minority of these patients.[51] The indication for pTIPS in CTP-B patients still requires further investigation. Interestingly, when using MELD score, pTIPS was found to be associated with improved survival in patients with MELD of at least 19, with no survival benefit if MELD less than 12.[52]

Other Considerations to Help Plan for Further Treatment

Diagnostic paracentesis to evaluate for spontaneous bacterial peritonitis that could have precipitated variceal bleeding should be performed before starting antibiotics.

Doppler ultrasound to assess the presence of hepatocellular carcinoma and portal vein patency should be performed prior to TIPS. Portal vein thrombosis can further increase portal pressure, and anticoagulation is of benefit to prevent recurrent variceal hemorrhage, but should not be initiated in the setting of active or recent hemorrhage. In fact, a recent trial showed that TIPS placement was more effective than EVL plus propranolol in preventing variceal rebleeding in patients with cirrhosis and PVT occluding greater than 50% of the lumen.[49]

For patients with GEV requiring enteral feeding, there is reluctance to insert nasogastric or enteric tubes, especially early after endoscopic treatment, out of fear that it may precipitate variceal (re)bleeding. While the mere presence of varices is not considered a contraindication, most hepatology/gastroenterology providers wait 24 to 48 hours after endoscopic treatment, although there are limited data in this regard. A recent retrospective chart review on patients requiring enteric feeding with known EV but no recent bleeding or endoscopic treatment reported that 14% of patients developed hematemesis, bloody nasogastric aspirate, or melena within 48 hours from tube placement,[53] but it did not offer details regarding the source of bleeding. A small randomized study[54] looked at enteral feeding versus no feeding after variceal hemorrhage and found no differences in outcomes, including gastrointestinal hemorrhage; however, the study was underpowered to detect a statistically significant difference.

Risk stratification of early rebleeding or death using CTP score and MELD score is essential, as it modifies the therapeutic strategy for high-risk patients.

TIPS considerations include

- Adjunctive embolization of esophageal and/or gastric collaterals at the time of TIPS placement is routinely performed by many interventional radiologists, as it was shown to decrease short-term rebleeding rate[55,56]
- Discontinue vasoactive medication (once TIPS is in place, octreotide or other vasoactive medication is of no benefit, as pressure reduction achieved by TIPS is much greater than reduction with pharmacologic therapy)
- Secondary prophylaxis with NSBBs and EVL is not recommended as long as TIPS remains patent with a gradient less than 12 mm Hg (the threshold associated with complications secondary to portal hypertension)
- TIPS will need evaluation with ultrasound Doppler every 6 months to check for patency; if suspicion for stenosis, TIPS interrogation/revision is necessary to make sure the gradient remains less than 12 mm Hg

ACUTE VARICEAL BLEEDING FROM FUNDAL VARICES

Although the general management is similar, endoscopic treatment of bleeding fundal varices does not rely upon EVL as complete suction of the varix into the ligator is difficult (fundal varices are usually larger than esophageal varices and the gastric mucosa is thicker), and postbanding ulcers can lead to severe hemorrhage.[1] More efficient endoscopic methods to control bleeding from GOV2/IGV1 include obliteration with cyanoacrylate glue or endoscopic ultrasound with combined coil insertion and cyanoacrylate or other adjuncts such as Gelfoam,[57–62] although not approved in the United States and currently used off-label. Interventional radiology treatments include TIPS and BRTO.[63–66] TIPS has a greater than 90% success rate in achieving initial hemostasis,[67] and it is recommended by the AASLD as the treatment of choice for bleeding from fundal varices.[1] As fundal varices may bleed at lower portosystemic pressure gradient than esophageal varices and may persist post-TIPS, BRTO is an attractive alternative in patients with a patent gastro- or splenorenal shunt. Furthermore, combining TIPS and BRTO may be an effective approach in selected patients with bleeding gastric varices.[68,69] Given the complexity of care and the high expertise required for optimal treatment, patients with bleeding fundal varices should be treated in a tertiary center by a multidisciplinary team.

In conclusion, several interventions are recommended for the outpatient and inpatient management of esophageal and gastric varices. Although a select group of patients is best served by a multidisciplinary portal hypertension treatment team in a tertiary center, most patients can and should receive optimal treatment from practicing gastroenterologists.

DISCLOSURE

The authors have nothing to disclose. Supported by the Yale Liver Center (National Institutes of Health grant P30 DK34989).

REFERENCES

1. Garcia-Tsao G, Abraldes JG, Berzigotti A, et al. Portal hypertensive bleeding in cirrhosis: risk stratification, diagnosis, and management: 2016 practice guidance by the American Association for the study of liver diseases. Hepatology 2017;65: 310–35.

2. Sarin SK, Kumar A. Gastric varices: profile, classification, and management. Am J Gastroenterol 1989;84:1244–9.

3. Kanwal F, Tapper EB, Ho C, et al. Development of quality measures in cirrhosis by the practice metrics committee of the American Association for the Study of Liver Diseases. Hepatology 2019;69:1787–97.

4. Villanueva C, Albillos A, Genesca J, et al. Beta blockers to prevent decompensation of cirrhosis in patients with clinically significant portal hypertension (PREDESCI): a randomised, double-blind, placebo-controlled, multicentre trial. Lancet 2019;393:1597–608.

5. De Franchis R, Abraldes JG, Bajaj J, et al. Expanding consensus in portal hypertension report of the Baveno VI Consensus Workshop: stratifying risk and individualizing care for portal hypertension. J Hepatol 2015;63:743–52.

6. North Italian Endoscopic Club for the S, Treatment of Esophageal V. Prediction of the first variceal hemorrhage in patients with cirrhosis of the liver and esophageal varices. A prospective multicenter study. N Engl J Med 1988;319:983–9.

7. Ripoll C, Groszmann R, Garcia-Tsao G, et al. Hepatic venous pressure gradient predicts clinical decompensation in patients with compensated cirrhosis. Gastroenterology 2007;133:481–8.

8. Abraldes JG, Bureau C, Stefanescu H, et al. Noninvasive tools and risk of clinically significant portal hypertension and varices in compensated cirrhosis: the "Anticipate" study. Hepatology 2016;64:2173–84.

9. Augustin S, Pons M, Maurice JB, et al. Expanding the Baveno VI criteria for the screening of varices in patients with compensated advanced chronic liver disease. Hepatology 2017;66:1980–8.

10. Thabut D, Bureau C, Layese R, et al. Validation of Baveno VI criteria for screening and surveillance of esophageal varices in patients with compensated cirrhosis and a sustained response to antiviral therapy. Gastroenterology 2019;156: 997–1009.e5.

11. Berzigotti A, Seijo S, Arena U, et al. Elastography, spleen size, and platelet count identify portal hypertension in patients with compensated cirrhosis. Gastroenterology 2013;144:102–11.e1.

12. Takuma Y, Nouso K, Morimoto Y, et al. Measurement of spleen stiffness by acoustic radiation force impulse imaging identifies cirrhotic patients with esophageal varices. Gastroenterology 2013;144:92–101.e2.

13. Petta S, Sebastiani G, Bugianesi E, et al. Non-invasive prediction of esophageal varices by stiffness and platelet in non-alcoholic fatty liver disease cirrhosis. J Hepatol 2018;69:878–85.

14. Patanwala I, McMeekin P, Walters R, et al. A validated clinical tool for the prediction of varices in PBC: the Newcastle varices in PBC score. J Hepatol 2013;59: 327–35.

15. Colecchia A, Ravaioli F, Marasco G, et al. A combined model based on spleen stiffness measurement and Baveno VI criteria to rule out high-risk varices in advanced chronic liver disease. J Hepatol 2018;69:308–17.

16. Jangouk P, Turco L, De Oliveira A, et al. Validating, deconstructing and refining Baveno criteria for ruling out high-risk varices in patients with compensated cirrhosis. Liver Int 2017;37:1177–83.

17. Turco L, Villanueva C, La Mura V, et al. Lowering portal pressure improves outcomes of patients with cirrhosis, with or without ascites: a meta-analysis. Clin Gastroenterol Hepatol 2020;18(2):313–27.e6.

18. Yang J, Ge K, Chen L, et al. The efficacy comparison of carvedilol plus endoscopic variceal ligation and traditional, nonselective β-blockers plus endoscopic variceal ligation in cirrhosis patients for the prevention of variceal rebleeding: a meta-analysis. Eur J Gastroenterol Hepatol 2019;31(12):1518–26.

19. Zacharias AP, Jeyaraj R, Hobolth L, et al. Carvedilol versus traditional, nonselective beta-blockers for adults with cirrhosis and gastroesophageal varices. Cochrane Database Syst Rev 2018;(10):CD011510.

20. Schwarzer R, Kivaranovic D, Paternostro R, et al. Carvedilol for reducing portal pressure in primary prophylaxis of variceal bleeding: a dose-response study. Aliment Pharmacol Ther 2018;47:1162–9.

21. Abd ElRahim AY, Fouad R, Khairy M, et al. Efficacy of carvedilol versus propranolol versus variceal band ligation for primary prevention of variceal bleeding. Hepatol Int 2018;12:75–82.

22. Gupta V, Rawat R, Shalimar, et al. Carvedilol versus propranolol effect on hepatic venous pressure gradient at 1 month in patients with index variceal bleed: RCT. Hepatol Int 2017;11:181–7.

23. Reiberger T, Ulbrich G, Ferlitsch A, et al. Carvedilol for primary prophylaxis of variceal bleeding in cirrhotic patients with haemodynamic non-response to propranolol. Gut 2013;62:1634–41.

24. Poynard T, Cales P, Pasta L, et al. Beta-adrenergic-antagonist drugs in the prevention of gastrointestinal bleeding in patients with cirrhosis and esophageal varices. An analysis of data and prognostic factors in 589 patients from four randomized clinical trials. Franco-Italian Multicenter Study Group. N Engl J Med 1991;324:1532–8.

25. Tripathi D, Ferguson JW, Kochar N, et al. Randomized controlled trial of carvedilol versus variceal band ligation for the prevention of the first variceal bleed. Hepatology 2009;50:825–33.

26. Shah HA, Azam Z, Rauf J, et al. Carvedilol vs. esophageal variceal band ligation in the primary prophylaxis of variceal hemorrhage: a multicentre randomized controlled trial. J Hepatol 2014;60:757–64.

27. Mandorfer M, Bota S, Schwabl P, et al. Nonselective beta blockers increase risk for hepatorenal syndrome and death in patients with cirrhosis and spontaneous bacterial peritonitis. Gastroenterology 2014;146:1680–16890.e1.

28. Serste T, Melot C, Francoz C, et al. Deleterious effects of beta-blockers on survival in patients with cirrhosis and refractory ascites. Hepatology 2010;52: 1017–22.

29. Bossen L, Krag A, Vilstrup H, et al. Nonselective beta-blockers do not affect mortality in cirrhosis patients with ascites: post hoc analysis of three randomized controlled trials with 1198 patients. Hepatology 2016;63:1968–76.

30. Mookerjee RP, Pavesi M, Thomsen KL, et al. Treatment with non-selective beta blockers is associated with reduced severity of systemic inflammation and improved survival of patients with acute-on-chronic liver failure. J Hepatol 2016;64:574–82.

31. Tergast TL, Kimmann M, Laser H, et al. Systemic arterial blood pressure determines the therapeutic window of non-selective beta blockers in decompensated cirrhosis. Aliment Pharmacol Ther 2019;50:696–706.

32. Gluud LL, Krag A. Banding ligation versus beta-blockers for primary prevention in oesophageal varices in adults. Cochrane Database Syst Rev 2012;(8):CD004544.

33. Sharma M, Singh S, Desai V, et al. Comparison of therapies for primary prevention of esophageal variceal bleeding: a systematic review and network meta-analysis. Hepatology 2019;69:1657–75.

34. Mishra SR, Sharma BC, Kumar A, et al. Primary prophylaxis of gastric variceal bleeding comparing cyanoacrylate injection and beta-blockers: a randomized controlled trial. J Hepatol 2011;54:1161–7.

35. Albillos A, Zamora J, Martinez J, et al. Stratifying risk in the prevention of recurrent variceal hemorrhage: results of an individual patient meta-analysis. Hepatology 2017;66:1219–31.

36. Fukuda T, Hirota S, Sugimura K. Long-term results of balloon-occluded retrograde transvenous obliteration for the treatment of gastric varices and hepatic encephalopathy. J Vasc Interv Radiol 2001;12:327–36.

37. Hung HH, Chang CJ, Hou MC, et al. Efficacy of non-selective beta-blockers as adjunct to endoscopic prophylactic treatment for gastric variceal bleeding: a randomized controlled trial. J Hepatol 2012;56:1025–32.

38. Lo GH, Liang HL, Chen WC, et al. A prospective, randomized controlled trial of transjugular intrahepatic portosystemic shunt versus cyanoacrylate injection in the prevention of gastric variceal rebleeding. Endoscopy 2007;39:679–85.

39. Mishra SR, Chander Sharma B, Kumar A, et al. Endoscopic cyanoacrylate injection versus beta-blocker for secondary prophylaxis of gastric variceal bleed: a randomised controlled trial. Gut 2010;59:729–35.

40. Ardevol A, Ibanez-Sanz G, Profitos J, et al. Survival of patients with cirrhosis and acute peptic ulcer bleeding compared with variceal bleeding using current first-line therapies. Hepatology 2018;67:1458–71.
41. Vuachet D, Cervoni JP, Vuitton L, et al. Improved survival of cirrhotic patients with variceal bleeding over the decade 2000-2010. Clin Res Hepatol Gastroenterol 2015;39:59–67.
42. Villanueva C, Colomo A, Bosch A, et al. Transfusion strategies for acute upper gastrointestinal bleeding. N Engl J Med 2013;368:11–21.
43. Seo YS, Park SY, Kim MY, et al. Lack of difference among terlipressin, somato-statin, and octreotide in the control of acute gastroesophageal variceal hemor-rhage. Hepatology 2014;60:954–63.
44. Chavez-Tapia NC, Barrientos-Gutierrez T, Tellez-Avila F, et al. Meta-analysis: anti-biotic prophylaxis for cirrhotic patients with upper gastrointestinal bleeding - an updated Cochrane review. Aliment Pharmacol Ther 2011;34:509–18.
45. Escorsell A, Pavel O, Cardenas A, et al. Esophageal balloon tamponade versus esophageal stent in controlling acute refractory variceal bleeding: a multicenter randomized, controlled trial. Hepatology 2016;63:1957–67.
46. Ibrahim M, El-Mikkawy A, Abdel Hamid M, et al. Early application of haemostatic powder added to standard management for oesophagogastric variceal bleeding: a randomised trial. Gut 2019;68:844–53.
47. Garcia-Pagan JC, Caca K, Bureau C, et al. Early use of TIPS in patients with cirrhosis and variceal bleeding. N Engl J Med 2010;362:2370–9.
48. Hernandez-Gea V, Procopet B, Giraldez A, et al. Preemptive-TIPS improves outcome in high-risk variceal bleeding: an observational study. Hepatology 2019;69:282–93.
49. Lv Y, Qi X, He C, et al. Covered TIPS versus endoscopic band ligation plus pro-pranolol for the prevention of variceal rebleeding in cirrhotic patients with portal vein thrombosis: a randomised controlled trial. Gut 2018;67:2156–68.
50. Lv Y, Yang Z, Liu L, et al. Early TIPS with covered stents versus standard treat-ment for acute variceal bleeding in patients with advanced cirrhosis: a rando-mised controlled trial. Lancet Gastroenterol Hepatol 2019;4:587–98.
51. Thabut D, Pauwels A, Carbonell N, et al. Cirrhotic patients with portal hypertension-related bleeding and an indication for early-TIPS: a large multi-centre audit with real-life results. J Hepatol 2017;68:73–81.
52. Lv Y, Zuo L, Zhu X, et al. Identifying optimal candidates for early TIPS among pa-tients with cirrhosis and acute variceal bleeding: a multicentre observational study. Gut 2019;68:1297–310.
53. Al-Obaid L, Bazarbashi AN, Cohen ME, et al. Enteric tube placement in patients with esophageal varices: Risks and predictors of postinsertion gastrointestinal bleeding. JGH Open 2019;4(2):256–9.
54. de Ledinghen V, Beau P, Mannant PR, et al. Early feeding or enteral nutrition in patients with cirrhosis after bleeding from esophageal varices? A randomized controlled study. Dig Dis Sci 1997;42:536–41.
55. Gaba RC. Transjugular intrahepatic portosystemic shunt creation with emboliza-tion or obliteration for variceal bleeding. Tech Vasc Interv Radiol 2016;19:21–35.
56. Qi X, Liu L, Bai M, et al. Transjugular intrahepatic portosystemic shunt in combi-nation with or without variceal embolization for the prevention of variceal rebleed-ing: a meta-analysis. J Gastroenterol Hepatol 2014;29:688–96.
57. Al-Ali J, Pawlowska M, Coss A, et al. Endoscopic management of gastric variceal bleeding with cyanoacrylate glue injection: safety and efficacy in a Canadian population. Can J Gastroenterol 2010;24:593–6.

58. Kahloon A, Chalasani N, DeWitt J, et al. Endoscopic therapy with 2-octyl-cyano-acrylate for the treatment of gastric varices. Dig Dis Sci 2014;59:2178–83.
59. Rios Castellanos E, Seron P, Gisbert JP, et al. Endoscopic injection of cyanoac-rylate glue versus other endoscopic procedures for acute bleeding gastric vari-ces in people with portal hypertension. Cochrane Database Syst Rev 2015;(5):CD010180.
60. Bhat YM, Weilert F, Fredrick RT, et al. EUS-guided treatment of gastric fundal vari-ces with combined injection of coils and cyanoacrylate glue: a large U.S. expe-rience over 6 years (with video). Gastrointest Endosc 2016;83:1164–72.
61. Weil D, Cervoni JP, Fares N, et al. Management of gastric varices: a French na-tional survey. Eur J Gastroenterol Hepatol 2016;28:576–81.
62. Lee HA, Chang JM, Goh HG, et al. Prognosis of patients with gastric variceal bleeding after endoscopic variceal obturation according to the type of varices. Eur J Gastroenterol Hepatol 2019;31:211–7.
63. Imai Y, Nakazawa M, Ando S, et al. Long-term outcome of 154 patients receiving balloon-occluded retrograde transvenous obliteration for gastric fundal varices. J Gastroenterol Hepatol 2016;31:1844–50.
64. Lee SJ, Kim SU, Kim MD, et al. Comparison of treatment outcomes between balloon-occluded retrograde transvenous obliteration and transjugular intrahe-patic portosystemic shunt for gastric variceal bleeding hemostasis. J Gastroenterol Hepatol 2017;32:1487–94.
65. Chu HH, Kim M, Kim HC, et al. Long-term outcomes of balloon-occluded retro-grade transvenous obliteration for the treatment of gastric varices: a comparison of ethanolamine oleate and sodium tetradecyl sulfate. Cardiovasc Interv Radiol 2018;41:578–86.
66. Stein DJ, Salinas C, Sabri S, et al. Balloon retrograde transvenous obliteration versus endoscopic cyanoacrylate in bleeding gastric varices: comparison of re-bleeding and mortality with extended follow-up. J Vasc Interv Radiol 2019;30: 187–94.
67. Chau TN, Patch D, Chan YW, et al. "Salvage" transjugular intrahepatic portosys-temic shunts: gastric fundal compared with esophageal variceal bleeding. Gastroenterology 1998;114:981–7.
68. Lakhoo J, Bui JT, Lokken RP, et al. Transjugular intrahepatic portosystemic shunt creation and variceal coil or plug embolization ineffectively attain gastric variceal decompression or occlusion: results of a 26-patient retrospective study. J Vasc Interv Radiol 2016;27:1001–11.
69. Saad WE. Combining transjugular intrahepatic portosystemic shunt with balloon-occluded retrograde transvenous obliteration or augmenting tips with variceal embolization for the management of gastric varices: an evolving middle ground? Semin Intervent Radiol 2014;31:266–8.

Cutaneous Manifestations of Chronic Liver Disease

Ashaki D. Patel, MD*, Kimberly Katz, MD, Kenneth B. Gordon, MD

KEYWORDS

- Cutaneous manifestations • Liver disease • Cirrhosis • Pruritus • Jaundice

KEY POINTS

- Although chronic liver disease can be caused by multiple different etiologies, cutaneous physical examination findings seen in patients with chronic liver disease are often nonspecific.
- Pruritus, jaundice, and spider angiomas are common skin findings seen in many patients with hepatic dysfunction.
- Specific cutaneous signs of chronic liver disease are commonly seen in the setting of untreated hepatitis.

INTRODUCTION

There are many cutaneous manifestations of liver disease. Recognition of various skin associations of liver disease can not only help guide diagnosis but may help with management of the underlying liver disease as well. Cutaneous manifestations can be divided into general cutaneous signs and symptoms that may manifest in cirrhosis, and other, more specific cutaneous signs that are associated with distinct chronic liver diseases. General cutaneous signs include pruritus, jaundice, xanthomas, spider angiomas, palmar erythema, hair loss, and nail changes. Liver diseases with more specific cutaneous signs that are reviewed here include primary biliary cholangitis, hepatitis B, hepatitis C, hemochromatosis, and alcoholic liver disease.

GENERAL CUTANEOUS SIGNS OF HEPATIC DISEASE
Pruritus

Pruritus is defined as an unpleasant sensation that prompts a response to scratch.[1] Overall, it is the most common skin-related complaint and the most common cutaneous manifestation of liver disease. In patients with liver disease, pruritus is often associated with cholestasis in conditions like primary biliary cholangitis, primary

Department of Dermatology, Medical College of Wisconsin, 8701 Watertown Plank Road, Milwaukee, WI 53226, USA
* Corresponding author.
E-mail address: aspatel@mcw.edu

Clin Liver Dis 24 (2020) 351–360
https://doi.org/10.1016/j.cld.2020.04.003
1089-3261/20/© 2020 Elsevier Inc. All rights reserved.

sclerosing cholangitis, obstructive choledocholithiasis, carcinoma of the bile duct, and chronic viral hepatitis.

The sensation of itch is primarily mediated by unmyelinated C-fibers with nerve endings in the epidermis. Various itch mediators act on these nerve endings and transmit the sensation of itch through the ascending spinothalamic nerve tract, resulting in the perception of itch. There are various itch mediators in the skin, and several are thought to play a role in liver disease, including bile acids, endogenous opioids, lysophosphatidic acid, and autotaxin.[2,3] Bile acids (BAs) accumulate in patients with liver disease resulting in cholestasis. It is known that injection of bile acids into the skin of healthy individuals produces the sensation of itch.[4] However, pruritus does not always happen in all patients with cholestatic liver disease; thus, implying that BA levels do not always correlate with intensity of pruritus. In addition, BA resins do not always successfully diminish itch in patients with cholestasis.[5] Nevertheless, BA resins remain a mainstay of therapy in cholestatic patients. Although some studies have demonstrated that endogenous opioids also may play a role mediating itch, the relationship between endogenous opioids and itch intensity has not been fully elucidated.[6] Lysophosphatidic acid (LPA), a phospholipid produced by the enzyme autotaxin (ATX), is another endogenous molecule that has been found to play a significant role in cholestatic pruritus.[6,7] Unlike endogenous opioids, serum LPA levels and ATX activity does correlate with intensity of pruritus.

Pruritus has a significant impact on patient-reported quality of life and is often the reason patients seek medical care.[8] Currently, cholestyramine, an anion exchange resin, is the only medication approved by the Food and Drug Administration for cholestatic pruritus.[9] There are several additional agents that have been studied as treatment for cholestatic pruritus. A meta-analysis of five prospective randomized clinical trials showed that rifampicin is effective in treating cholestatic pruritus as well. However, administration for longer than 2 weeks is not recommended because of side effects including potential hepatotoxicity.[10] Sertraline, a serotonin reuptake inhibitor, has also shown to be moderately effective in cholestatic pruritus.[11] Because sertraline is metabolized by the liver caution should be used when administering this agent in patients with liver disease. The fourth line of therapy is opioid antagonists. Both μ-opioid receptor antagonists, naltrexone and naloxone, have been effective in treating cholestatic pruritus; however, they should be avoided in patients with acute liver injury or severe liver insufficiency.[12–14] Further research investigating LPA antagonists and ATX blockers as future therapeutic agents is still required. Additional nonpharmacological treatments may be used in combination with these oral therapies or as second-line treatments if the usual oral therapies fail. These include narrowband ultraviolet B therapy (nbUVB), plasmapheresis, nasobiliary drainage, albumin dialysis, and biliary diversion procedures. Of these, nbUVB therapy is commonly used in the dermatologic setting to treat itch and inflammatory disorders of the skin. The antipruritic effect of phototherapy may be due to an alteration of cytokine release, depletion of Langerhans cells, chemical modification of pruritogens in the skin, and the reduction of skin sensitivity to pruritogens.[15]

Nevus Araneus

Nevus araneus, commonly known as a spider angioma, is a cutaneous vascular manifestation that can be seen in 10% to 15% of healthy individuals. However, when multiple spider angiomas are seen, they can be a manifestation of liver disease, especially alcoholic cirrhosis and hepatopulmonary syndrome.[16,17] Spider angiomas are so named because they consist of an ascending spiraling arteriole, ending in the superficial epidermis, with numerous branching capillaries radiating peripherally in the papillary dermis, revealing the configuration of a spider.[18] They are classically non-palpable, blanching lesions approximately 1 to 10 mm in size, usually dispersed over the face, chest, arms, and hands. However, atypical lesions have been described in conjunction with liver disease, including larger spider angiomas, papillary spider angiomas, and mucocutaneous spider angiomas.[19–21] Spider angiomas are dilations of preexisting arterioles in the skin, thought to be mediated by various factors including increased estrogen levels, increased vascular endothelial growth factor, basic fibroblastic growth factor, and even substance P.[22,23] Spider angiomas tend to resolve as the underlying liver disease is treated.

Palmar Erythema

Palmar erythema refers to a nontender, blanching, symmetric redness of both palms, and sometimes soles. Erythema is most commonly seen on the thenar and hypothenar eminences of the palmar surface.[24] Although palmar erythema can be seen in many clinical states, palmar erythema of hepatic disease should not be confused with physiologic erythema of the palms, which often presents over the entire palm due to positioning, temperature, or pressure. Palmar erythema seen in hepatic disease has been observed to be caused by increased free estrogen levels, which leads to vasodilation of surface capillaries in the hands.[24]

Xanthomas

Xanthomas are yellow-orange papules or plaques that form around the eyes due to the deposition of lipids in the dermis, specifically macrophages. They can develop due to either a primary or secondary lipid disorder, but in the setting of hepatic disease, xanthomas are most commonly seen secondary to primary biliary cholangitis (PBC).[25,26] Total cholesterol is often elevated in PBC[27], and abnormal cholesterol metabolism in hepatic disease contributes to formation of xanthomas. It is thought that approximately 15% to 50% of patients with PBC have xanthomas[25]. Xanthelasmas, or plane xanthomas of the eyelids, are believed to occur in approximatley 5-10% of patients with PBC.[28] Xanthomas tend to regress with treatment of the underlying hyperlipidemia.

Jaundice

Jaundice refers to a yellow to brown discoloration of the skin and/or mucous membranes secondary to hyperbilirubinemia, often exceeding the range of 2.5 to 3.0 mg/dL. The color change often corresponds to the level of bilirubin with mild hyperbilirubinemia causing mild yellow color change all the way to brown, indicating more severe hyperbilirubinemia.[29] When present, it is important to establish the cause of jaundice, including conjugated or unconjugated and prehepatic, intrahepatic, or posthepatic.[30]

CUTANEOUS PATTERNS SEEN IN SPECIFIC HEPATIC DISEASES
Primary Biliary Cholangitis

PBC is an autoimmune disease leading to the progressive destruction of the small bile ducts of the liver. In 50% of patients, the presenting symptom is pruritus. Pruritus when accompanied by jaundice, hyperpigmentation, and xanthomas is specific for PBC.[31] However, PBC can present with a variety of other cutaneous manifestations. In a prospective case control study looking at dermatologic manifestations in 49 patients with PBC, a total of 330 different skin disorders were identified and more than one-third of these patients presented initially with a cutaneous finding of PBC. The most common cutaneous presentation of PBC in this cohort was fungal infections including tinea pedis and onychomycosis. Pruritus and xerosis (dry skin) were found in 69.3% of patients.[32] In addition, because PBC is an autoimmune disorder, it can be seen in conjunction with other autoimmune disorders that affect the skin, including Sjögren syndrome, and morphea.[33–35]

Hepatitis B

Hepatitis B is a chronic liver infection caused by the hepatitis B virus. The infection is often divided into the pre-icteric (prodromal) phase and the icteric phase. Urticarial lesions are common during the prodromal phase and are thought to be due to immune-complex deposition.[36] Urticaria is characterized as the development of wheals (itchy edematous papules or plaques in the superficial dermis, that typically develop acutely within 24 hours) and/or angioedema (more painful swelling that occurs deeper in the dermis and subcutaneous/submucosal tissue lasting longer than 24 hours).[1]

Hepatitis B infection can also present with various types of vasculitides, including small vessel vasculitis, urticarial vasculitis, and polyarteritis nodosa.[37] Small vessel vasculitis refers to immune-complex deposition in the dermal post-capillary venules, leading to cutaneous presentations with palpable purpura, erythematous papules, or hemorrhagic vesicles that range in size from 1 mm to several centimeters.[1] Urticarial vasculitis is a variant of small vessel vasculitis that presents with urticarial lesions rather than erythematous or purpuric lesions.

Polyarteritis nodosa (PAN), a type of medium-sized vasculitis, is most commonly associated with hepatitis B. In fact, approximately 7% to 8% of patients with hepatitis B have concomitant PAN.[38–40] PAN usually occurs approximately 6 months into a hepatitis B infection, likely due to immune-complex deposition. Interestingly, the treatment for hepatitis B–associated PAN is antiviral agents combined with plasma exchanges.[40]

In addition to vasculitis, metabolic disorders like porphyria cutanea tarda (PCT) also may be seen with hepatitis B. Porphyrias are metabolic disorders that arise from either inherited or acquired deficiencies in 1 of 8 heme synthesis enzymes. The disorder manifests on the skin as blisters, erosions, milia, or fragile skin in sun-exposed areas of the body, classically the dorsal hands. Of the various types of porphyrias, PCT is most commonly seen in hepatitis infections.[41] Although the exact etiology of this relationship is not clear yet, activation of the host immune system and complement system with heightened autoimmune phenomenon are thought to be contributing factors.[41,42] It is also important to mention that patients with PCT and chronic active hepatitis have an increased risk of developing hepatocellular carcinoma.[43]

Finally, hepatitis B infections have also been known to trigger a type of dermatitis called acrodermatitis papulosa, or Gianotti-Crosti syndrome. This is a symmetric, popular eruption on the face, extremities, and buttocks associated most commonly with viral infections.[44] Although it is more common to see Gianotti-Crosti syndrome in childhood, it has been reported several times in adults associated with concomitant hepatitis B infection.[45,46]

Hepatitis C

Although recent advances in hepatitis C treatment often cure patients of the infection, patients who do not receive or who fail treatment can go on to develop chronic infection, which is associated with multiple cutaneous manifestations. Some skin findings associated with chronic hepatitis C infection are also seen in patients with hepatitis B infection, including small vessel vasculitis, urticarial vasculitis, and PCT. Other cutaneous manifestations, such as cryoglobulinemia, necrolytic acral erythema, sarcoidosis, and lichen planus, are more specific to hepatitis C infection.

Cryoglobulinemia refers to the presence of cryoglobulins, or immunoglobulins with the ability to precipitate at temperatures less than 37 °C in the blood.[47] The presence of cryoglobulins in the blood leads to a systemic inflammatory syndrome that includes cryoglobulinemic vasculitis with cutaneous manifestations. Predisposing conditions for this type of vasculitis include hepatitis C infection.[48] In fact, approximately 80% of mixed cryoglobulinemia is secondary to hepatitis C virus (HCV) infection.[49] Cutaneous manifestations of this type of vasculitis include purpura, ulcers usually on distal extremities, livedo reticularis, and urticarial lesions. The treatment for cryoglobulinemia depends on the underlying cause. For hepatitis C–related cryoglobulinemia, treatment with direct-acting antiviral therapy is essential.[47]

Another common cutaneous manifestation seen in patients with hepatitis C is necrolytic acral erythema (NAE). NAE is even thought to be a cutaneous marker for hepatitis C infection.[50,51] Clinically, NAE presents as painful and/or pruritic well-circumscribed dark violet to black-colored plaques with hyperkeratosis on mostly acral skin. Although it can present clinically similar to necrolytic migratory erythema, positive HCV serology with normal glucagon levels can help make the diagnosis.[52] Treatment of NAE is also very closely related to treatment with hepatitis C. Several reports have shown resolution of NAE with interferon alfa and ribavirin.[53,54] Oral zinc, even in patients with normal zinc serum levels, has also shown to be effective, as it may enhance the effects of hepatitis C treatment.[55–57]

Lichen planus (LP) is a chronic autoimmune, inflammatory disorder that affects both the skin and mucous membranes. Its exact etiology is unknown; however, infectious triggers, especially hepatitis C, are known to be associated with LP. It is clinically characterized as having shiny, flat-topped, violaceous, polygonal-shaped papules up to a centimeter in size.[58] However, in the mouth, it manifests most commonly on the buccal mucosa as reticular white plaques, white papules, or atrophic erosions.[59] Many studies have shown a significant association between LP and HCV, more specifically erosive oral LP.[59] The prevalence of hepatitis C in patients with oral LP is high, and longstanding HCV infection has been observed to be a risk factor in development of oral LP.[60,61] A meta-analysis also showed significant association between oral LP and HCV, suggesting that it is reasonable to screen for hepatitis C in patients with oral LP. Of note, isolated cutaneous LP has not been shown to be significantly associated with HCV.[58]

Hemochromatosis

Hemochromatosis, and the state of iron overload it describes, is most commonly caused by an inherited disorder affecting iron transportation. Whereas PBC is most commonly seen in female individuals, 90% of patients with diagnosed with hemochromatosis are male.[31] Hereditary hemochromatosis is one of the most common genetic disorders in white individuals and often clinically manifests in those with underlying comorbid inflammatory liver conditions such as hepatic steatosis, alcoholic liver disease, and hepatitis.[62–64] In addition to nonspecific cutaneous stigmata associated with comorbid hepatic disease, one of the most commonly seen cutaneous findings in patients with excess iron deposition in the skin is hyperpigmentation.

Hyperpigmentation is the presenting symptom in one-third of patients with hemochromatosis and is usually generalized, yet prominence can be noted on exposed skin.[65] Skin often appears slate gray (due to dermal iron) or brown (due to increased melanin production).[66,67] In a minority of patients, the mucous membranes and conjunctiva are also affected. This hyperpigmentation is reflected in the description of hemochromatosis as "bronze diabetes."

Unlike most other causes of chronic liver disease, most systemic dysfunction due to iron deposition can be effectively treated. Phlebotomy usually reverses damage done to many organ systems, including the skin, and phlebotomy often leads to lightning of the skin.[62,67]

Cirrhosis and Alcohol Cirrhosis

Cirrhosis refers to the histology findings of hepatic nodules, fibrosis, and loss of functional hepatocytes that occurs in the setting of chronic liver disease.[67] Four of the most common liver diseases that lead to cirrhosis include alcoholic liver disease, chronic viral hepatitis, hemochromatosis, and nonalcoholic liver disease.[67,68]

Cutaneous manifestations of cirrhosis affect the skin, nails, and hair. Alterations in vascular physiology lead to the appearance of palmar erythema, spider angiomas, and paper money skin. Paper money skin is a rarer variant of spider angiomas that appear as diffuse, thin plaques of superficial capillaries usually on the trunk. These lesions blanch with diascopy and the wiry thin vessels resemble the silk threads seen on dollar bills in the United States.[69] Caput medusa describes the dilated and tortuous abdominal veins that occur due to portal hypertension.

Nail changes seen in the setting of cirrhosis include those caused by defects to the nail bed, such as Muerhcke lines and Terry nails. Muerhcke lines are characterized by double transverse lines that disappear when pressure is applied. These paired lines are due to decreased serum albumin and abnormal nail bed vasculature.[64,67] In Terry nails, the proximal two-thirds of the nail appears white with sparing of the distal nail that appears as a band of normal pink or brown color.[31,66,67] Clubbing, in which the angle between the proximal nail fold and nail plate is greater than 180°, is often seen in patients with pulmonary hypertension.[1] Although Terry nails are classically associated with cirrhosis, the nail findings in patients with cirrhosis are nonspecific and can be seen in a variety of other systemic conditions.

Diffuse thinning or loss of pubic and axillary hair or the development of female distribution of pubic hair is often seen in the setting of hyperestrinism. Cutaneous manifestations of liver disease are seen in nearly half of chronic alcoholics.[66,70] Nearly three-fourths of patients with alcohol cirrhosis have spider angiomas, palmar erythema, and Dupuytren contracture.[70]

SUMMARY

Ultimately, there are many cutaneous manifestations of liver disease. In some instances, cutaneous signs may be a marker of liver disease (ie, NAE) or may even be related to underlying severity of liver disease. In other cases, cutaneous signs may be more nonspecific (ie, pruritus, spider angiomas). Ultimately cutaneous manifestations are important to both recognize and treat. Recognition of these skin findings may aid in earlier diagnosis and management of chronic liver diseases, and treatment of cutaneous signs helps render a more complete approach to patient care.

DISCLOSURE

The authors have nothing to disclose.

REFERENCES

1. Bolognia JL, Schaffer JV, Cerroni L. Dermatology. 4th edition. Philadelphia: Elsevier; 2018.
2. Bernhard JD. Itch: mechanisms and management of pruritus. New York: McGraw-Hill; 1994.

3. Bunchorntavakul C, Reddy KR. Pruritus in chronic cholestatic liver disease. Clin Liver Dis 2012;16(2):331–46.
4. Varadi DP. Pruritus induced by crude bile and purified bile acids: experimental production of pruritus in human skin. Arch Dermatol 1974;109(5):678–81.
5. Kuiper EM, van Erpecum KJ, Beuers U, et al. The potent bile acid sequestrant colesevelam is not effective in cholestatic pruritus: results of a double-blind, randomized, placebo-controlled trial. Hepatology 2010;52(4):1334–40.
6. Kremer AE, Martens JJ, Kulik W, et al. Lysophosphatidic acid is a potential mediator of cholestatic pruritus. Gastroenterology 2010;139(3):1008–18, 1018.e1001.
7. Kremer AE, Bolier R, van Dijk R, et al. Advances in pathogenesis and management of pruritus in cholestasis. Dig Dis 2014;32(5):637–45.
8. Jin XY, Khan TM. Quality of life among patients suffering from cholestatic liver disease-induced pruritus: a systematic review. J Formos Med Assoc 2016; 115(9):689–702.
9. Duncan JS, Kennedy HJ, Triger DR. Treatment of pruritus due to chronic obstructive liver disease. Br Med J (Clin Res Ed) 1984;289(6436):22.
10. Bachs L, Pares A, Elena M, et al. Effects of long-term rifampicin administration in primary biliary cirrhosis. Gastroenterology 1992;102(6):2077–80.
11. Mayo MJ, Handem I, Saldana S, et al. Sertraline as a first-line treatment for cholestatic pruritus. Hepatology 2007;45(3):666–74.
12. Bergasa NV, Alling DW, Talbot TL, et al. Effects of naloxone infusions in patients with the pruritus of cholestasis. A double-blind, randomized, controlled trial. Ann Intern Med 1995;123(3):161–7.
13. Wolfhagen FH, Sternieri E, Hop WC, et al. Oral naltrexone treatment for cholestatic pruritus: a double-blind, placebo-controlled study. Gastroenterology 1997;113(4):1264–9.
14. Terg R, Coronel E, Sorda J, et al. Efficacy and safety of oral naltrexone treatment for pruritus of cholestasis, a crossover, double blind, placebo-controlled study. J Hepatol 2002;37(6):717–22.
15. Hussain AB, Samuel R, Hegade VS, et al. Pruritus secondary to primary biliary cholangitis: a review of the pathophysiology and management with phototherapy. Br J Dermatol 2019;181(6):1138–45.
16. Li CP, Lee FY, Hwang SJ, et al. Spider angiomas in patients with liver cirrhosis: role of alcoholism and impaired liver function. Scand J Gastroenterol 1999; 34(5):520–3.
17. Silverio Ade O, Guimaraes DC, Elias LF, et al. Are the spider angiomas skin markers of hepatopulmonary syndrome? Arq Gastroenterol 2013;50(3):175–9.
18. Khasnis A, Gokula RM. Spider nevus. J Postgrad Med 2002;48(4):307–9.
19. Yalcin K, Ekin N, Atay A. Unusual presentations of spider angiomas. Liver Int 2013;33(3):487.
20. Sharma A, Sharma V. Giant spider angiomas. Oxf Med Case Reports 2014; 2014(3):55.
21. Singh S, Sahoo AK, Ramam M, et al. Mucocutaneous spider angiomas in an adolescent with chronic liver disease. Arch Dis Child 2018;103(12):1145.
22. Li CP, Lee FY, Hwang SJ, et al. Spider angiomas in patients with liver cirrhosis: role of vascular endothelial growth factor and basic fibroblast growth factor. World J Gastroenterol 2003;9(12):2832–5.
23. Li CP, Lee FY, Hwang SJ, et al. Role of substance P in the pathogenesis of spider angiomas in patients with nonalcoholic liver cirrhosis. Am J Gastroenterol 1999; 94(2):502–7.

24. Serrao R, Zirwas M, English JC. Palmar erythema. Am J Clin Dermatol 2007;8(6): 347–56.
25. Purohit T, Cappell MS. Primary biliary cirrhosis: pathophysiology, clinical presentation and therapy. World J Hepatol 2015;7(7):926–41.
26. Baila-Rueda L, Mateo-Gallego R, Lamiquiz-Moneo I, et al. Severe hypercholesterolemia and phytosterolemia with extensive xanthomas in primary biliary cirrhosis: role of biliary excretion on sterol homeostasis. J Clin Lipidol 2014;8(5):520–4.
27. Longo M, Crosignani A, Battezzati PM, et al. Hyperlipidaemic state and cardiovascular risk in primary biliary cirrhosis. Gut 2002;51(2):265–9.
28. Kaplan MM, Gershwin ME. Primary biliary cirrhosis. N Engl J Med 2005;353(12): 1261–73.
29. Morioka D, Togo S, Kumamoto T, et al. Six consecutive cases of successful adult ABO-incompatible living donor liver transplantation: a proposal for grading the severity of antibody-mediated rejection. Transplantation 2008;85(2):171–8.
30. Fargo MV, Grogan SP, Saguil A. Evaluation of jaundice in adults. Am Fam Physician 2017;95(3):164–8.
31. Cherfane CE, Hollenbeck RD, Go J, et al. Hereditary hemochromatosis: missed diagnosis or misdiagnosis? Am J Med 2013;126(11):1010–5.
32. Koulentaki M, Ioannidou D, Stefanidou M, et al. Dermatological manifestations in primary biliary cirrhosis patients: a case control study. Am J Gastroenterol 2006; 101(3):541–6.
33. Murray-Lyon IM, Thompson RP, Ansell ID, et al. Scleroderma and primary biliary cirrhosis. Br Med J 1970;3(5717):258–9.
34. Marasini B, Gagetta M, Rossi V, et al. Rheumatic disorders and primary biliary cirrhosis: an appraisal of 170 Italian patients. Ann Rheum Dis 2001;60(11): 1046–9.
35. Powell FC, Schroeter AL, Dickson ER. Primary biliary cirrhosis and the CREST syndrome: a report of 22 cases. Q J Med 1987;62(237):75–82.
36. Cribier B. Urticaria and hepatitis. Clin Rev Allergy Immunol 2006;30(1):25–9.
37. Gower RG, Sausker WF, Kohler PF, et al. Small vessel vasculitis caused by hepatitis B virus immune complexes. Small vessel vasculitis and HBsAG. J Allergy Clin Immunol 1978;62(4):222–8.
38. Guillevin L, Lhote F, Cohen P, et al. Polyarteritis nodosa related to hepatitis B virus. A prospective study with long-term observation of 41 patients. Medicine (Baltimore) 1995;74(5):238–53.
39. Guillevin L, Mahr A, Callard P, et al. Hepatitis B virus-associated polyarteritis nodosa: clinical characteristics, outcome, and impact of treatment in 115 patients. Medicine (Baltimore) 2005;84(5):313–22.
40. Trepo C, Guillevin L. Polyarteritis nodosa and extrahepatic manifestations of HBV infection: the case against autoimmune intervention in pathogenesis. J Autoimmun 2001;16(3):269–74.
41. Pyrsopoulos NT, Reddy KR. Extrahepatic manifestations of chronic viral hepatitis. Curr Gastroenterol Rep 2001;3(1):71–8.
42. Akhter A, Said A. Cutaneous manifestations of viral hepatitis. Curr Infect Dis Rep 2015;17(2):452.
43. Baravelli CM, Sandberg S, Aarsand AK, et al. Porphyria cutanea tarda increases risk of hepatocellular carcinoma and premature death: a nationwide cohort study. Orphanet J Rare Dis 2019;14(1):77.
44. Marcassi AP, Piazza CAD, Seize M, et al. Atypical Gianotti-Crosti syndrome. An Bras Dermatol 2018;93(2):265–7.

45. Dikici B, Uzun H, Konca C, et al. A case of Gianotti Crosti syndrome with HBV infection. Adv Med Sci 2008;53(2):338–40.
46. Turhan V, Ardic N, Besirbellioglu B, et al. Gianotti-Crosti syndrome associated with HBV infection in an adult. Ir J Med Sci 2005;174(3):92–4.
47. Silva F, Pinto C, Barbosa A, et al. New insights in cryoglobulinemic vasculitis. J Autoimmun 2019;105:102313.
48. Levey JM, Bjornsson B, Banner B, et al. Mixed cryoglobulinemia in chronic hepatitis C infection. A clinicopathologic analysis of 10 cases and review of recent literature. Medicine (Baltimore) 1994;73(1):53–67.
49. Vleugels RA, Rosenbach MA, Zone JJ, et al. Dermatological Signs of Systemic Disease E-Book. Netherlands: Elsevier Health Sciences; 2016.
50. el Darouti M, Abu el Ela M. Necrolytic acral erythema: a cutaneous marker of viral hepatitis C. Int J Dermatol 1996;35(4):252–6.
51. Abdallah MA, Ghozzi MY, Monib HA, et al. Necrolytic acral erythema: a cutaneous sign of hepatitis C virus infection. J Am Acad Dermatol 2005;53(2):247–51.
52. Dogra S, Jindal R. Cutaneous manifestations of common liver diseases. J Clin Exp Hepatol 2011;1(3):177–84.
53. Hivnor CM, Yan AC, Junkins-Hopkins JM, et al. Necrolytic acral erythema: response to combination therapy with interferon and ribavirin. J Am Acad Dermatol 2004;50(5 Suppl):S121–4.
54. Khanna VJ, Shieh S, Benjamin J, et al. Necrolytic acral erythema associated with hepatitis C: effective treatment with interferon alfa and zinc. Arch Dermatol 2000; 136(6):755–7.
55. Abdallah MA, Hull C, Horn TD. Necrolytic acral erythema: a patient from the United States successfully treated with oral zinc. Arch Dermatol 2005; 141(1):85–7.
56. Takagi H, Nagamine T, Abe T, et al. Zinc supplementation enhances the response to interferon therapy in patients with chronic hepatitis C. J Viral Hepat 2001;8(5): 367–71.
57. Najarian DJ, Lefkowitz I, Balfour E, et al. Zinc deficiency associated with necrolytic acral erythema. J Am Acad Dermatol 2006;55(5 Suppl):S108–10.
58. Shengyuan L, Songpo Y, Wen W, et al. Hepatitis C virus and lichen planus: a reciprocal association determined by a meta-analysis. Arch Dermatol 2009; 145(9):1040–7.
59. Al Robaee AA, Al Zolibani AA. Oral lichen planus and hepatitis C virus: is there real association? Acta Dermatovenerol Alp Pannonica Adriat 2006;15(1):14–9.
60. Nagao Y, Sata M. A retrospective case-control study of hepatitis C virus infection and oral lichen planus in Japan: association study with mutations in the core and NS5A region of hepatitis C virus. BMC Gastroenterol 2012;12:31.
61. Lodi G, Giuliani M, Majorana A, et al. Lichen planus and hepatitis C virus: a multicentre study of patients with oral lesions and a systematic review. Br J Dermatol 2004;151(6):1172–81.
62. Chevrant-Breton J, Simon M, Bourel M, et al. Cutaneous manifestations of idiopathic hemochromatosis: study of 100 cases. Arch Dermatol 1977;113(2):161–5.
63. Koulaouzidis A, Bhat S, Moschos J. Skin manifestations of liver diseases. Ann Hepatol 2007;6(3):181–4.
64. Harrison-Findik DD. Role of alcohol in the regulation of iron metabolism. World J Gastroenterol 2007;13(37):4925–30.
65. Callen JP, Gruber GG, Hodge SJ, et al. Cutaneous manifestations of gastrointestinal disorders. J Ky Med Assoc 1978;76(12):603–7.

66. Wu GY, Selsky N, Grant-Kels JM. Atlas of dermatological manifestations of gastrointestinal disease. New York: Springer; 2013.

67. Smith LH Jr. Overview of hemochromatosis. West J Med 1990;153(3):296–308.

68. Irving MG, Halliday JW, Powell LW. Association between alcoholism and increased hepatic iron stores. Alcohol Clin Exp Res 1988;12(1):7–13.

69. Bean WB. Acquired palmar erythema and cutaneous vascular "spiders". Arch Intern Med 1943;134(5):846–53.

70. Hazin R, Abu-Rajab Tamimi TI, Abuzetun JY, et al. Recognizing and treating cutaneous signs of liver disease. Cleve Clin J Med 2009;76(10):599–606.

Pathology in Patients with Chronic Liver Disease

A Practical Approach to Liver Biopsy Interpretation in Patients with Acute and Chronic Liver Diseases

Audrey Deeken-Draisey, MD, Sambasiva M. Rao, MD, Guang-Yu Yang, MD, PhD*

KEYWORDS

- Chronic liver disease • Pathology • Acute liver disease • Liver biopsy • Treatment
- Staging

KEY POINTS

- Liver biopsy and histologic examination are the mainstay for the diagnosis of liver diseases, despite recent robust advances in imaging and molecular procedures.
- Liver biopsy can provide useful information regarding the structural integrity and type and degree of injury, disease activity, response to treatment, progression of disease and degree/staging of fibrosis.
- The caveat for liver biopsy is the limited size, possibly representing one 50,000th of whole organ, leading to sampling error.
- However, this issue is obviated to some extent by using ultrasound and computed tomography-guided biopsies.
- Liver biopsies are performed to evaluate both acute and chronic liver diseases, in addition to mass-forming lesions.

INTRODUCTION
Normal Liver Histology

The human liver is a complex organ performing a multitude of different functions that include specialized metabolic, synthetic, and secretory nature as well as uptake and detoxification of xenobiotics. Based on vascular anatomy and portal vein distribution liver is divided into 8 functionally independent segments. Each segment has its own vascular pedicle consisting of branches of portal vein, hepatic artery, and bile duct.

Department of Pathology, Northwestern University Feinberg School of Medicine, Northwestern Memorial Hospital, 251 East Huron Street, Feinberg 7-230, Chicago, IL 60611, USA
* Corresponding author.
E-mail address: g-yang@northwestern.edu

Clin Liver Dis 24 (2020) 361–372
https://doi.org/10.1016/j.cld.2020.04.001
1089-3261/20/© 2020 Elsevier Inc. All rights reserved.

Histologically, the liver cell organization is referred to as classical lobule or Rappaport's liver acinus. The classical lobule, which is considered a structural unit, is hexagonal, with terminal hepatic vein (central vein) in the center and portal triads, containing branches of hepatic artery, portal vein, and bile duct, are at the periphery (**Fig. 1**). In contrast with the classic lobule, Rappaport's acinus is based on functional microcirculatory pattern and contains portal triads in the center and hepatic vein radicals at the periphery. The liver acinus is arbitrarily subdivided into zones 1, 2, and 3 corresponding to periportal, mid portion, and perihepatic venular areas, respectively. Hepatocytes in zone 1 (periportal area) receives blood rich in oxygen and nutrients and cells in zones 2 and 3 receive blood that is progressively depleted of energy resources, making hepatocytes in zone 3 particularly vulnerable to circulatory insults. In the lobule, hepatocytes are arranged in rows of single cell cords separated by sinusoids. Although under light microscopy all the hepatocytes in the lobule seem to be homogeneous, it is well-recognized that cells in different zones exhibit structural and functional heterogeneity.

ADEQUACY OF LIVER BIOPSY

Irrespective of the route by which liver biopsy is performed, the goal is to obtain a fragment(s) of tissue measuring 1 to 2 cm in length, preferably using a broader gauge needle so that a minimum of 10 to 20 portal areas are included for proper evaluation of rejection, biliary tract diseases, and acute and chronic liver diseases.[1-3] With an adequate liver biopsy specimen, it is the responsibility of the pathologist to systematically analyze both the lobules and portal areas for parenchymal diseases, biliary tract diseases, sinusoidal changes, and mass lesions.

USEFULNESS OF SPECIAL STAINS

Throughout the years, the use of special stains in histopathologic evaluation of liver biopsies has been refined to accommodate a varied set of diagnostic problems in liver function and disease state. Special stains help to increase the diagnostic accuracy of the grading and staging of chronic hepatitis; diagnosing cirrhosis and biliary tract disorders; and assessing fatty liver disease, iron and copper overload, and neoplastic process.[4] Although the exact methods vary between institutions, many hospitals have a standardized set of stains for each liver biopsy. These stains include hematoxylin and eosin, trichrome, reticulin, iron, periodic acid-Schiff (PAS), and diastase pretreated PAS.[4]

Masson trichrome staining helps to identify fibrosis and is the standard method for demonstrating the extent of fibrosis including cirrhosis (**Fig. 2**). Pathologist should be

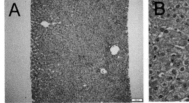
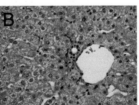
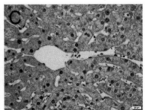

Fig. 1. Morphology of the liver. (*A*) Liver biopsy with normal architecture of central vein to portal triads, (*B*) normal portal tract showing interlobular bile duct, arteriole and portal-vein branch, and (*C*) normal central vein and liver parenchyma.

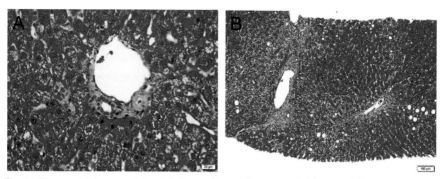

Fig. 2. Masson trichrome stain. (*A*) Normal portal tract and (*B*) portal fibrosis with thin fibrous bridging.

very cautious in interpreting trichrome stain, because collapse owing to necrosis may be interpreted as fibrosis. It is always important to compare the intensity of staining in the portal areas and other areas (see **Fig. 2**A). True fibrosis should show same dark blue stain (see **Fig. 2**B), whereas collapsed areas show a pale blue staining pattern. Reticulin stain is useful in evaluating architecture, collapse, necrosis, fibrosis, and thickness of hepatic plates. Normally, hepatic plates are 1 cell thick (and, rarely, 2 cells thick; **Fig. 3**A), whereas in regeneration and nodular regenerative hyperplasia, the plates are usually 2 to 3 cells thick and in neoplastic lesions they are more than 3 cells thick. In hepatocellular carcinomas, the reticulin fibers are markedly decreased or completely lost (**Fig. 3**B).

PAS stain demonstrates hepatocellular glycogen stores (**Fig. 4**A). Decreased PAS staining can be seen in ischemic damage or necrosis of hepatocytes that have lost their glycogen stores (**Fig. 4**B). Diastase pretreated PAS stains nonglycogen glycoproteins, which has strong usefulness in the identification of phagocytic material within histiocytes (**Fig. 4**C), alpha-1-antritrypsin globules in hepatocytes (**Fig. 4**D), and basement membrane surrounding the bile ducts and ductules.

Iron stain (Perls' Prussian blue stain) identifies hemosiderin and is useful in assessing the amount of iron in both hepatocytes, bile duct epithelium, histiocytes, and Kupffer cells (**Fig. 5**). Hemosiderin with Perls' stain appear as bluish granular material, whereas ferritin appears as a faint blue blush and should not be interpreted as iron.

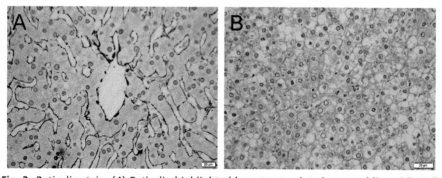

Fig. 3. Reticulin stain. (*A*) Reticulin-highlighted hepatocyte plate in normal liver. (*B*) Well-differentiated hepatocellular carcinoma with loss of reticuline fiber.

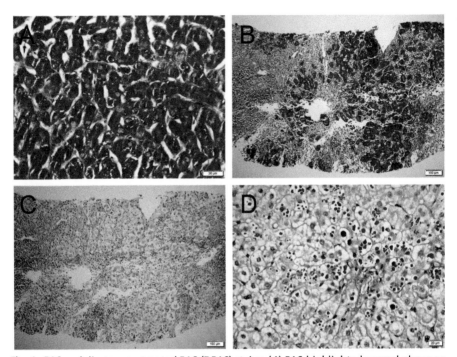

Fig. 4. PAS and diastase pretreated PAS (DPAS) stains. (*A*) PAS-highlighted normal glycogen-rich hepatocytes, (*B*) Liver with bridging necrosis and PAS-highlighted hepatocytes, (*C*) DPAS highlighted clusters of histocytes surrounding necrotic hepatocytes, (*D*) DPAS highlighted alpha-1-antritrypsin globules in hepatocytes.

Iron stain is also helpful in differentiating hemosiderin from other brown or tan staining pigments seen on hematoxylin and eosin, particularly lipofuscin.

PIGMENTS IN LIVER

Commonly observed pigments in the liver include lipofuscin, bile, and hemosiderin. Other rare pigments include Dubin-Johnson pigment and black granules of gold in patients receiving gold chloride for rheumatoid arthritis. Lipofuscin pigment is usually present in perivenular areas and increases with advancing age (**Fig. 6**A) and usually stains with diastase PAS stain and Ziehl-Neelsen stain. A ground glass hepatocyte is a hepatocyte with a flat, hazy, and uniformly dull appearing cytoplasm, commonly owing to either glycogene accumulation or hepatitis viral B surface antigen inclusion (**Fig. 6**B). Hemosiderin is usually first accumulates in zone 1 (see **Fig. 5**C, D) and gradually extends to zones 2 and 3 (see **Fig. 5**A, B). Hemosiderin is a golden brown refractile pigment and easily differentiated from other pigments by Perls' stain (see **Fig. 5**A). Bile pigment is yellow or green and present in hepatocyte cytoplasm and in the canaliculi (**Fig. 6**C, D). Bland cholestasis that is associated with anabolic steroid or estrogen therapy is mostly confined to the perivenular area (**Fig. 6**E, F). Similarly, in the early stages of bile duct obstruction, cholestasis is mostly confined to the perivenular area. The pigment in hepatocytes in Dubin-Johnson syndrome is granular dark brown lipomelanin and stained with Ziehl-Neelsen stain.

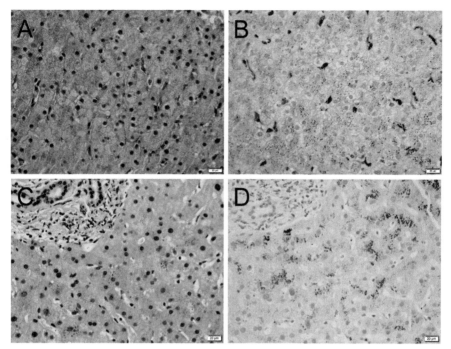

Fig. 5. Perls' iron stain. (*A*) Liver with hemosiderin laden Kupffer cells in the sinusoid space, (*B*) intensely iron-stained Kupffer cells and iron deposition in the hepatocytes, (*C*) hematoxylin and eosin stain showing cytoplasmic hemosiderin granules, and (*D*) iron deposition in the hepatocytes.

COMMON MORPHOLOGIC CHANGES: CLUES TO DISEASE RECOGNITION

Some of the commonly used buzz words that are diagnostically and clinically relevant include macrovesicular fatty change, microvascular fatty change, ballooning change of hepatocytes, lobular disarray, and interface hepatitis.

Macrovesicular Fatty Change

Cytoplasmic fat accumulation in the liver is in the form of either a macrovesicular or microvesicular type. Macrovesicular fatty change can be either in the form of single large fat droplet or several small droplets (**Fig. 7A**). Macrovesicular fatty change is the most common type and represents an excess accumulation of triglycerides in the hepatocytes secondary to diverse etiologies, including alcohol and the metabolic syndrome. Morphologically, the large droplet type is characterized by a large single vacuole in the cytoplasm displacing the nucleus to the periphery. Small droplet fatty change appears as multiple small droplets with centrally located nucleus. Fatty change is (grading of steatosis) scored as mild (6%–33%), moderate (34%–66%), or marked (>67%).[5–7] Less than 5% is consider as normal. Scoring should be on a low power objective (4× or 10×). Pathologists are often asked to evaluate the percentage of fat in the donor liver and should report only the amount of macrovesicular fat.

Microvesicular Fatty Change

In this category, cytoplasm is replete with tiny vesicles appearing foamy and nucleus retained in the center. Sometimes, it is difficult to identify microvesicular fatty change

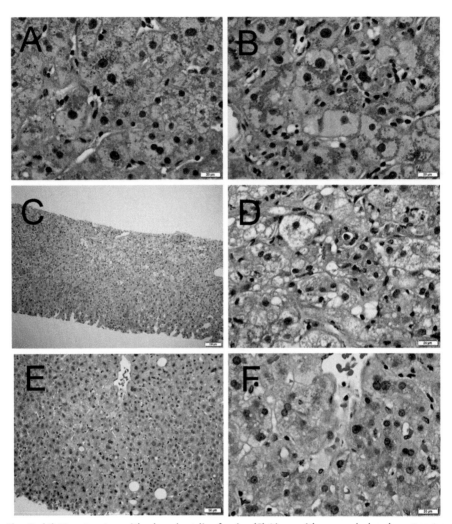

Fig. 6. (*A*) Hepatocytes with abundant lipofuscin. (*B*) Liver with ground-glass hepatocytes and lipofuscin. (*C*) Zone 3 hepatocytes showing ballooning change and cholestasis. (*D*) Canaliculi cholestasis. (*E, F*) Numerous bile plugs are present in canaliculi.

necessitating the use of specific fat stains on frozen sections. Microvesicular fatty change is due to genetic or toxin-induced abnormalities in peroxisomal and mitochondrial fatty acid oxidation.[8–10]

Ballooning Change of Hepatocytes

One of the key histologic components to make a diagnosis of steatohepatitis is the identification of ballooned hepatocytes along with lobular inflammation and pericellular fibrosis.[5–7] Ballooning change is characterized by markedly swollen hepatocytes, 2 to 3 times larger than normal hepatocytes with clear or rarefied cytoplasm secondary to intracellular fluid accumulation (**Fig. 7**B). Cells without these classic features should not be classified as ballooned cells. In case of uncertainty, ballooned cells can be easily confirmed by demonstration of loss of intermediate filaments, cytokeratins

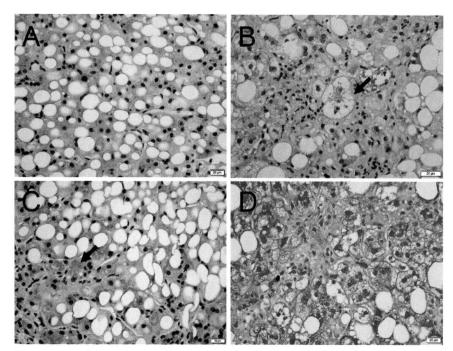

Fig. 7. Steatohepatitis. (*A*) Macrovesicular steatosis, (*B*) macrovesicular steatosis with ballooning hepatocytes (*arrow*), (*C*) macrovesicular steatosis with Mallory body (*arrow*), and (*D*) trichrome stain highlighted pericellular fibrosis.

8/18, by immunohistochemistry. Mallory-Denk bodies, when present, are seen only in ballooned cells (**Fig. 7**C).

Lobular Disarray

Normally, hepatocytes are arranged in single cell cords surrounded by sinusoids. However, in acute hepatitis, irrespective of etiology, hepatocytes with ballooning change, individual (apoptotic bodies) or focal cell necrosis, regenerating cells and condensed reticulin resulting in disorganized appearance of cords (**Fig. 8**A). In addition, there is associated inflammatory infiltrate and may be canalicular cholestasis. Recognition of this histologic pattern (lobular disarray) is very helpful in the diagnosis of acute hepatitis.

Interface Hepatitis

Limiting plate or membrane is an imaginary line where the hepatic parenchyma comes in contact with portal mesenchyme. Usually, this stromal–parenchymal interface is well-defined (see **Fig. 1**B). In the event of acute or chronic hepatitis, this interface is distorted by inflammatory infiltrate with an extension of portal inflammation into the adjacent parenchyma causing hepatocyte loss (apoptosis) and eventually fibrosis.[11] Interface activity can be mild, moderate, or severe and is seen commonly with autoimmune hepatitis (AIH), chronic viral infection, Wilson's disease, and biliary tract diseases (**Fig. 8**). An appreciation of interface activity is very helpful in the diagnosis of chronic hepatitis.[11–13]

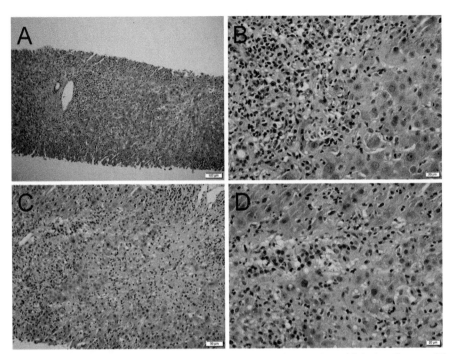

Fig. 8. (*A*) AIH with portal inflammation, minimal central necrosis and lobular disarray, (*B*) portal inflammation with interface activity and numerous plasma cells, (*C*) central and bridging necrosis, and (*D*) bridging necrosis and cluster of plasma cells.

DISEASE PATTERN RECOGNITION

Some novel or specific disease pattern(s) can be recognized morphologically. Particularly, with this background information, we provide clues and guidelines for the diagnosis of most common liver diseases for which biopsies are performed.

Fatty Liver Disease

Although varied etiologies cause fatty liver, the 2 most common causes in the contemporary period are alcohol and obesity (the metabolic syndrome) referred to as alcoholic and nonalcoholic fatty liver disease, respectively.[5] Both alcoholic and nonalcoholic fatty liver disease cause macrovesicular fatty changes that usually start in zone 3 and extend to the other zones with increasing severity. Fatty change should be reported as mild, moderate, or severe, depending on the percentage of hepatocytes with macrovesicular fat.[6] If there is lobular or portal inflammation, it should be included in the report. Fatty change, irrespective of the grade, is a benign and reversible condition with the cessation of underlying cause(s). However, if the inciting cause persists, steatosis progresses to steatohepatitis. Interestingly, there are no identifiable morphologic features that indicate progression or the underlying cause of steatosis. In addition to macrovesicular fatty change, diagnostic criteria for steatohepatitis are ballooned hepatocytes with or without Mallory-Denk bodies, necroinflammatory changes in the lobules, and pericellular (chicken-wire type) fibrosis (**Fig. 7**D).[6] Inflammatory infiltrate secondary to hepatocyte injury includes lymphocytes, histiocytes, and neutrophils. It is generally believed that the number of neutrophils are greater in alcoholic steatohepatitis than in nonalcoholic steatohepatitis. However, satellitosis (neutrophils surrounding ballooned cells with Mallory-Denk bodies) is seen in both alcoholic and nonalcoholic steatohepatitis (see **Fig. 7**). To indicate the disease activity and fibrosis, the NASH [Nonalcoholic Steatohepatitis] Clinical Research Network developed a scoring system based on fatty change, ballooning change, lobular inflammation (**Tables 1** and **2**).[6] Although this scoring system was developed for nonalcoholic fatty liver disease, it can be used for scoring both alcoholic and nonalcoholic fatty liver disease.

Autoimmune Hepatitis

AIH is an immune-mediated liver disease that can present either as acute onset hepatitis mimicking acute viral hepatitis or as chronic hepatitis. Patients with a chronic form of AIH may present with nonspecific clinical symptoms, advanced liver disease, or after having been diagnosed during routine laboratory evaluation for liver enzymes.

Morphologic features of acute autoimmune hepatitis
Lobular disarray consisting of plasma cell infiltrate, apoptotic bodies, ballooning change, Kupffer cell hyperplasia, and variable degrees of necrosis, ranging from perivenular areas to submassive necrosis (see **Fig. 8**).[11–14] In addition, portal inflammation with predominant plasma cell infiltrate and interface activity usually seen (see **Fig. 8**B, D). Canalicular cholestasis and hepatocyte resetting can be seen. In true acute AIH, no portal fibrosis is seen.

Morphologic features of chronic autoimmune hepatitis
The key histologic features are portal inflammation with interface activity, hepatocyte rosette formation, emperipolesis, variable lobular necroinflammatory activity and fibrosis.[11–14] Portal inflammation with predominant plasma cell infiltrate (>70%) or clusters of plasma cells (groups of 5–10 plasma cells) with interface activity is a good diagnostic indicator of AIH (see **Fig. 8**B, D). In chronic AIH portal fibrosis is a consistent finding and the degree of fibrosis depends on the duration and severity of disease. Fibrosis should be staged as portal expansion (stage 1), periportal septa (stage 2), bridging septa (stage 3), and obvious cirrhosis (stage 4). Similar morphologic features can be seen in chronic hepatitis caused by several etiologies including viral infection and drugs. A definitive diagnosis of AIH is possible and should be rendered only after correlating with levels of serum IgG, antinuclear antibodies, anti-smooth muscle antibodies, and liver/kidney microsomal antibodies.

Table 1
Nonalcoholic fatty liver disease activity score system from the nonalcoholic steatohepatitis clinical research network

Score	Fat	Ballooning Cells	Lobular Inflammation
0	Minimal (<5%)	None	None
1	6%–33%	Few	<2 foci per 20× field
2	33%–66%	Many	2–4 foci per 20× field
3	>67%	–	>4 foci per 20× field

From Klein DE, Brunt EM, Van Natta M, et al. Design and validation of a histological scoring system for nonalcoholic fatty liver disease. *Hepatology.* 2005;41(6):1313-1321; with permission.

Table 2
Nonalcoholic steatohepatitis clinical research network scoring system

Fibrosis Stage	Histologic Findings
0	None
1A	Mild zone 3, perisinusoidal
1B	Moderate zone 3, perisinusoidal
1C	Portal/periportal
2	Perisinusoidal and periportal
3	Bridging fibrosis
4	Cirrhosis

From Klein DE, Brunt EM, Van Natta M, et al. Design and validation of a histological scoring system for nonalcoholic fatty liver disease. *Hepatology.* 2005;41(6):1313-1321; with permission.

Drug-Induced Liver Injury

More than 350 drugs have been implicated in causing liver injury, and this number is progressively increasing with the use of immunomodulatory drugs in the treatment of different malignant neoplasms.[8] Drugs can cause acute or chronic liver injury that can simulate any type of liver disease. Usually, drug-induced liver injury is either due to a direct toxic effect (predictable) or an idiosyncratic effect (unpredictable), the latter being the most common type.[8] The direct toxic effect is dose dependent (acetaminophen, some chemotherapeutic drugs) and idiosyncratic through an immunologic idiosyncrasy or an immunoallergic injury (drug hypersensitivity). The pattern of liver injury caused by drugs include zonal necrosis, hepatitis (acute or chronic) with or without cholestasis, granulomas, bland cholestasis, reactive hepatitis, steatosis/steatohepatitis, and sinusoidal obstruction syndrome.[8,9,15] Findings of zonal necrosis or submassive necrosis, predominant eosinophilic infiltrate in the portal areas (**Fig. 9**) and lobules and sinusoidal obstruction syndrome are highly suggestive of drug-induced liver injury. However, in a majority of cases the diagnosis of drug-induced liver injury depends on good clinical history and elimination of viral and autoimmune etiologies.

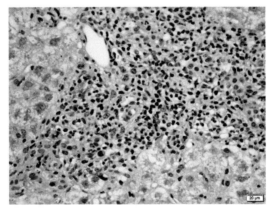

Fig. 9. Drug-induced portal inflammation with dominant lymphocytes and a few of eosinophils.

Immune Checkpoint Inhibitor-Induced Liver Injury

Immune checkpoint inhibitors are currently used in the treatment of different types of malignancies that can cause adverse liver effects. Liver biopsy findings are variable and include lobular hepatitis with or without focal necrosis, sinusoidal macrophage infiltrate with microgranulomas, perivenular hepatitis, portal infiltrate with interface activity, and rarely only bile duct injury with ductular proliferation.[16–18] Lymphoid infiltrates consists of mostly CD3- and CD8-positive cells and fewer CD20- or CD4-positive cells.[17] There are no specific immune checkpoint inhibitor-induced morphologic changes, and requires differentiation from acute and chronic viral diseases and AIH.[16,18]

Sinusoidal Obstruction Syndrome

Sinusoidal obstruction syndrome, previously referred to as veno-occlusive disease, is seen in patients with bone marrow transplantation, hematopoietic stem cell transplantation, and patients receiving chemotherapy for metastatic colorectal carcinoma to the liver.[8,19] Sinusoidal obstruction syndrome is due to toxic injury to sinusoidal endothelial cells and hepatic vein endothelial cells resulting in swelling and the rounding up of endothelial cells. Morphologically, sinusoidal obstruction syndrome is characterized by sinusoidal dilatation, congestion, leakage of blood into space of Disse, atrophy of liver cords, and necrosis of hepatocytes. In severe cases, perisinusoidal fibrosis, nodular regenerative hyperplasia and fibrous obliteration of central vein can be seen.

A PRACTICAL APPROACH TO BIOPSY INTERPRETATION AND CONCLUSION

As discussed elsewhere in this article, there is tremendous overlap in the cellular alterations and morphologic changes caused by virus infection, autoimmunity, drug- and toxin-induced injury, or metabolic diseases. No single morphologic finding can point to a definitive diagnosis. Pathologists should first identify the cellular alterations, pattern of injury, and severity of injury. After a thorough evaluation of the biopsy, and based on histologic findings, a proper differential diagnosis should be formulated. A final diagnosis should be rendered only after evaluating detailed clinical history and laboratory and serologic studies. Without such correlation, the diagnosis will be incomplete or inaccurate.

DISCLOSURE

The authors have disclosed that they have no significant relationships with or financial interest in any commercial companies pertaining to this article.

REFERENCES

1. Fryer E, Wang LM, Verrill C, et al. How often do our liver core biopsies reach current definitions of adequacy? J Clin Pathol 2013;66(12):1087–9.
2. Schiano TD, Azeem S, Bodian CA, et al. Importance of specimen size in accurate needle liver biopsy evaluation of patients with chronic hepatitis C. Clin Gastroenterol Hepatol 2005;3(9):930–5.
3. Bedossa P, Dargere D, Paradis V. Sampling variability of liver fibrosis in chronic hepatitis C. Hepatology 2003;38(6):1449–57.
4. Lefkowitch JH. Special stains in diagnostic liver pathology. Semin Diagn Pathol 2006;23(3–4):190–8.
5. Ong JP, Younossi ZM. Epidemiology and natural history of NAFLD and NASH. Clin Liver Dis 2007;11(1):1–16, vii.

6. Kleiner DE, Brunt EM, Van Natta M, et al. Design and validation of a histological scoring system for nonalcoholic fatty liver disease. Hepatology 2005;41(6): 1313–21.

7. Sorrentino P, Tarantino G, Conca P, et al. Silent non-alcoholic fatty liver disease-a clinical-histological study. J Hepatol 2004;41(5):751–7.

8. Kleiner DE. Recent advances in the histopathology of drug-induced liver injury. Surg Pathol Clin 2018;11(2):297–311.

9. Ramachandran R, Kakar S. Histological patterns in drug-induced liver disease. J Clin Pathol 2009;62(6):481–92.

10. Kleiner DE. The pathology of drug-induced liver injury. Semin Liver Dis 2009; 29(4):364–72.

11. Balitzer D, Shafizadeh N, Peters MG, et al. Autoimmune hepatitis: review of histologic features included in the simplified criteria proposed by the international autoimmune hepatitis group and proposal for new histologic criteria. Mod Pathol 2017;30(5):773–83.

12. Gurung A, Assis DN, McCarty TR, et al. Histologic features of autoimmune hepatitis: a critical appraisal. Hum Pathol 2018;82:51–60.

13. Nguyen Canh H, Harada K, Ouchi H, et al. Acute presentation of autoimmune hepatitis: a multicentre study with detailed histological evaluation in a large cohort of patients. J Clin Pathol 2017;70(11):961–9.

14. Roberts EA. Autoimmune hepatitis from the paediatric perspective. Liver Int 2011;31(10):1424–31.

15. Russo MW, Scobey M, Bonkovsky HL. Drug-induced liver injury associated with statins. Semin Liver Dis 2009;29(4):412–22.

16. Zen Y, Yeh MM. Checkpoint inhibitor-induced liver injury: a novel form of liver disease emerging in the era of cancer immunotherapy. Semin Diagn Pathol 2019; 36(6):434–40.

17. Zen Y, Yeh MM. Hepatotoxicity of immune checkpoint inhibitors: a histology study of seven cases in comparison with autoimmune hepatitis and idiosyncratic drug-induced liver injury. Mod Pathol 2018;31(6):965–73.

18. Karamchandani DM, Chetty R. Immune checkpoint inhibitor-induced gastrointestinal and hepatic injury: pathologists' perspective. J Clin Pathol 2018;71(8): 665–71.

19. Stevenson HL, Prats MM, Sasatomi E. Chemotherapy-induced Sinusoidal Injury (CSI) score: a novel histologic assessment of chemotherapy-related hepatic sinusoidal injury in patients with colorectal liver metastasis. BMC Cancer 2017; 17(1):35.

Transjugular Intrahepatic Portosystemic Shunts

Advances and New Uses in Patients with Chronic Liver Disease

Justin R. Boike, MD, MPH[a],*, Steven L. Flamm, MD[b]

KEYWORDS

- Transjugular intrahepatic portosystemic shunt • Portal hypertension • Ascites
- Varices • Portal vein thrombosis • Spontaneous portal systemic shunts
- Hepatorenal syndrome • Hepatopulmonary syndrome

KEY POINTS

- Transjugular intrahepatic portosystemic shunts have had significant advancements with the introduction of covered, controlled expansion stents resulting in improvement control of ascites and variceal bleeding.
- Transjugular intrahepatic portosystemic shunts are an effective treatment for portal vein thrombosis and can allow for recanalization of the portal vein to permit liver transplantation.
- Transjugular intrahepatic portosystemic shunts and embolization of spontaneous portal systemic shunts is an effective therapy for refractory hepatic encephalopathy.
- Transjugular intrahepatic portosystemic shunts for hepatopulmonary syndrome results in improvement in arterial oxygenation and patient symptoms; however, these results are not sustained after 3 months.
- Transjugular intrahepatic portosystemic shunts is an effective treatment of hepatorenal syndrome with improved mortality in a select patient group however this is not a primary indication for Transjugular intrahepatic portosystemic shunts based on limited data.

INTRODUCTION

Chronic liver disease is the most common cause for clinically significant portal hypertension. Portal hypertension is accompanied most often by the development of ascites and variceal bleeding.[1] These complications lead to significant morbidity and

---

[a] Department of Medicine, Northwestern Feinberg School of Medicine, 676 North St. Clair Street, Suite 1400, Chicago, IL 60611, USA; [b] Hepatology Program, Department of Medicine, Northwestern Feinberg School of Medicine, Chicago, IL, USA
* Corresponding author.
E-mail address: justin.boike@northwestern.edu
Twitter: @justinboike (J.R.B.)

Clin Liver Dis 24 (2020) 373–388
https://doi.org/10.1016/j.cld.2020.04.007
1089-3261/20/© 2020 Elsevier Inc. All rights reserved.

liver.theclinics.com

mortality among patients with cirrhosis. Since the introduction of transjugular intrahepatic portosystemic shunts (TIPS) in 1988, its use has been supported by clinical practice guidelines for the treatment of portal hypertensive complications.[2–5] Presently the primary indications for TIPS have been for the treatment of ascites refractory to medical management and bleeding gastrointestinal varices refractory to endoscopic therapies (**Table 1**).[3,5] Recently, there have been significant advances in TIPS stent technology as well as improvements in placement technique.[6–9] This has resulted in expanded use of TIPS beyond traditional indications supported by well-established guidelines. This article reviews the advances in TIPS and the evidence supporting emerging indications.

Table 1
Indications for TIPS

Indications for TIPS	Clinical Scenario
Traditional	
Esophageal varices	Bleeding refractory to endoscopic therapy
Gastric varices	Primary treatment of bleeding event
Ascites	Ascites refractory to diuretics
Hepatic hydrothorax	Hydrothorax refractory to diuretics
Budd-Chiari syndrome	Not responsive to anticoagulation
Novel	
Early management of ascites	Consideration after 2–3 large volume paracentesis
Before abdominal surgery	Decrease portal hypertension to permit safely performing surgery (ie, laparoscopic cholecystectomy)
Recanalization of portal vein thrombosis	Chronically occluded portal vein thrombosis with portal hypertensive complications and/or to facilitate liver transplant
Embolization of clinically significant spontaneous portosystemic shunts	Refractory hepatic encephalopathy from spontaneous portosystemic shunts
Treatment of hepatopulmonary syndrome	Treatment of moderate-severe hepatopulmonary syndrome
Treatment of hepatorenal syndrome	Treatment of hepatorenal syndrome refractory to medical therapy

PORTAL HYPERTENSION PHYSIOLOGY AND PLACEMENT
Portal Hypertension

Portal hypertension is characterized by an increase in the portal venous pressure in relation to the systemic pressure. This portosystemic gradient (PSG) leads to a pressure difference across the liver. This is typically driven by advanced fibrosis or cirrhosis but can also occur in the setting of portal vein thrombosis (PVT). TIPS placement effectively reduces portal pressure by creating a shunt from the portal venous system (portal vein), through the liver, to the systemic system (hepatic vein). This effectively reduces the PSG alleviating the increased hydrostatic pressure of the portal system. A normal PSG is 5 mm Hg or less. Clinically significant portal hypertension with formation of ascites and varices occurs when the PSG increases to greater than 10 mm Hg. Esophageal varices are at risk for bleeding with a PSG of greater than 12 mm Hg.

Evaluation for Transjugular Intrahepatic Portosystemic Shunt Candidacy

Recipients for TIPS should be formally evaluated by a gastroenterologist or hepatologist to determine if TIPS is appropriate and the benefits outweigh the risks. Liver transplantation candidacy is an important consideration because many traditional indications for TIPS (ascites, hepatic hydrothorax, and bleeding varices) are also indications for liver transplantation. If a patient is a candidate for liver transplantation, this evaluation should occur before the placement of the TIPS to ensure appropriate coordination with the transplantation center in the rare event TIPS leads to worsening hepatic function or liver failure. Considerations include the Model for End-stage Liver Disease (MELD) score, which prognosticates survival after TIPS. Recipients with MELD scores ranging from 6 to 14 generally are not impacted by TIPS, whereas MELD scores of greater than 19 have significantly decreased survival after TIPS, and placement of TIPS should be considered in conjunction with liver transplantation evaluation. Placement of a TIPS should also be performed by an Interventional Radiologist with sufficient expertise in the deployment of TIPS. Recipients should undergo cross-sectional imaging of the liver and portal system with intravenous contrast (either computed tomography or MRI) to assist with procedural planning. Liver ultrasound examination with Doppler imaging of the vessels is an alternative when contrasted cross-sectional imaging it contraindicated. Other pre-TIPS evaluation includes echocardiography to evaluate for underlying congestive heart failure and pulmonary heart failure to ensure cardiovascular reserve with the anticipated large volume of venous return to the heart after TIPS.

Contraindications and Considerations to Transjugular Intrahepatic Portosystemic Shunts

Absolute and relative contraindications to placement of a TIPS are listed in **Table 2**. Absolute contraindications include significant heart failure and/or severe pulmonary hypertension.[3] At the time of TIPS placement, there is a rapid increase in blood volume return to the right heart from portal system. This dynamic shift can result in severe acute decompensated heart failure and be an ongoing issue in those with baseline heart failure. Patients without heart failure but with severe volume overload and elevated right atrial pressures should ideally be adequately diuresed to a euvolemic state before TIPS placement to avoid triggering acute decompensated heart failure after TIPS. Similarly, significant valvular heart disease can result in cardiac decompensation after TIPS and these patients should be managed with the consultation of a cardiologist.[10] Other absolute contraindications to TIPS include ongoing bacteremia or uncontrolled infections because this could lead to seeding of the TIPS prosthesis and serve as a nidus for ongoing infection known as TIPSitis.[11]

Table 2 Absolute and relative contraindications to TIPS	
Absolute	**Relative**
Congestive heart failure	Refractory hepatic encephalopathy
Severe pulmonary hypertension	End-stage liver disease (MELD >19)
Bacteremia/infection	Volume overloaded state
Biliary obstruction	Centrally located liver mass (hepatocellular carcinoma, metastatic disease)
Large liver cysts	Valvular heart disease

The most important relative contraindication to consider is the patient's history of hepatic encephalopathy (HE). HE arises from spontaneous portosystemic shunting (ie, varices or other intra-abdominal collateral veins) of blood combined with underlying hepatic dysfunction from chronic liver disease. Placement of a TIPS can further exacerbate HE owing to increased shunting of portal blood flow through the liver. Approximately 35% of patients experience transient HE after TIPS.[1,3] In some patients (<5%), HE can be refractory thereafter and require permanent occlusion of the TIPS. Thus, a patient with ongoing baseline HE that is not controlled with medical therapy is unlikely a TIPS candidate owing to risk of debilitating HE after TIPS.

Although the placement of a TIPS is a single procedure, there are considerations for its management thereafter. Recipients require monitoring of the TIPS stent with ultrasound doppler imaging at a minimum every 6 months to ensure patency.[3] If ultrasound examination suggests TIPS dysfunction or if there is clinical evidence to suggest occlusion, such as recurrent ascites, then a TIPS revision by interventional radiology is indicated.

Advances in Transjugular Intrahepatic Portosystemic Shunt Stents and Procedural Technique

Until the early 2001, TIPS stents were exclusively bare metal or uncovered stents. These stents unfortunately had high rates failure characterized by stent thrombosis requiring multiple revisions for repeat dilations.[12] Polytetrafluoroethylene-covered stents, or covered stents were introduced in 2001 in the United States and now have entirely replaced bare metal stents in clinical use.[13] Covered stents are associated with lower rates of thrombosis and improved efficacy, as well as improved survival compare to traditional bare metal stents.[12] Covered stents were further improved in 2017 with the introduction of controlled expansion stents (Viatorr CX; W. L. Gore & Associates, Flagstaff, Ariz).[7] These covered, controlled expansion stents allow the operator to dilate the stent diameter to a fixed value of 8 mm. If necessary, then or at a future date, the stent could be further dilated to 10 mm to further decrease the PSG. Of note, noncontrolled expansion stents passively dilate over time to their nominal diameter regardless of initial dilation size. For example, a 10-mm diameter stent would continue to passively dilate even if was dilated to a diameter of 8 mm at the time of placement.[8,14] When compared with traditional covered stents, controlled expansion stents have been shown to result in significantly fewer admissions for ascites (6% vs 14%; $P = .006$) in the first 3 months as well as lower rates of HE when stents are dilated to 8 mm versus 10 mm (26.6% vs 43.2%) with a benefit seen up to 2 years after TIPS.[7,14]

Placement of TIPS has also greatly improved with the assistance of intravascular ultrasound-guided portal vein access. This technique involves the use of an intravascular ultrasound probe positioned in the inferior vena cava and allows for better visualization of the portal veins for guiding the operator.[15] Traditionally, the use of the ultrasound probe was limited to cases with challenging anatomy or hepatic masses. However, it has now gained widespread use because it significantly reduces the fluoroscopy time, volume of iodinated contrast, and overall procedure time.[6,16] This advancement has permitted placement of stents directly across the inferior vena cava into the portal veins when the hepatic veins are completely occluded such as in Budd-Chiari syndrome.[15,17,18] Similarly, in the setting of chronic PVT, placement of a TIPS via the hepatic vein approach to reestablish portal vein blood flow is technically challenging. Transhepatic and trans-splenic approach permits successful cannulation of the portal vein and placement of TIPS along with establishment of portal vein flow.[19–22]

EMERGING INDICATIONS FOR TRANSJUGULAR INTRAHEPATIC PORTOSYSTEMIC SHUNTS

Transjugular Intrahepatic Portosystemic Shunts for Early-Onset Ascites

Ascites that fails to respond to traditional diuretic therapy and dietary sodium restriction (<2 g/d) has been shown to be successfully treated with TIPS, with resolution of ascites approaching 60% to 80% compared with repeated large volume paracentesis (LVP).[3,5,23] Early randomized controlled trials (RCTs) of TIPS for ascites demonstrated these benefits with the use of primarily bare metal (uncovered) stents.[24–30] There were, however, conflicting data on the survival benefit of TIPS compared with LVP. These initial RCTs, using bare metal stents, were composed of heterogenous patient populations with a significant number of patients with decompensated liver disease (Child-Pugh C cirrhosis).[23,31–35] In the most recent multicenter RCT from 2017, the authors used covered stents (not newer controlled expansion stents) in patients with Child-Pugh Scores of less than 12 who were defined as having early ascites by needing 2 LVP within 3 weeks.[36] The authors compared TIPS (n = 29) with LVP with albumin infusions (n = 33).[36] They demonstrated a significant transplant free survival benefit of TIPS (93%) compared with LVP (52%) (P<.003) at 1 year. In multivariate analysis, the only factor associated with improved transplant-free survival was the placement of a TIPS. Among those receiving a TIPS, 52% did not require any further paracentesis compared with none in the LVP group. The average number of paracentesis after TIPS was only 1.0 ± 1.6 per patient in the TIPS group compared with 10.1 ± 7.0 per patient in the LVP group (P<.001). The rates of HE at 1 year were similar among the TIPS and LVP groups at 65%, whereas the number of days of hospitalization were significantly higher in the LVP group (35 ± 40) versus the TIPS group (17 ± 28) (P = .04).[36] These recent data suggest that patients with compensated cirrhosis (Childs-Pugh Score of <12) would benefit from placement of TIPS, both with improved transplant-free survival but also with decreased hospitalization without the added risk of increase HE. These findings, combined with early studies using bare metal stents, suggest that earlier intervention with TIPS at the onset of ascites before further hepatic decompensation likely confers a survival benefit along with improved quality of life from decreased paracentesis without added increase in rates of HE.

Transjugular Intrahepatic Portosystemic Shunts for Treatment of Portal Vein Thrombosis

PVT can be acute or chronic and often occurs in the setting of cirrhosis. Among patients without cirrhosis and PVT, patients frequently have an hypercoagulable state such as in an inherited genetic mutation (ie, factor V Leiden or prothrombin mutations) or in the setting of a myeloproliferative disorder (ie, polycythemia vera).[37,38]

Acute portal vein thrombosis

Acute PVT is typically best managed with therapeutic anticoagulation; however, success rates are only 38% to 44% after at least 6 months of treatment.[37,39] The use of TIPS with portal vein thrombectomy or thrombolysis was shown to be successful with recanalization of the portal vein in 16 of 17 (94%) noncirrhotic patients with acute PVT. Subsequent portal vein patency was 88% at 2 years.[40]

Chronic portal vein thrombosis

Among patients with chronic PVT, the occluded portal vein undergoes cavernous transformation, which leads to the formation of vascular channels. Yet, this transformation is often insufficient to decompress the portal system, and gastroesophageal varices can form with clinically significant bleeding.[41] Treatment of chronic PVT with therapeutic anticoagulation is also fairly unsuccessful with resolution rates of less than 5%, and associated variceal bleeding rates of greater than 50%.[41–43] Aside from variceal bleeding, the presence of chronic PVT has frequently been a contraindication to liver transplantation, given the inadequacy of the native portal vein for anastomosis to the recipient portal vein.[44] Using transhepatic and trans-splenic access as described elsewhere in this article, a TIPS can be placed and allow recanalization of the portal vein, a technique described as a TIPS portal vein reconstruction.[19] Rates of successful recanalization of the portal vein have historically ranged from 57% to 84% (**Table 3**). In the most recent report, among patients listed for liver transplantation at a single center, TIPS portal vein reconstruction was technically successful in 98% of patients, with 39% undergoing successful liver transplantation without subsequent PVT or portal vein complications after transplantation.[45]

Table 3 Reports of TIPS for the treatment and recanalization of chronic PVT				
Author, Year	Study Period	Portal Vein Recanalization	Duration of Follow-up	Portal Vein Patency Rate
Luca et al,[46] 2011	2003–2010	57% (40/70)	20.7 mo	95% (38/40)
Qi et al,[47] 2015	2009–2011	84% (43/51)	40.07 mo	76% (33/43)
Han et al,[48] 2011	2001–2008	75% (43/57)	24 mo	68% (29/43)
Thornberg et al,[45] 2015	2009–2015	98% (60/61)	19.2 mo	92% (50/60)

Transjugular Intrahepatic Portosystemic Shunts for the Treatment of Spontaneous Portosystemic Shunts

HE in cirrhosis often occurs in two situations, episodic HE or refractory HE. Episodic HE is thought to be related to an acute precipitant, such as infection or gastrointestinal bleeding, whereas refractory HE is characterized by ongoing mental disturbance, typically with continuously elevated ammonia levels but without precipitating triggers. Medical therapy of refractory encephalopathy is often ineffective.[49] Refractory encephalopathy is thought to be related to spontaneous portosystemic shunts that divert substantial portal blood flow away from the liver and result in poor hepatic clearance of toxins. Shunting can occur via small collaterals; however, large shunts may be present that can be detected on cross-sectional imaging. Large spontaneous portosystemic shunts typically include mesoentericorenal or mesoentericocaval shunts and can occur in the setting of relatively preserved hepatic synthetic function. This preserved hepatic function results in low MELD scores; hence, patients often have low priority for liver transplantation despite debilitating HE. These spontaneous portosystemic shunts are estimated to contribute to shunting and persistent HE in 46% to 70% of cases.[50–52] As such, these spontaneous portosystemic shunts have been a therapeutic target for embolization and treatment of refractory HE. The use of TIPS grants access into the portal system and easily permits both embolization of culprit shunts and offers portal decompression through the TIPS to prevent future spontaneous portosystemic shunt formation through reduction in the PSG. The published evidence on the embolization of spontaneous portosystemic shunts for treatment of HE has been limited to small case reports with varying approaches at embolization and varying use of TIPS.[53] The largest retrospective multicenter case series to date using TIPS to embolize spontaneous portosystemic shunts to treat refractory HE involved 37 cirrhotic patients, excluding patients with Child-Pugh C (>13).[54] Refractory HE was defined as at least 2 hospital admissions for HE (grade 2 or higher based on the West Haven classification) despite at least 30 days of maximal medical therapy (daily lactulose with or without an oral antibiotic). The average MELD score among TIPS recipients was 13. Within the first 100 days after TIPS and embolization, 59.4% of patients (22/37) remained free of HE. Eighteen patients (48.6% overall) remained free of any HE for the duration of follow-up (mean, 697 ± 157 days). After embolization of the spontaneous portosystemic shunts, there was a significant decrease in the severity of HE and, when it did recur, in the number of hospitalizations and length of stay (**Fig. 1**). Four patients (11%) required repeat embolization based on recurrence of HE. In multivariate analysis, the MELD score was found to be the most predictive of post-TIPS HE with a cutoff score of 11, yielding the highest discrimination (sensitivity of 68.4% and specificity of 77.6%) for recurrent HE.

Transjugular Intrahepatic Portosystemic Shunts to Facilitate an Abdominal Surgery

Extrahepatic intra-abdominal surgery in the setting of cirrhosis and portal hypertension has been associated with a significant risk for postoperative mortality (10%–76%) and postoperative complications, including intraoperative bleeding related to portal hypertension, persistent ascites, and even hepatic decompensation manifest by liver failure.[55–57] The Child-Pugh score is a well-validated tool to predict postoperative mortality after abdominal surgery in patients with cirrhosis.[56,58] Although patients with Child-Pugh C cirrhosis have the worst prognosis, patients with Child-Pugh score A and B are at risk for poor postoperative outcomes. Intraoperative bleeding related to portal hypertension is often problematic. Ascites in the postoperative period can prohibit surgical wound healing and result in abdominal wound infections and even dehiscence.[59,60] The placement of a surgical drain to permit drainage of ascites is not ideal, given risk for bacterial peritonitis along with the likelihood of continued drainage. Placement of a preoperative TIPS to effectively reduce the portal pressure gradient and decrease intraoperative bleeding complications, as well as prevent postoperative ascites, is appealing. There have been multiple reports of success in using TIPS to facilitate abdominal surgery; however, there are no RCTs.[61–66] One group within the context of a case-controlled retrospective study examined 18 patients with cirrhosis who underwent a TIPS compared with 17 historical controls matched on age, etiology of cirrhosis, indication for surgery, and type of surgery to assess potential survival differences.[67] No significant differences in survival were observed at 1 month (83% vs 88%) or 1 year (54% vs 63%), although the Child-Pugh score was higher in the TIPS group compared with the control group (7.7 vs 6.2; $P<.05$). A subsequent larger study assessed 66 preoperative TIPS recipients compared with 68 non-TIPS operative patients across 4 institutions.[68] The groups were matched on etiology of cirrhosis and surgical procedures, and the categories of Child-Pugh score (6 vs 6) and MELD scores (11 vs 11) were similar among the 2 groups. The preoperative TIPS group had lower intraoperative RBC transfusions (8 vs 1; $P = .015$) and lower rates of postoperative ascites (20.4% vs 38.2%; $P = .012$); however, the 30-day and 90-day postoperative mortality rates were similar (1.8% vs 3% [$P = .355$] and 7.5% vs 7.8% [$P = .644$], respectively). Yet, although no difference in survival was observed, survival rates in both groups outperformed traditional mortality estimates after extrahepatic intra-abdominal surgery, suggesting the control group patients perhaps were otherwise optimal candidate for surgery resulting in improved survival rates (**Table 4**).

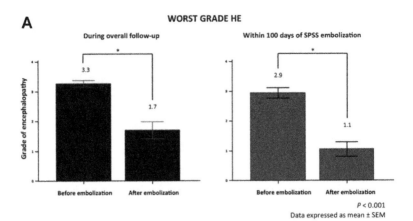

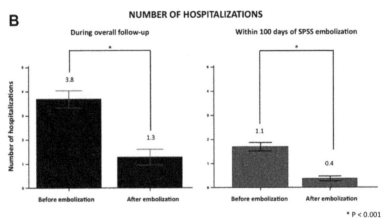

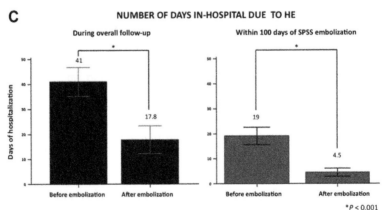

Fig. 1. Short- and long-term changes before versus after embolization in terms of the most severe grade of HE (*A*), number of hospitalizations (*B*), and days spent in the hospital (*C*) because of HE. SEM, standard error of the mean. (*From* Laleman W, Simon-Talero M, Maleux G, et al. Embolization of large spontaneous portosystemic shunts for refractory hepatic encephalopathy: a multicenter survey on safety and efficacy. *Hepatology.* 2013;57(6):2448-2457; with permission.)

Table 4
Preoperative TIPS before abdominal surgery

Author, Year	Number of Patients	Abdominal Surgery	Child-Pugh Score	Time from TIPS to Surgery (Range)	Pre-TIPS PSG Post-TIPS PSG (mm Hg)	Surgical/TIPS Complications	Postoperative Mortality, n (%)
Azoulay et al,[61] 2001	7	Tumor resection AAA repair Hartmann's reversal	A–C	1–5 mo	18 ± 5 9 ± 5	1 liver failure 1 postoperative ascites	1 (17%)
Grübel et al,[62] 2002	2	Colectomy Nephrectomy	C	3–8 wk	17–26 8–14	None	0 (0%)
Gil et al,[63] 2004	3	Tumor resection	A–B	14–45 d	20–28 6–7	1 encephalopathy 1 CHF	0 (0%)
Schlenker et al,[64] 2009	7	Abdominal and pelvic resection	A–B	1–32 d	9–22 3–10	1 postoperative ascites 2 encephalopathy 1 liver failure	1 (17%)
Kim et al[65]	6	AVR Colectomy	A–C	6–46 d	Not reported	1 renal failure 3 encephalopathy	0 (0%)
Menahem et at,[66] 2015	8	Colon resections	A–C	1–9 wk	15.5 ± 2.9 7.5 ± 1.9	1 bacterial peritonitis 1 encephalopathy 3 ascites 1 hemorrhage 3 liver failure	2 (25%)

Abbreviations: AAA, abdominal aortic aneurysm; AVR, aortic valve replacement; CHF, congestive heart failure.
Adapted from Philip M. Thornburg B. Preoperative Transjugular Intrahepatic Portosystemic Shunt Placement for Extrahepatic Abdominal Surgery. In: *Seminars in Interventional Radiology.* Vol 35. Thieme Medical Publishers; 2018:203-205; with permission.

Transjugular Intrahepatic Portosystemic Shunts for Hepatopulmonary Syndrome

Hepatopulmonary syndrome (HPS) is a disorder of pulmonary oxygenation that occurs in the setting of portal hypertension with or without cirrhosis with a severity that is independent of the severity of underlying liver disease.[69,70] The pathophysiology of HPS consists of inappropriate vasodilation of the pulmonary capillaries that results in a ventilation–perfusion mismatch from increased shunting of pulmonary blood flow, leading to a decrease in arterial oxygen tension. The inappropriate vasodilation is suspected to relate to an increased release of nitric oxide from the pulmonary endothelium in combination with genetic polymorphisms associated with proinflammatory mediators released by circulating macrophage in response to portal hypertension.[71,72] Unfortunately, there is no proven medical therapy for HPS, and treatment is supportive with oxygen supplementation.[73] Prompt referral for liver transplantation evaluation is recommended because transplantation ameliorates the problem.[73] TIPS has been assessed as a potential treatment of HPS within the context of 11 case reports and series. A meta-analysis of the reports of 12 patients who underwent TIPS for the treatment of HPS reported on a mean duration of follow-up of 9.3 months.[74] Improvement in arterial oxygenation was observed in 9 patients immediately after TIPS; however, this finding was not sustained in 2 patients. Of the remaining 3 patients, 2 remained unchanged after TIPS and 1 had worsening oxygenation 4 months after TIPS. Interestingly, 1 patient had recurrence of subjective pulmonary symptoms in the setting of TIPS stenosis that resolved with TIPS revision. The same authors published a follow-up report among TIPS recipients at their institution over a 1-year period.[75] They identified 23 TIPS recipients meeting the diagnostic criteria for HPS who were undergoing TIPS for another indication, such as variceal bleeding, ascites, or Budd-Chiari syndrome. Of the 23 patients with HPS, dyspnea was reported in 5 patients. After TIPS, 4 of 5 patients (80%) reported improvement in dyspnea immediately after TIPS. However, 50% reported return of dyspnea after 3 months. Improvements in measured arterial oxygen tension were also observed at 1 month after TIPS, but this improvement was not sustained at 3 months. These data combined with previous case reports suggest that TIPS may have a role for transient improvement in symptoms and oxygenation in HPS, with success in 75% to 80% of patients. However, improvement is not sustained after 3 months. Until additional data are available, there is no definitive role for TIPS placement in the setting of HPS at present.

Transjugular Intrahepatic Portosystemic Shunts for the Hepatorenal Syndrome

The hepatorenal syndrome (HRS) has long been thought to be a form of functional renal failure that occurs in the setting of intense renal vasoconstriction among patients with cirrhosis or acute liver failure.[76] More recently, that concept has been challenged by emerging data suggesting HRS is likely multifactorial with a contribution from proinflammatory cytokines resulting in cellular changes at the renal tubular level that result in decreases in the glomerular filtration rate.[5,77] Nonetheless, the current mainstay of treatment for HRS has been volume expansion of the intravascular space, and splanchnic and arterial vasoconstrictors in an effort to increase renal perfusion. Placement of a TIPS has the potential to redistribute portal blood volume to the systemic circulation, thereby increasing renal perfusion and decreasing the effects of the renin–angiotensin–aldosterone system.[78] TIPS has been assessed for the treatment of HRS; however, the reports are few owing to the unique patient profile who would benefit from a TIPS. The largest prospective study using TIPS for the treatment of HRS among nonliver transplantation candidates involved 31 patients. Patients with documented HRS unresponsive to standard volume-expanding medical therapy received TIPS on average 3.4 weeks after the onset of renal insufficiency. The average portal to systemic gradient pressures decreased from 21 to 13 mm Hg after TIPS. **Table 5** demonstrates baseline laboratory parameters including renal function and urine volume. There was a significant improvement in serum creatinine, the glomerular filtration rate, and urine output after TIPS.

Of the 31 patients, 4 of 7 on hemodialysis before TIPS were able to stop dialysis following return of renal recovery. After TIPS, survival at 3, 6, and 12 months was 81%, 71%, and 48% respectively, a dramatic improvement compared with historical reports of 10% survival at 3 months after the onset of HRS. The greatest survival benefit was seen among patients with type 2 HRS and those who had resolution of ascites with TIPS. Of note, improved renal function among non-HRS patients undergoing TIPS for refractory ascites have also been reported.[23] Despite these promising results, further RCTs have not been conducted among patients with HRS. In lieu of additional data, there is as of yet not a defined role for TIPS in the setting of HRS.

Table 5
Liver and renal function after TIPS

Characteristic (Mean)	Baseline (n = 31)	Week 1 (n = 30)	Week 2 (n = 30)	Week 4 (n = 29)	P value
Child-Pugh score	9.5	9.4	9.3	8.8	NS
Bilirubin (mg/dL)	3.1	4.4	4.1	3.2	NS
Albumin (g/dL)	2.9	2.9	3.4*	3.3	*<.05
Serum creatinine (mg/mL)	2.3	1.7	1.6	1.5	<.01
Creatinine clearance (mL/min)	18	42	48	44	<.001
Urine volume (mL/24 h)	544	788	1041	1248	<.05

Values displayed are averages and P values represent comparison with baseline values.
  * Week 2 compared to Baseline.
  Adapted from Brensing KA, Textor J, Perz J, et al. Long term outcome after transjugular intrahepatic portosystemic stent-shunt in non-transplant cirrhotics with hepatorenal syndrome: a phase II study. https://doi.org/10.1136/gut.47.2.288; with permission.

SUMMARY

TIPS has been an established treatment for portal hypertensive complications, including refractory ascites and variceal bleeding. Advancements in TIPS stent technology and improvements in technique of placement have led to novel indications for TIPS beyond traditional guideline-supported indications. These emerging indications include the treatment of chronic PVT and the use of TIPS before abdominal surgery to alleviate portal hypertensive complications. The use of TIPS can also facilitate the embolization of large portal systemic shunts to alleviate refractory HE owing to excessive portal shunting. Along with these novel indications and expanded use, additional data are awaited to determine if TIPS for other indications such as HPS and HRS is safe and effective. Despite these advances, TIPS remains an invasive procedure with risks for complications, hence the evaluation and decision to place a TIPS should be made in conjunction with an experienced gastroenterologist/hepatologist and performed at a center with expertise to ensure a successful patient outcome.

DISCLOSURE

Dr J. Boike receives investigator-initiated grant support from W. L. Gore & Associates, the Manufacturer of the TIPS Viatorr® stent.

REFERENCES

1. D'Amico G, Garcia-Tsao G, Pagliaro L. Natural history and prognostic indicators of survival in cirrhosis: a systematic review of 118 studies. J Hepatol 2006;44(1): 217–31.
2. Rossle M, Richter GM, Noldge G, et al. Performance of an intrahepatic portacaval-shunt (PCS) using a catheter technique-a case-report. Hepatology 1988;8:1348. WB SAUNDERS CO INDEPENDENCE SQUARE WEST CURTIS CENTER, STE 300, PHILADELPHIA.
3. Boyer TD, Haskal ZJ. The role of transjugular intrahepatic portosystemic shunt (TIPS) in the management of portal hypertension: update 2009. Hepatology 2010;51(1):306.
4. Runyon BA. Introduction to the revised American Association for the Study of Liver Diseases Practice Guideline management of adult patients with ascites due to cirrhosis 2012. Hepatology 2013;57(4):1651–3.
5. European Association for the Study of the Liver. Electronic address: easloffice@easloffice.eu, European Association for the Study of the Liver. EASL Clinical Practice Guidelines for the management of patients with decompensated cirrhosis. J Hepatol 2018;69(2):406–60.
6. Gipson MG, Smith MT, Durham JD, et al. Intravascular US–guided portal vein access: improved procedural metrics during TIPS creation. J Vasc Interv Radiol 2016;27(8):1140–7.
7. Praktiknjo M, Lehmann J, Fischer S, et al. Novel diameter controlled expansion TIPS (Viatorr CX ®)graft reduces readmission compared to regular covered TIPS graft and bare metal graft. J Hepatol 2017;66(1):S48–9.
8. Miraglia R, Maruzzelli L, Di Piazza A, et al. Transjugular intrahepatic portosystemic shunt using the new Gore Viatorr controlled expansion endoprosthesis: prospective, single-center, preliminary experience. Cardiovasc Intervent Radiol 2019;42(1):78–86.
9. Miraglia R, Maruzzelli L, Tuzzolino F, et al. Transjugular intrahepatic portosystemic shunts in patients with cirrhosis with refractory ascites: comparison of clinical outcomes by using 8- and 10-mm PTFE-covered stents. Radiology 2017;284(1):281–8.
10. Billey C, Billet S, Robic MA, et al. A prospective study identifying predictive factors of cardiac decompensation after TIPS: the Toulouse algorithm. Hepatology 2019. https://doi.org/10.1002/hep.30934.
11. Kochar N, Tripathi D, Arestis NJ, et al. Tipsitis: incidence and outcome-a single centre experience. Eur J Gastroenterol Hepatol 2010;22(6):729–35.
12. Angermayr B, Cejna M, Koenig F, et al. Survival in patients undergoing transjugular intrahepatic portosystemic shunt: ePTFE-covered stent grafts versus bare stents. Hepatology 2003;38(4):1043–50.
13. Bureau C, Carlos Garcia-Pagan J, Otal P, et al. Improved clinical outcome using polytetrafluoroethylene-coated stents for TIPS: results of a randomized study. Gastroenterology 2004;126(2):469–75.
14. Wang Q, He C, Yin Z, et al. Small-diameter covered stents do not affect efficacy but reduce hepatic encephalopathy in transjugular intrahepatic portosystemic shunt for the prevention of variceal rebleeding in cirrhosis. J Hepatol 2017;66(1):S47–8.
15. Petersen B. Intravascular ultrasound-guided direct intrahepatic portacaval shunt: description of technique and technical refinements. J Vasc Interv Radiol 2003;14(1):21–32.
16. Farsad K, Fuss C, Kolbeck KJ, et al. Transjugular intrahepatic portosystemic shunt creation using intravascular ultrasound guidance. J Vasc Interv Radiol 2012;23(12):1594–602.

17. Boyvat F, Aytekin C, Harman A, et al. Transjugular intrahepatic portosystemic shunt creation in Budd-Chiari syndrome: percutaneous ultrasound-guided direct simultaneous puncture of the portal vein and vena cava. Cardiovasc Intervent Radiol 2006;29(5):857–61.
18. Petersen BD, Clark TWI. Direct intrahepatic portocaval shunt. Tech Vasc Interv Radiol 2008;11(4):230–4.
19. Salem R, Vouche M, Baker T, et al. Pretransplant portal vein recanalization—transjugular intrahepatic portosystemic shunt in patients with complete obliterative portal vein thrombosis. Transplantation 2015;99(11):2347–55.
20. Thornburg B, Desai K, Hickey R, et al. Portal vein recanalization and transjugular intrahepatic portosystemic shunt creation for chronic portal vein thrombosis: technical considerations. Tech Vasc Interv Radiol 2016;19(1):52–60.
21. Haddad MM, Fleming CJ, Thompson SM, et al. Comparison of bleeding complications between transplenic versus transhepatic access of the portal venous system. J Vasc Interv Radiol 2018;29(10):1383–91.
22. Habib A, Desai K, Hickey R, et al. Portal vein recanalization-transjugular intrahepatic portosystemic shunt using the transsplenic approach to achieve transplant candidacy in patients with chronic portal vein thrombosis. J Vasc Interv Radiol 2015;26(4):499–506.
23. Ginès P, Uriz J, Calahorra B, et al. Transjugular intrahepatic portosystemic shunting versus paracentesis plus albumin for refractory ascites in cirrhosis. Gastroenterology 2002;123(6):1839–47.
24. Deltenre P, Mathurin P, Dharancy S, et al. Transjugular intrahepatic portosystemic shunt in refractory ascites: a meta-analysis. Liver Int 2005;25(2):349–56.
25. Chen R, Ge X, Huang Z, et al. XY-J of clinical, 2014 undefined. Prophylactic use of transjugular intrahepatic portosystemic shunt aids in the treatment of refractory ascites: metaregression and trial sequential meta-analysis. journals.lww.com. Available at: https://journals.lww.com/jcge/FullText/2014/03000/Prophylactic_Use_of_Transjugular_Intrahepatic.17.aspx. Accessed November 24, 2019.
26. Bai M, Qi X, Yang Z, et al. DF-W journal of, 2014 undefined. TIPS improves liver transplantation-free survival in cirrhotic patients with refractory ascites: an updated meta-analysis. ncbi.nlm.nih.gov. Available at: https://www.ncbi.nlm.nih.gov/pmc/articles/PMC3949280/. Accessed November 24, 2019.
27. Albillos A, Bañares R, González M, et al. MC-J of, 2005 undefined. A meta-analysis of transjugular intrahepatic portosystemic shunt versus paracentesis for refractory ascites. Elsevier. Available at: https://www.sciencedirect.com/science/article/pii/S0168827805004307. Accessed November 24, 2019.
28. Gaba RC, Parvinian A, Casadaban LC, et al. Survival benefit of TIPS versus serial paracentesis in patients with refractory ascites: a single institution case-control propensity score analysis. Clin Radiol 2015;70(5):e51–7.
29. Salerno F, Cammà C, Enea M, et al. 2007 undefined. Transjugular intrahepatic portosystemic shunt for refractory ascites: a meta-analysis of individual patient data. Elsevier. Available at: https://www.sciencedirect.com/science/article/pii/S0016508507011614. Accessed November 24, 2019.
30. Saab S, Nieto JM, Lewis SK, et al. TIPS versus paracentesis for cirrhotic patients with refractory ascites. Cochrane Database Syst Rev 2006. https://doi.org/10.1002/14651858.cd004889.pub2.
31. Lebrec D, Giuily N, Hadengue A, et al. Transjugular intrahepatic portosystemic shunts: comparison with paracentesis in patients with cirrhosis and refractory ascites: a randomized trial. J Hepatol 1996;25(2):135–44.

32. Rössle M, Ochs A, Gülberg V, et al. A comparison of paracentesis and transjugular intrahepatic portosystemic shunting in patients with ascites. N Engl J Med 2000;342(23):1701–7.
33. Sanyal AJ, Genning C, Reddy KR, et al. The North American study for the treatment of refractory ascites. Gastroenterology 2003;124(3):634–41.
34. Salerno F, Merli M, Riggio O, et al. Randomized controlled study of TIPS versus paracentesis plus albumin in cirrhosis with severe ascites. Hepatology 2004; 40(3):629–35.
35. Narahara Y, Kanazawa H, Fukuda T, et al. Transjugular intrahepatic portosystemic shunt versus paracentesis plus albumin in patients with refractory ascites who have good hepatic and renal function: a prospective randomized trial. J Gastroenterol 2011;46(1):78–85.
36. Bureau C, Thabut D, Oberti F, et al. Transjugular intrahepatic portosystemic shunts with covered stents increase transplant-free survival of patients with cirrhosis and recurrent ascites. Gastroenterology 2017;152(1):157–63.
37. Plessier A, Darwish-Murad S, Hernandez-Guerra M, et al. Acute portal vein thrombosis unrelated to cirrhosis: a prospective multicenter follow-up study. Hepatology 2010;51(1):210–8.
38. Garcia-Pagán JC, Buscarini E, Janssen HLA, et al. EASL clinical practice guidelines: vascular diseases of the liver. J Hepatol 2016;64(1):179–202.
39. Turnes J, García-Pagán JC, González M, et al. Portal hypertension-related complications after acute portal vein thrombosis: impact of early anticoagulation. Clin Gastroenterol Hepatol 2008;6(12):1412–7.
40. Klinger C, Riecken B, Schmidt A, et al. Transjugular local thrombolysis with/without TIPS in patients with acute non-cirrhotic, non-malignant portal vein thrombosis. Dig Liver Dis 2017;49(12):1345–52.
41. Noronha Ferreira C, Seijo S, Plessier A, et al. Natural history and management of esophagogastric varices in chronic noncirrhotic, nontumoral portal vein thrombosis. Hepatology 2016;63(5):1640–50.
42. Orr DW, Harrison PM, Devlin J, et al. Chronic mesenteric venous thrombosis: evaluation and determinants of survival during long-term follow-up. Clin Gastroenterol Hepatol 2007;5(1):80–6.
43. Spaander MCW, Hoekstra J, Hansen BE, et al. Anticoagulant therapy in patients with non-cirrhotic portal vein thrombosis: effect on new thrombotic events and gastrointestinal bleeding. J Thromb Haemost 2013;11(3):452–9.
44. Lladó L, Fabregat J, Castellote J, et al. Management of portal vein thrombosis in liver transplantation: influence on morbidity and mortality. Clin Transplant 2007. https://doi.org/10.1111/j.1399-0012.2007.00728.x.
45. Thornburg B, Desai K, Hickey R, et al. Pretransplantation portal vein recanalization and transjugular intrahepatic portosystemic shunt creation for chronic portal vein thrombosis: final analysis of a 61-patient cohort. J Vasc Interv Radiol 2017; 28(12):1714–21.e2.
46. Luca A, Miraglia R, Caruso S, et al. Short- and long-term effects of the transjugular intrahepatic portosystemic shunt on portal vein thrombosis in patients with cirrhosis. Gut 2011;60(6):846–52.
47. Qi X, He C, Guo W, et al. Transjugular intrahepatic portosystemic shunt for portal vein thrombosis with variceal bleeding in liver cirrhosis: outcomes and predictors in a prospective cohort study. Liver Int 2016;36(5):667–76.
48. Han G, Qi X, He C, et al. Transjugular intrahepatic portosystemic shunt for portal vein thrombosis with symptomatic portal hypertension in liver cirrhosis. J Hepatol 2011;54(1):78–88.

49. Córdoba J, Mínguez B. Hepatic encephalopathy. Semin Liver Dis 2008;28(1):70–80.
50. Lam KC, Juttner HU, Reynolds TB. Spontaneous portosystemic shunt - relationship to spontaneous encephalopathy and gastrointestinal hemorrhage. Dig Dis Sci 1981;26(4):346–52.
51. Ohnishi K, Sato S. MS-AJ of, 1986 undefined. Clinical and portal hemodynamic features in cirrhotic patients having a large spontaneous splenorenal and/or gastrorenal shunt. search.ebscohost.com. Available at: http://search.ebscohost. com/login.aspx?direct=true&profile=ehost&scope=site&authtype= crawler&jrnl=00029270&AN=16221007&h=YieGjkGmOEDO8452QBGp34y% 2BXYcMwJPSOH%2BBg0PQD4sAvbB2iAzf1bGK%2B2rNivskp T1OMqaIVRdRdvtJOLkaZA%3D%3D&crl=c. Accessed November 26, 2019.
52. Riggio O, Efrati C, Catalano C, et al. High prevalence of spontaneous portal-systemic shunts in persistent hepatic encephalopathy: a case-control study. Hepatology 2005;42(5):1158–65.
53. Zidi SH, Zanditenas D, Gelu-Siméon M, et al. Treatment of chronic portosystemic encephalopathy in cirrhotic patients by embolization of portosystemic shunts. Liver Int 2007;27(10):1389–93.
54. Laleman W, Simon-Talero M, Maleux G, et al. Embolization of large spontaneous portosystemic shunts for refractory hepatic encephalopathy: a multicenter survey on safety and efficacy. Hepatology 2013;57(6):2448–57.
55. Wong R, Rappaport W, Witte C, et al. GH-J of the, 1994 undefined. Risk of non-shunt abdominal operation in the patient with cirrhosis. Available at: https:// europepmc.org/abstract/med/7921390. Accessed November 25, 2019.
56. Ziser A, Plevak D. TJ of, 1999 undefined. Morbidity and mortality in cirrhotic patients undergoing anesthesia and surgery. Available at: anesthesiology.pubs. asahq.org http://anesthesiology.pubs.asahq.org/article.aspx?articleid=1947432. Accessed November 25, 2019.
57. Aranha GV, Sontag SJ, Greenlee HB. Cholecystectomy in cirrhotic patients: a formidable operation. Am J Surg 1982;143(1):55–60.
58. Durand F, Valla D. Assessment of the prognosis of cirrhosis: Child-Pugh versus MELD. J Hepatol 2005;42(SUPPL. 1).
59. Bruix J, Castells A, Bosch J, et al. Surgical resection of hepatocellular carcinoma in cirrhotic patients: prognostic value of preoperative portal pressure. Gastroenterology 1996;111(4):1018–22.
60. Aranha GV, Greenlee HB. Intra-abdominal surgery in patients with advanced cirrhosis. Arch Surg 1986;121(3):275–7.
61. Azoulay D, Buabse F, Damiano I, et al. Neoadjuvant transjugular intrahepatic portosystemic shunt: a solution for extrahepatic abdominal operation in cirrhotic patients with severe portal hypertension. J Am Coll Surg 2001;193(1):46–51.
62. Grübel P, Pratt DS, Elhelw T. Transjugular intrahepatic portosystemic shunt for portal decompression before abdominal and retroperitoneal surgery in patients with severe portal hypertension [3]. J Clin Gastroenterol 2002;34(4):489–90.
63. Gil A, Martınez-Regueira F, Hernandez-Lizoain JL, et al. The role of transjugular intrahepatic portosystemic shunt prior to abdominal tumoral surgery in cirrhotic patients with portal hypertension. Eur J Surg Oncol 2004;30(1):46–52.
64. Schlenker C, Johnson S, Trotter JF. Preoperative transjugular intrahepatic portosystemic shunt (TIPS) for cirrhotic patients undergoing abdominal and pelvic surgeries. Surg Endosc 2009;23(7):1594–8.
65. Kim J, Dasika N. EY-J of clinical, 2009 undefined. Cirrhotic patients with a transjugular intrahepatic portosystemic shunt undergoing major extrahepatic surgery.

Available at: journals.lww.com https://journals.lww.com/jcge/fulltext/2009/07000/Cirrhotic_Patients_With_a_Transjugular.13.aspx. Accessed November 25, 2019.

66. Menahem B, Lubrano J, Desjouis A, et al. Transjugular intrahepatic portosystemic shunt placement increases feasibility of colorectal surgery in cirrhotic patients with severe portal hypertension. Dig Liver Dis 2015;47(1):81–4.

67. Vinet E, Perreault P, Bouchard L, et al. Transjugular intrahepatic portosystemic shunt before abdominal surgery in cirrhotic patients: a retrospective, comparative study. Can J Gastroenterol 2006;20(6):401–4.

68. Tabchouri N, Barbier L, Menahem B, et al. Original study: transjugular intrahepatic portosystemic shunt as a bridge to abdominal surgery in cirrhotic patients. J Gastrointest Surg 2019;23(12):2383–90.

69. Rodriguez-Roisin R, Krowka MJ, Herve PH, et al. Pulmonary-hepatic vascular disorders (PHD). European Respiratory Journal 2004;24(5):861–80.

70. Kaymakoglu S, Kahraman T, Kudat H, et al. Hepatopulmonary syndrome in non-cirrhotic portal hypertensive patients. Dig Dis Sci 2003;48(3):556–60.

71. Roberts K, Kawut S, Krowka M, et al. 2010 undefined. Genetic risk factors for hepatopulmonary syndrome in patients with advanced liver disease. Elsevier. Available at: https://www.sciencedirect.com/science/article/pii/S0016508510004634. Accessed November 27, 2019.

72. Fallon MB, Abrams GA, Luo B, et al. The role of endothelial nitric oxide synthase in the pathogenesis of a rat model of hepatopulmonary syndrome. Gastroenterology 1997;113(2):606–14.

73. Rodríguez-Roisin R, Krowka MJ. Hepatopulmonary syndrome - a liver-induced lung vascular disorder. N Engl J Med 2008;358(22):2378.

74. Tsauo J, Weng N, Ma H, et al. HZ-J of V and, 2015 undefined. Role of transjugular intrahepatic portosystemic shunts in the management of hepatopulmonary syndrome: a systemic literature review. Elsevier. Available at: https://www.sciencedirect.com/science/article/pii/S105104431500411X. Accessed November 27, 2019.

75. Tsauo J, Zhao H, Zhang X, et al. Effect of transjugular intrahepatic portosystemic shunt creation on pulmonary gas exchange in patients with hepatopulmonary syndrome: a prospective study. J Vasc Interv Radiol 2019;30(2):170–7.

76. Arroyo V, Ginès P, Gerbes AL, et al. Definition and diagnostic criteria of refractory ascites and hepatorenal syndrome in cirrhosis. Hepatology 1996;23(1):164–76.

77. de Seigneux S, Martin P-Y. Preventing the Progression of AKI to CKD: the role of mitochondria. J Am Soc Nephrol 2017;28:1327–36.

78. Guevara M, Ginès P, Bandi JC, et al. Transjugular intrahepatic portosystemic shunt in hepatorenal syndrome: effects on renal function and vasoactive systems. Hepatology 1998;28(2):416–22.

Focal Nodular Hyperplasia and Hepatic Adenoma
Evaluation and Management

Lauren Myers, PA-C*, Joseph Ahn, MD

KEYWORDS

- Focal nodular hyperplasia • Hepatic adenoma • Hepatocellular adenoma
- Liver lesion

KEY POINTS

- Focal nodular hyperplasia (FNH) is a common benign liver lesion that rarely requires intervention.
- Hepatocellular adenomas (HCAs) are benign lesions commonly associated with obesity and oral contraceptive use in women.
- HCAs may be at risk for malignant transformation to hepatocellular carcinoma; risk of rupture is greatest in lesions over 5 cm in size.
- Molecular subtyping may be helpful to characterize and guide treatment decisions in HCA lesions.

FOCAL NODULAR HYPERPLASIA

Focal nodular hyperplasia (FNH) is the second most common benign hepatic lesion seen with a previously reported prevalence on ultrasound of 0.03%.[1] FNH lesions are typically discovered incidentally, and 74% of cases are asymptomatic. Those who present with symptoms may have mild epigastric abdominal pain or discomfort.[2] FNH may be seen in conjunction with elevations in alkaline phosphatase and/or gamma-glutamyl transferase (GGT) levels, or no abnormalities in liver biochemistries.[3] These lesions are most commonly seen in young and middle-aged women (ages 20–50 years) with a prevalence ratio of 8 women to every man diagnosed.[4–7] FNH lesions are generally solitary but may be associated with hepatic hemangiomas in about 20% of cases.[8]

Focal nodular hyperplasia are characterized by densely packed functioning hepatocytes fed by an enlarged artery with a central scar of fibrous tissue and malformed bile ductules. These are thought to reflect a hyperplastic response to a congenital or

Division of Gastroenterology and Hepatology, Oregon Health and Science University, 3181 Southwest Sam Jackson Park Road, MNP 4112, Portland, OR 97239, USA
* Corresponding author.
E-mail address: myersla@ohsu.edu

Clin Liver Dis 24 (2020) 389–403
https://doi.org/10.1016/j.cld.2020.04.013
1089-3261/20/© 2020 Elsevier Inc. All rights reserved.

acquired vascular abnormality. The background liver histology is otherwise normal.[9] It has been hypothesized there is a genetic component to their formation with noted activation of genes seen in vascular remodeling.[9] When FNH lesions are sampled, they are noted to have a characteristic map-like pattern of glutamine synthetase staining.[10,11]

Occasionally, FNH lesions are seen in an atypical form such as without a central scar (in which lesions are usually <3 cm in size), or associated with significant steatosis, intralesional fat; these constitute about 85% of atypical FNH lesions.[12,13] Multiple FNH lesions may be seen in patients with vascular disease such as Budd-Chiari syndrome or obliterative portal venopathy. In rare cases, FNH has been reported to cause Budd-Chiari.[12]

Because of the high prevalence of FNH lesions in women, it was initially thought there was a link between FNH and female hormones. Several studies have looked into both exogenous hormone administration and pregnancy. Neither oral contraceptive pills (OCPs) nor pregnancy were associated with FNH prevalence nor FNH progression.[14,15] As such, it is felt that FNH lesions are not hormonally sensitive.

Recently there have been studies of the possible association of FNH with prior chemotherapy exposure. Benign regenerative lesions have been noted in children with a history of malignancy receiving high-dose chemotherapy or a hematopoietic stem cell transplant. This is thought to be potentially a late manifestation of prior injury from chemotherapy or radiation therapy.[16,17] In adults, a case series identified 14 patients previously treated with oxaliplatin who developed new FNH lesions. The pathogenesis of this remains unknown.[18]

Diagnosis of Focal Nodular Hyperplasia

FNH lesions seen on ultrasound imaging appear slightly hypoechoic or isoechoic to the background liver tissue (**Table 1**). The surrounding liver tissue may often be seen as steatotic.[12,19,20] With Doppler ultrasound, there may be the presence of multiple well-defined arterial vessels originating from the center of the lesion traveling to the periphery and the presence of feeding vessels from the hepatic arterial tree.[12,21]

Table 1
Imaging characteristics of focal nodular hyperplasia lesions

	Ultrasound	CEUS	CT	MRI
FNH	Homogenous mostly isoechoic	Spoke wheel centrifugal pattern enhancement	Unenhanced phase: hypointense/isointense with surrounding liver	Iso/hypointense in T1 weighted
	On Doppler: centrifugal arterial flow, radiating central vessel	Enhancement in arterial phase	Homogenous enhancement of lesion on arterial phase, hyperintense except central scar	Hyper/isointense Central hyperintense scar on T2 weighted
		Remaining hyper/isointense in portal and late phases	Isointense on portal and late phases	Homogenous -enhancement arterial phase
				Enhancement of lesion in later phase with hepatobiliary gadolinium

Contrast-enhanced ultrasound (CEUS) may be helpful in diagnosing small FNH lesions (**Fig. 1**). The use of intravenous microbubbles in the early arterial phase gives an enhancement in a centrifugal appearance in FNH lesions that closely corresponds with lesion size.[12,22] CEUS has a reported 93% sensitivity and 100% specificity in diagnosing FNH lesions smaller than 35 mm in size. MRI is less accurate in diagnosing small FNH lesions, and as such, it is has been recommended that CEUS, where available, be used to diagnose FNH lesions less than 3 cm.[23,24]

Cross-sectional imaging including computed tomography (CT) and MRI with the addition of extracellular contrast may be used to noninvasively diagnose FNH. Five imaging criteria may be used to guide diagnosis:

1. Signal intensity of the lesion is similar to surrounding liver tissue
2. Homogeneity of the lesion.
3. Strong enhancement in the arterial phase without washout
4. Presence of a central scar
5. Lesion may be lobulated but lacks a capsule

In the absence of abnormal liver biochemistries, chronic liver disease, and extrahepatic malignancy, this is 98% specific and 70% sensitive to diagnose FNH.[2,12,24]

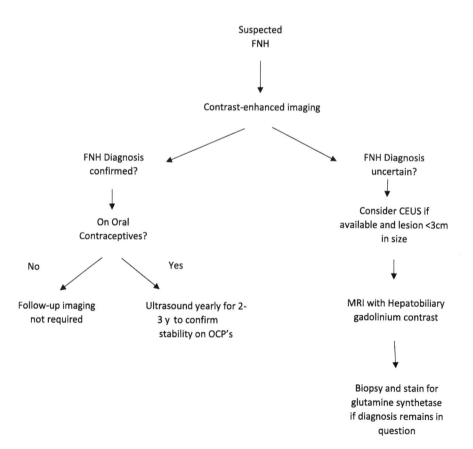

Fig. 1. Diagnosis and management of FNH.

MRI with extracellular contrast utilizes gadolinium-based chelate agents that shorten the longitudinal relaxation time (T1) and have similar pharmacokinetics of iodinated contrast for CT that rely on differential blood flow between liver and lesion for lesion detection.[25] FNH lesions are best seen on MRI in the arterial phase in which the lesion is noted to have intense enhancement given its predominant arterial blood supply. The FNH lesion appears consistent with background liver in post-contrast imaging, and its characteristic central scar is T2 hyperintense. For lesions smaller than 3 cm, 40% of FNH lesions are inconclusive on standard MRI.[26] MRI is felt to be less accurate in diagnosing small FNH lesions because of the lack of central stellate scarring seen.[23] On standard extracellular contrast MRI, hepatocellular adenoma (HCA) and FNH may both have overlapping imaging features with arterial enhancement.[27] As management of these lesions is distinct, further differentiation of these lesions is crucial. The addition of specific MR hepatobiliary gadolinium contrast agent increases the ability to differentiate these lesions. Hepatobiliary gadolinium agents gadoxetate disodium and gadobenate dimeglumine have selective uptake in functioning hepatocytes and are secreted in bile in the hepatobiliary phase. Gadoxetate disodium is most commonly used in clinical practice, as it has a higher percentage of excretion of the agent into the biliary system and a faster time for accumulation of contrast agent into hepatocytes over gadobenate dimeglumine.[26] FNH lesions are thought to have abnormal drainage from bile calculi because of ductular reaction along the septa, while an HCA lesion has few to no bile ducts, resulting in increased accumulation of hepatobiliary gadolinium contrast agent in FNH lesions during hepatobiliary phase of MRI.[26,28] With the addition of hepatobiliary gadolinium, over 90% of FNH lesions are noted to be either hyperintense or isointense on the hepatobiliary phase, while solid components of most HCA lesions appear hypointense.[29,30] In cases where FNH cannot be distinguished from HCA, the lesion should be biopsied and stained for glutamine synthetase to improve diagnostic certainty.[31]

Management of Focal Nodular Hyperplasia

Approximately 70% of cases of FNH are asymptomatic and do not require intervention. There is no malignant transformation potential. Several case reports have been published highlighting the spontaneous rupture of larger FNH lesions.[32,33] However, most FNH lesions followed over time were either stable or found to have regressed in size.[34]

Symptoms can occur in approximately 20% of patients with FNH thought caused by the increased size of the mass causing liver capsular stretch. Surgical resection may be a consideration for symptomatic individuals unresponsive to analgesia.[2,35–37] The most common indications for resection were symptoms or diagnostic uncertainty and suspicion for cancer.[38] Surgery for FNH lesions was more frequently performed in men, for smaller lesions and for atypical FNH lesions.[5] For minimally invasive treatment approaches for FNH, there are limited data, but studies are predominantly focused on transarterial embolization.[39] This is predominantly considered for individuals who are not surgical candidates or if the resection site is difficult.[40] Overall, there is poor correlation between FNH lesions and symptoms, and even if a patient is symptomatic, treatment is rarely recommended.[24]

For those individuals with a firm diagnosis of FNH and who are not on OCPs, ongoing follow-up imaging is not recommended. There is no indication to discontinue OCPs or discourage pregnancy in individuals with FNH. Ongoing follow-up for FNH lesions is not necessary in pregnancy, but it has been recommended for those who continue OCPs to have an ultrasound annually for 2 to 3 years to ensure stability.[4,24]

Focal nodular hyperplasia features

- 8:1 young female predominance
- Typically, not clinically significant
- Common imaging characteristics include a homogenous, hypervascular lesion with a central scar
- Map-like pattern of glutamine synthetase staining on biopsy
- Not hormonally sensitive
- Ongoing imaging surveillance is not recommended in the absence of OCP use with the firm diagnosis FNH

HEPATOCELLULAR ADENOMA

HCA is seen 10 times less frequently than FNH, with a prevalence of 0.001% to 0.004% in the general population. On ultrasound studies, the prevalence has been noted to be 7 cases per 100,000 populuation.[1,24,41] HCA has a female-to-male ratio 10:1, with the most common presentation in women of child-bearing age in their third and fourth decade.[24,41] HCAs are most often a solitary lesion in the right hepatic lobe found as an incidental finding in 12% to 25% of cases. In cases that present with symptoms, they may range from chronic right upper quadrant pain/epigastric pain to acute pain associated with anemia or even circulatory collapse in settings of acute HCA rupture or hemorrhage.[41]

Historically, HCAs were identified in women of childbearing age with approximately 1 case per 100,000 population without the use of OCPs. With the increasing utilization of early generation OCPs in the 1960s and 1970s, there was an increase in prevalence to 3 to 4 cases per 100,000 population in women who used OCPs.[42] The risks of HCAs are increased 30- to 40-fold for those on OCPs.[24] This hormonal association is seen also in the setting of HCA enlargement during pregnancy.[41] It has been noted that lesion size can regress with the removal of exogenous hormones/OCPs.[43] Additionally, there is an increased association of HCA lesions with androgenic steroid use. The risk of androgen-associated lesions correlates with cumulative androgen dosing, and those who are suspected for abusing androgenic steroids should be monitored for liver risks.[44] In cases of endogenously increased androgens or sex hormone imbalances such as polycystic ovarian syndrome (PCOS) or Klinefelter syndrome, HCA prevalence is also increased.[24]

Obesity, along with the associated risk factors of the metabolic syndrome, has been found to be linked with the development and progression of HCAs.[45,46] Increased levels of adipokines circulating in obesity trigger the release of interleukin (IL)-6 by adipocytes. IL-6 has been previously identified as a risk factor for malignant transformation[47]

Glycogen storage disease (GSD) is linked with an increased prevalence of HCAs and greater risk of malignant transformation to hepatocellular carcinoma (HCC), particularly with GSD types Ia, III, and IV. The frequency of reported HCA in this population is 16% to 74%, with HCA typically occurring in the second and third decade of life with a male predominance. Hepatomegaly in these cases is near universal, and the presence of bilobar HCA lesions is seen more commonly than in the general population. There is a 50% risk of developing at least 1 HCA lesion by age 25 in GSD with an associated increased risk of HCC. At least half of GSD-associated HCAs tend to be of the inflammatory subtype. Management with frequent ultrasound surveillance and early consideration of surgical resection is recommended in this population.[41,48]

The complications arising from the presence of HCA lesions are risk of hemorrhage of the lesion and malignant transformation to HCC. The risk of hemorrhage occurs in

11% to 29% of cases, but it typically occurs in lesions larger than 5 cm.[41] Over 50% of histologically examined HCA lesions were noted to have bleeding, but the cases of symptomatic bleeding were again associated with lesion size greater than 5 cm.[49,50] The risk of malignant transformation of HCA is 5% to 10% overall and also increases with lesion size.[47] Thus with increased risk of these complications, resection is recommended for lesions over 5 cm in size.

Molecular Subtypes of Hepatocellular Adenoma

HCA is a benign neoplasm of hepatocyte proliferation in response to a hormonal or metabolic abnormality.[41] These lesions may be further classified by molecular subtypes to describe disease risk factors and associated complications.

Hepatocyte nuclear factor 1α

Hepatocyte nuclear factor 1α (HNF1α) inactivating mutation account for 34% to 46% of all HCAs.[49,51] Most of these lesions are highly steatotic because of the biallelic inactivating mutations of the HNF1α gene. This abnormal HNF1α gene silences expression of liver fatty acid binding protein (LAFBP), which impairs fatty acid movement in the hepatocytes leading to intracellular fat deposition.[10,51,52] Ninety percent of HCA lesions with HNF1α inactivating mutation are found in women who use OCPs. Hormones are felt to act as endogenous genotoxic agents that may partly be responsible for somatic mutations in HNF1α- mutated HCA.[51,53] Familial hepatic adenomatosis with multiple lesions and maturity-onset diabetes mellitus of the young (MODY) have been associated with this molecular subtype.[54] Malignant transformation of these lesions is rare.[24,52]

Inflammatory

The inflammatory subtype of HCA lesions is seen in approximately 18% to 44% of cases and is typically asymptomatic.[49,51] This subtype arises from the sustained activation of the Janus Kinase (JAK) signal transducer and activation transcription (STAT) pathway, resulting in hepatocellular proliferation.[49,51] On histopathology, the inflammatory subtype is noted to have inflammatory infiltrates, sinusoidal dilatation, and dystrophic vessels with immunostaining noting the expression of serum amyloid protein (SAA) and C-reactive protein (CRP).[52,53] These lesions are prone to bleeding because of their dilated sinusoids and abnormal arteries. They tend to be more subcapsular in location and larger in size..[52] Inflammatory HCAs are associated with a high body mass index (BMI) and excessive alcohol consumption.[10] They may be associated with chronic anemia, elevated CRP, or alkaline phosphatase/GGT elevations.[49]

Telangiectatic hepatocellular adenoma

Telangiectatic HCA (formerly known as telangiectatic FNH) has been reclassified under the inflammatory hepatocellular adenoma subtype based on molecular similarities. These lesions have been associated with OCP/hormonal therapy, and patients are more likely to be overweight, with 15%–40% of cases presenting with another benign liver lesion.[55,56] Telangiectatic HCAs are also more likely to be symptomatic because of increased risks of intralesional hemorrhage and necrosis.[56,57]

β-catenin

The sustained activation of β-catenin gene leads to uncontrolled hepatocyte formation and constitutes a molecular subtype classification of HCAs. β-catenin activation is noted with cytologic abnormalities of increased nuclear cytoplasmic ratio, nuclear atypia and an acinar pattern of staining.[52] This subtype of HCA is more frequently found in men, associated with GSD, male hormone administration, and familial adenomatous polyposis. β-catenin is the most frequently activated oncogene in HCCs, and this sub-type has a greater likelihood of malignant transformation to HCC.[10,51,53] Recently, β-catenin associated HCAs have been further divided into 2 subtypes: mutations of cadherin-associated protein β1 (CTNNB1) exon 3 activating β-catenin and mutations of CTNNB1 exon 7 or 8, which mildly activate the Wnt/β-catenin pathway. Clinically, these 2 subtypes differ in their risk of HCC malignant transformation. CTNNB1 muta-tions exon 7 and 8 account for approximately 3% of HCAs, are found at a young age, and are not associated with an increased risk of malignant transformation. Conversely, CTNNB1 mutations exon 3 are approximately 7% of lesions and have the highest risk of malignant transformation because of the full β-catenin pathway activation. These are associated with androgens and vascular liver disease and have a 10% malig-nant/premalignant risk.[49]

Mixed inflammatory and β-catenin
Upon review of HCA lesions, 2 additional subtypes have been noted to share both the inflammatory and either CTNNB1 exon 3 or CTNNB1 exon 7,8 β-catenin pheno-types.[49] Although β-catenin and inflammatory pathways may be found in mixed HCA lesions, β-catenin and the biallelic inactivation of HNF1α pathways are mutually exclusive.[53] In cases of mixed and multiple lesions, β-catenin and exon 3 were asso-ciated with the largest nodule.[49]

Sonic hedgehog
Activation of the sonic hedgehog pathway leads to benign hepatocyte proliferation and has been newly characterized as a subtype of hepatocellular adenoma account-ing for approximately 4% of lesions in the study population. This has been associated with higher BMI and OCP use in the population. The sonic hedgehog subtype was more frequently associated with symptomatic bleeding.[49]

Unclassified
There are 7% to 23% of hepatocellular adenoma lesions that remain unclassified without specific genetic or pathologic abnormalities found at this time.[49,53]

Diagnosis of Hepatocellular Ademona

HCAs may be seen as a heterogenous lesion on ultrasound that may be hyperechoic if steatotic, with an anechoic center if any prior hemorrhage. CEUS may note hyperen-hancement with the arterial phase, hypoenhancement in the portal phase, and no enhancement in late phase. The diagnosis of HCA may be made by CT imaging, noting that if a lesion is more often homogenous than heterogenous, it may be hypodense appearing if steatotic or hyperdense in the presence of hemorrhage.[41]

Although MRI is helpful in diagnosing HCA, it may also be useful in identifying different subtypes of HCA lesions. Inflammatory HCA lesions appear hyperintense on T2 weighted MR images with arterial hyperenhancement that persists into the por-tal venous phase. With the high T2 signal intensity, there is increased T2 signal along the peripheral rim noted as the atoll sign.[52,53,58,59] HNF1α HCA lesions are noted by their diffuse intralesional fat deposition diagnosed on in- and opposed-phase imaging. They have a nonpersistent arterial enhancement.[58] β-catenin has been found to acti-vate the organic anion transporting polypeptide (OATP) B1/B3 and as a consequence allows for uptake of the hepatobiliary contrast gadolinium. β-catenin HCA, particularly CTNNB1 exon 3 subtype lesions have been found to uptake contrast and are iso- to hyperintense relative to liver parenchyma in the hepatobiliary phase of MRI. Caution should be used in interpreting this, as both FNH lesions and some HCC lesions enhance in the presence of hepatobiliary contrast agent.[59,60] Sonic hedgehog HCA lesions have not been associated with particular MRI characteristics; however, it is hypothesized this subtype may be characterized by the presence of hemorrhage on imaging.[59]

At this time, there are no recommendations for histopathology or molecular subtyping of HCA in routine clinical practice. The identification of subtypes on imaging is not currently a driving factor in HCA management.[24,59] It has been proposed, however, that molecular classification may be most helpful in women, particularly those with small lesions (<5 cm) to help guide treatment and surveillance[49] (**Table 2**).

The most common differential diagnosis for HCA is FNH; however, HCA may share imaging characteristics with HCC such as washout or the presence of a capsule. The clinical context in which these lesions occur is important to consider: the presence of underlying liver disease, postmenopausal state, or use of anabolic steroids, all of which may increase the potential of malignancy.[61,62] As the management for HCA, FNH, and HCC differs significantly, in cases for which imaging is inconclusive and further data will have an impact on treatment, a biopsy can be obtained.[4]

Management of Hepatocellular Ademona

Upon the diagnosis of HCA, all OCPs and other forms of exogenous hormones (ie, intrauterine device [IUD], androgens) should be stopped (**Fig. 2**). Regardless of size, all HCA lesions diagnosed in men are recommended to be surgically resected or treated with a curative intent because of the increased risk of malignancy.[4,24] Weight reduction should be encouraged, as weight loss has demonstrated lesion stability and/or reduction in the size of HCA lesions.[45,63]

Women who are diagnosed with HCA lesions smaller than 5 cm may be managed conservatively. Follow-up imaging is recommended every 6 months (for a 1 year based on European guidelines, for 2 years based on US guidelines) to establish growth patterns and monitor for malignant transformation.[4,24] Alpha-fetoprotein (AFP) may be trended but has not been found to be a reliable marker for malignant transformation, as it is often normal even in cases of transformation.[64] Long-term observation of HCA lesions suggests that most lesions are stable (58%) or decrease in size (37%). Fat-containing lesions are significantly less likely to decrease in size than lesions without fat. After an initial size decrease was seen within 5 years, no further changes in size were seen beyond 5 years, suggestive that lesions typically remain stable beyond a 5-year timeframe.[65]

Surgical resection

Given the increased risk of rupture and risks of malignancy associated with growing size, HCA lesions greater than 5 cm are recommended to be surgically resected.[4] Additionally, growth seen on surveillance of an HCA lesion of at least 20% would prompt recommendation for surgical excision.[24] Laparoscopic excision of the HCA is ideal if lesion location and patient comorbidities permit. In cases of hemodynamic instability associated with HCA hemorrhage/rupture, transarterial embolization and abdominal packing with initial laparotomy are recommended to stop hemorrhage and allow for stabilization. A plan for more definitive resection is then recommended 24 to 48 hours later.[66] For adenomas seen in GSD patients, surgical resection is an effective step in HCC prevention until consideration for definitive liver transplant. However, partial hepatectomy is more morbid in GSD than the general population.[48]

Indications for surgical resection in hepatocellular adenomas include lesion size of at least 5 cm, HCAs in males, HCAs that grow at least 20% on surveillance, any instance of biopsy-proven β-catenin mutation, HCAs associated with GSD.

Table 2
Hepatocellular ademona molecular classifications

| | | | Mixed Inflammatory/B-catenin | | | |
| | | | B-Catenin | | | |
	HNF1A	Inflammatory	b-catenin Exon 3	b-catenin Exon 7,8	Sonic Hedgehog	Unclassified
	HNF1A mutations	Sustained JAK/STAT pathway activation	Mutation CTNNB1 exon 3	Mutation CTNNB1 exon 7,8	Activation Sonic Hedgehog pathway	Unknown
Prevalence of lesions	~34%–46%	~18%–44%	~7%	~3%	~4%	~7%–23%
OCP association?	Yes	Yes			Yes	
Risk associations	MODY	Alcohol, elevated BMI	Androgen use, GSD, familial adenomatous polyposis, vascular liver disease		Elevated BMI	
Presentation	Female, hepatic adenomatosis	Elevated alk phos/GGT/CRP, anemia	Male, malignant transformation	Young patient	Symptomatic bleeding	
Risk of malignancy	Rare		High risk	Less risk		
Histology	Intracellular fat deposits	Inflammatory infiltrates, sinusoidal dilatation, abnormal vessels	Increased nuclear ratio, nuclear atypia, large lesions	Nuclear atypia		
MRI characteristics	Intralesional fat deposition, nonpersistent arterial enhancement	Hyperintense on T2 weighted, increased T2 signal along rim of lesion atoll sign	Uptake gadolinium contrast, iso- or hyperintense on hepatobiliary phase		Possible findings of hemorrhage	

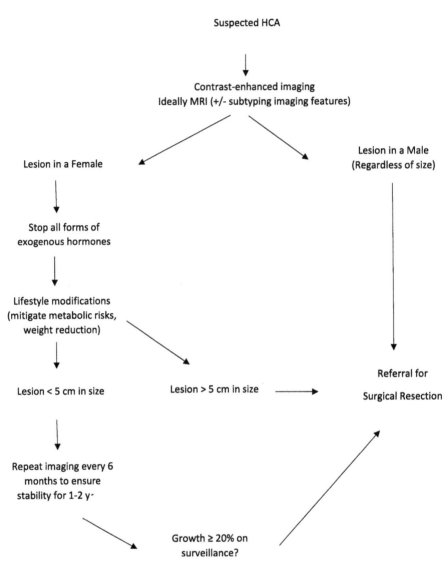

Fig. 2. Management of HCA.

Minimally Invasive Treatments

Transarterial embolization and ablation may be pursued in settings of poor surgical candidacy, in cases of acute hemorrhage, or as a bridge to surgical resection to decrease the size and bleeding potential of HCA lesions. Embolization monotherapy may be limited in treatment of HCA as it may not eradicate all the cells in adenoma and has been found to require retreatment in 25% of cases. There are limited data on the use of microwave ablation in the treatment of HCA. Radiofrequency ablation (RFA) has been used in small unresectable HCA and may impede growth in settings of pregnancy or hormones when a patient may be unable to stop therapy. RFA is mostly used in lesions less than 5 cm, and decreased effectiveness is seen with increasing lesion size.[67–69]

Liver Transplantation

Liver transplantation may be considered in the treatment of HCAs, and transplantation has been performed for the presence of multiple adenoma lesions, suspicious or biopsy-proven malignant transformation, or the presence of portosystemic venous shunts. Specifically, criteria have been proposed for transplant for HCA that include histologic proof of malignant transformation or the presence of 3 of the 5 minor criteria:

More than 2 previous life-threatening hemorrhage
More than 2 prior hepatectomies
β-catenin mutated/inflammatory adenoma
Underlying liver disease such as major steatosis or vascular abnormalities
Age greater than 30 years old[70]

Liver transplantation may be considered in patients with multifocal, growing HCA lesions that do not regress with dietary improvements in GSD and as such would be curative of the underlying enzymatic defect in GSD.[48]

Pregnancy

Managing pregnant women with HCA should be individualized. Ideally there would be prepregnancy intervention (such as resection, ablation, or embolization) of large lesions or for lesions with complications during prior pregnancy.[71] Pregnancy is not contraindicated for those lesions less than 5 cm, and it is recommended to monitor for the potential of growth with ultrasound every 6 to 12 weeks during pregnancy.[4,24] Because of elevated levels of circulating estrogens, hyperdynamic circulation, and increased vascularity of the liver, the greatest risk of rupture is in the third trimester of pregnancy. Women with HCA can deliver vaginally in lieu of cesarean section if there are no other complicating factors. Surgical resection of HCA lesions may be considered in pregnant women who are under 24 weeks of pregnancy; however, general anesthesia risks are greatest in the second trimester, and abdominal surgery becomes more difficult in late second trimester because of the gravid uterus; thus it is generally avoided. Selective arterial embolization is only recommended if needed for lifesaving purposes during pregnancy because of increased risk of radiation exposure to the fetus (particularly before 26 weeks of gestation).[71]

Liver Adenomatosis

Liver adenomatosis is recognized as its own entity and characterized as the presence of multiple HCAs with more than 3 to 10 lesions present in normal liver parenchyma.[72] These lesions are associated with the metabolic syndrome hepatic steatosis and are thought to be as a result of congenital or acquired hepatic vascular abnormalities and mutations in the HNF1α germline.[49,51,73] Upon retrospective analysis, liver adenomatosis was found to be stable or regress in size of lesions with weight loss.[45] Because of the presence of multiple lesions, partial resection is challenging; thus liver adenomatosis is managed based on targeting the largest/dominant lesion.[24] Liver transplantation may be considered in select cases of liver adenomatosis.

SUMMARY

FNH and HCA lesions continue to pose diagnostic and management challenges despite improvements in imaging and refinements in therapeutic approaches. Given that focal liver lesions continue to evoke fear and uncertainty regarding the possibility of malignancy in patients and providers, it is important to understand the advances made in diagnostic and management approaches of FNH and HCA as outlined in this article. Clear understanding of FNH and HCA imaging features and molecular subtyping will prove useful in alleviating uncertainty and reducing fear in the practical care of these patients seen commonly in clinical practice. Finally, a more precise risk stratification of HCA lesions for progression to HCC will allow a more nuanced approach to refined management with more definitive decision making toward surgical or radiological therapy.

DISCLOSURE

The authors have nothing to disclose.

REFERENCES

1. Buscarini L, Fornari F, Civardi G, et al. Laparoscopy integrates ultrasound and ultrasound guided biopsy for diagnosis of benign liver tumors. Acta Endoscopica 1993;(23):27–36.
2. Cherqui D, Rahmouni A, Charlotte F, et al. Management of focal nodular hyperplasia and hepatocellular adenoma in young women: a series of 41 patients with clinical, radiological, and pathological correlations. Hepatology 1995;22(6): 1674–81.
3. Belghiti J, Cauchy F, Paradis V, et al. Diagnosis and management of solid benign liver lesions. Nat Rev Gastroenterol Hepatol 2014;11(12):737–49.
4. Marrero JA, Ahn J, Rajender Reddy K. ACG clinical guideline: the diagnosis and management of focal liver lesions. Am J Gastroenterol 2014;109(9):1328–47 [quiz: 1348].
5. Luciani A, Kobeiter H, Maison P, et al. Focal nodular hyperplasia of the liver in men: is presentation the same in men and women? Gut 2002;50(6):877–80.
6. Vilgrain V. Focal nodular hyperplasia. Eur J Radiol 2006;58(2):236–45.
7. Nguyen BN, Flejou JF, Terris B, et al. Focal nodular hyperplasia of the liver: a comprehensive pathologic study of 305 lesions and recognition of new histologic forms. Am J Surg Pathol 1999;23(12):1441–54.
8. Mathieu D, Zafrani ES, Anglade MC, et al. Association of focal nodular hyperplasia and hepatic hemangioma. Gastroenterology 1989;97(1):154–7.
9. Hussain SM, Terkivatan T, Zondervan PE, et al. Focal nodular hyperplasia: findings at state-of-the-art MR imaging, US, CT, and pathologic analysis. Radiographics 2004;24(1):3–17 [discussion: 18–9].
10. van Aalten SM, Verheij J, Terkivatan T, et al. Validation of a liver adenoma classification system in a tertiary referral centre: implications for clinical practice. J Hepatol 2011;55(1):120–5.
11. Roncalli M, Sciarra A, Tommaso LD. Benign hepatocellular nodules of healthy liver: focal nodular hyperplasia and hepatocellular adenoma. Clin Mol Hepatol 2016;22(2):199–211.
12. Dioguardi Burgio M, Ronot M, Salvaggio G, et al. Imaging of hepatic focal nodular hyperplasia: pictorial review and diagnostic strategy. Semin Ultrasound CT MR 2016;37(6):511–24.
13. Ronot M, Paradis V, Duran R, et al. MR findings of steatotic focal nodular hyperplasia and comparison with other fatty tumours. Eur Radiol 2013;23(4):914–23.
14. Mathieu D, Kobeiter H, Cherqui D, et al. Oral contraceptive intake in women with focal nodular hyperplasia of the liver. Lancet 1998;352(9141):1679–80.
15. Mathieu D, Kobeiter H, Maison P, et al. Oral contraceptive use and focal nodular hyperplasia of the liver. Gastroenterology 2000;118(3):560–4.

16. Gobbi D, Dall'Igna P, Messina C, et al. Focal nodular hyperplasia in pediatric patients with and without oncologic history. Pediatr Blood Cancer 2010;55(7):1420–2.

17. Pillon M, Carucci NS, Mainardi C, et al. Focal nodular hyperplasia of the liver: an emerging complication of hematopoietic SCT in children. Bone Marrow Transplant 2015;50(3):414–9.

18. Furlan A, Brancatelli G, Dioguardi Burgio M, et al. Focal nodular hyperplasia after treatment with oxaliplatin: a multiinstitutional series of cases diagnosed at MRI. AJR Am J Roentgenol 2018;210(4):775–9.

19. Bartolotta TV, Midiri M, Scialpi M, et al. Focal nodular hyperplasia in normal and fatty liver: a qualitative and quantitative evaluation with contrast-enhanced ultrasound. Eur Radiol 2004;14(4):583–91.

20. Shamsi K, De Schepper A, Degryse H, et al. Focal nodular hyperplasia of the liver: radiologic findings. Abdom Imaging 1993;18(1):32–8.

21. Bertin C, Egels S, Wagner M, et al. Contrast-enhanced ultrasound of focal nodular hyperplasia: a matter of size. Eur Radiol 2014;24(10):2561–71.

22. Wang W, Chen LD, Lu MD, et al. Contrast-enhanced ultrasound features of histologically proven focal nodular hyperplasia: diagnostic performance compared with contrast-enhanced CT. Eur Radiol 2013;23(9):2546–54.

23. Roche V, Pigneur F, Tselikas L, et al. Differentiation of focal nodular hyperplasia from hepatocellular adenomas with low-mechanical-index contrast-enhanced sonography (CEUS): effect of size on diagnostic confidence. Eur Radiol 2015; 25(1):186–95.

24. European Association for the Study of the Liver (EASL). EASL Clinical Practice Guidelines on the management of benign liver tumours. J Hepatol 2016;65(2): 386–98.

25. Seale MK, Catalano OA, Saini S, et al. Hepatobiliary-specific MR contrast agents: role in imaging the liver and biliary tree. Radiographics 2009;29(6):1725–48.

26. Bieze M, van den Esschert JW, Nio CY, et al. Diagnostic accuracy of MRI in differentiating hepatocellular adenoma from focal nodular hyperplasia: prospective study of the additional value of gadoxetate disodium. AJR Am J Roentgenol 2012;199(1):26–34.

27. Grazioli L, Bondioni MP, Haradome H, et al. Hepatocellular adenoma and focal nodular hyperplasia: value of gadoxetic acid–enhanced MR imaging in differential diagnosis. Radiology 2012;262(2):520–9.

28. Bioulac-Sage P, Balabaud C, Bedossa P, et al. Pathological diagnosis of liver cell adenoma and focal nodular hyperplasia: Bordeaux update. J Hepatol 2007;46(3):521–7.

29. Grazioli L, Morana G, Kirchin MA, et al. Accurate differentiation of focal nodular hyperplasia from hepatic adenoma at gadobenate dimeglumine–enhanced MR imaging: prospective study. Radiology 2005;236(1):166–77.

30. Grazioli L, Olivetti L, Mazza G, et al. MR imaging of hepatocellular adenomas and differential diagnosis dilemma. Int J Hepatol 2013;2013:374170.

31. Bioulac-Sage P, Cubel G, Taouji S, et al. Immunohistochemical markers on needle biopsies are helpful for the diagnosis of focal nodular hyperplasia and hepatocellular adenoma subtypes. Am J Surg Pathol 2012;36(11):1691–9.

32. Demarco MP, Shen P, Bradley RF, et al. Intraperitoneal hemorrhage in a patient with hepatic focal nodular hyperplasia. Am Surg 2006;72(6):555–9.

33. Rahili A, Cai J, Trastour C, et al. Spontaneous rupture and hemorrhage of hepatic focal nodular hyperplasia in lobus caudatus. J Hepatobiliary Pancreat Surg 2005; 12(2):138–42.

34. Kuo YH, Wang JH, Lu SN, et al. Natural course of hepatic focal nodular hyperplasia: a long-term follow-up study with sonography. J Clin Ultrasound 2009;37(3):132–7.

35. Krige JEJ, Jonas E, Beningfield SJ, et al. Resection of benign liver tumours: an analysis of 62 consecutive cases treated in an academic referral centre. S Afr J Surg 2017;55(3):27–34.

36. Descottes B, Glineur D, Lachachi F, et al. Laparoscopic liver resection of benign liver tumors. Surg Endosc 2003;17(1):23–30.

37. Kammula US, Buell JF, Labow DM, et al. Surgical management of benign tumors of the liver. Int J Gastrointest Cancer 2001;30(3):141–6.

38. Navarro AP, Gomez D, Lamb CM, et al. Focal nodular hyperplasia: a review of current indications for and outcomes of hepatic resection. HPB (Oxford) 2014; 16(6):503–11.

39. Virgilio E, Cavallini M. Managing focal nodular hyperplasia of the liver: surgery or minimally-invasive approaches? a review of the preferable treatment options. Anticancer Res 2018;38(1):33–6.

40. Amesur N, Hammond JS, Zajko AB, et al. Management of unresectable symptomatic focal nodular hyperplasia with arterial embolization. J Vasc Interv Radiol 2009;20(4):543–7.

41. Shaked O, Siegelman ES, Olthoff K, et al. Biologic and clinical features of benign solid and cystic lesions of the liver. Clin Gastroenterol Hepatol 2011;9(7): 547–62.e1-4.

42. Rooks JB, Ory HW, Ishak KG, et al. Epidemiology of hepatocellular adenoma. The role of oral contraceptive use. JAMA 1979;242(7):644–8.

43. Buhler H, Pirovino M, Akobiantz A, et al. Regression of liver cell adenoma. A follow-up study of three consecutive patients after discontinuation of oral contraceptive use. Gastroenterology 1982;82(4):775–82.

44. Martin NM, Abu Dayyeh BK, Chung RT. Anabolic steroid abuse causing recurrent hepatic adenomas and hemorrhage. World J Gastroenterol 2008;14(28):4573–5.

45. Bunchorntavakul C, Bahirwani R, Drazek D, et al. Clinical features and natural history of hepatocellular adenomas: the impact of obesity. Aliment Pharmacol Ther 2011;34(6):664–74.

46. Bioulac-Sage P, Taouji S, Possenti L, et al. Hepatocellular adenoma subtypes: the impact of overweight and obesity. Liver Int 2012;32(8):1217–21.

47. Stoot JH, Coelen RJ, De Jong MC, et al. Malignant transformation of hepatocellular adenomas into hepatocellular carcinomas: a systematic review including more than 1600 adenoma cases. HPB (Oxford) 2010;12(8):509–22.

48. Reddy SK, Kishnani PS, Sullivan JA, et al. Resection of hepatocellular adenoma in patients with glycogen storage disease type Ia. J Hepatol 2007;47(5):658–63.

49. Nault JC, Couchy G, Balabaud C, et al. Molecular classification of hepatocellular adenoma associates with risk factors, bleeding, and malignant transformation. Gastroenterology 2017;152(4):880–94.e6.

50. Dokmak S, Paradis V, Vilgrain V, et al. A single-center surgical experience of 122 patients with single and multiple hepatocellular adenomas. Gastroenterology 2009;137(5):1698–705.

51. Katabathina VS, Menias CO, Shanbhogue AK, et al. Genetics and imaging of hepatocellular adenomas: 2011 update. Radiographics 2011;31(6):1529–43.

52. Ronot M, Bahrami S, Calderaro J, et al. Hepatocellular adenomas: accuracy of magnetic resonance imaging and liver biopsy in subtype classification. Hepatology 2011;53(4):1182–91.

53. Laumonier H, Bioulac-Sage P, Laurent C, et al. Hepatocellular adenomas: magnetic resonance imaging features as a function of molecular pathological classification. Hepatology 2008;48(3):808–18.

54. Bacq Y, Jacquemin E, Balabaud C, et al. Familial liver adenomatosis associated with hepatocyte nuclear factor 1alpha inactivation. Gastroenterology 2003; 125(5):1470–5.
55. Attal P, Vilgrain V, Brancatelli G, et al. Telangiectatic focal nodular hyperplasia: US, CT, and MR imaging findings with histopathologic correlation in 13 cases. Radiology 2003;228(2):465–72.
56. Paradis V, Champault A, Ronot M, et al. Telangiectatic adenoma: an entity associated with increased body mass index and inflammation. Hepatology 2007; 46(1):140–6.
57. Bioulac-Sage P, Rebouissou S, Sa Cunha A, et al. Clinical, morphologic, and molecular features defining so-called telangiectatic focal nodular hyperplasias of the liver. Gastroenterology 2005;128(5):1211–8.
58. Fowler KJ, Brown JJ, Narra VR. Magnetic resonance imaging of focal liver lesions: approach to imaging diagnosis. Hepatology 2011;54(6):2227–37.
59. Zulfiqar M, Sirlin CB, Yoneda N, et al. Hepatocellular adenomas: understanding the pathomolecular lexicon, MRI features, terminology, and pitfalls to inform a standardized approach. J Magn Reson Imaging 2019. https://doi.org/10.1002/jmri.26902.
60. Sciarra A, Schmidt S, Pellegrinelli A, et al. OATPB1/B3 and MRP3 expression in hepatocellular adenoma predicts Gd-EOB-DTPA uptake and correlates with risk of malignancy. Liver Int 2019;39(1):158–67.
61. Quaglia A. Hepatocellular carcinoma: a review of diagnostic challenges for the pathologist. J Hepatocell Carcinoma 2018;5:99–108.
62. O'Neill EK, Cogley JR, Miller, F.H.. The ins and outs of liver imaging. Clin Liver Dis 2015;19(1):99–121.
63. Dokmak S, Belghiti J. Will weight loss become a future treatment of hepatocellular adenoma in obese patients? Liver Int 2015;35(10):2228–32.
64. Farges O, Dokmak S. Malignant transformation of liver adenoma: an analysis of the literature. Dig Surg 2010;27(1):32–8.
65. Shao N, Pandey A, Ghasabeh MA, et al. Long-term follow-up of hepatic adenoma and adenomatosis: analysis of size change on imaging with histopathological correlation. Clin Radiol 2018;73(11):958–65.
66. Cho SW, Marsh JW, Steel J, et al. Surgical management of hepatocellular adenoma: take it or leave it? Ann Surg Oncol 2008;15(10):2795–803.
67. Smolock AR, Cristescu MM, Potretzke TA, et al. Microwave ablation for the treatment of hepatic adenomas. J Vasc Interv Radiol 2016;27(2):244–9.
68. Silva JP, Klooster B, Tsai S, et al. Elective regional therapy treatment for hepatic adenoma. Ann Surg Oncol 2019;26(1):125–30.
69. van Rosmalen BV, Coelen RJS, Bieze M, et al. Systematic review of transarterial embolization for hepatocellular adenomas. Br J Surg 2017;104(7):823–35.
70. Chiche L, David A, Adam R, et al. Liver transplantation for adenomatosis: European experience. Liver Transpl 2016;22(4):516–26.
71. Broker ME, Ijzermans JN, van Aalten SM, et al. The management of pregnancy in women with hepatocellular adenoma: a plea for an individualized approach. Int J Hepatol 2012;2012:725735.
72. Flejou JF, Barge J, Menu Y, et al. Liver adenomatosis. An entity distinct from liver adenoma? Gastroenterology 1985;89(5):1132–8.
73. Greaves WO, Bhattacharya B. Hepatic adenomatosis. Arch Pathol Lab Med 2008;132(12):1951–5.

Viral Hepatitis Other than A, B, and C

Evaluation and Management

Amanda Cheung, MD*, Paul Kwo, MD

KEYWORDS

- Hepatitis D • Hepatitis E • Hepatotropic viruses • Human herpesvirus
- Viral hepatitis

KEY POINTS

- Hepatitis D virus (HDV) requires hepatitis B virus for replication and is more likely to cause chronic infection in the setting of HDV superinfection in hepatitis B surface antigen–positive individuals. Treatment of HDV remains limited, with ongoing need for new therapies.
- Hepatitis E is an increasingly recognized cause of chronic infection in immunocompromised individuals and is more common in genotypes 3 and 4, with sporadic cases occurring worldwide.
- Human herpesviruses are commonly benign infections in immunocompetent individuals but cause significant morbidity and mortality in immunocompromised hosts.

INTRODUCTION

The term viral hepatitis refers to liver inflammation that occurs because of a viral infection. There are 5 hepatotropic viruses (hepatitis A, B, C, D, and E) that selectively infect the liver. Acute hepatitis caused by these viruses may resolve without intervention or may develop into chronic infection in some instances. Nonhepatotropic viruses target different organs in the body but are also known to cause hepatitis, although these infections are typically mild in immunocompetent hosts. The significance of nonhepatotropic viruses is most notable in immunocompromised hosts, particularly in transplant recipients.

HEPATITIS D

Hepatitis D virus (HDV), also called delta virus, was first described in 1977 in a group of patients infected with hepatitis B virus (HBV) who were found to have more severe

Division of Gastroenterology and Hepatology, Stanford University School of Medicine, 750 Welch Road, Suite 210, Palo Alto, CA 94304, USA
* Corresponding author.
E-mail address: cheungac@stanford.edu

Clin Liver Dis 24 (2020) 405–419
https://doi.org/10.1016/j.cld.2020.04.008
1089-3261/20/© 2020 Elsevier Inc. All rights reserved.

hepatitis than their counterparts.[1] The hepatitis D virion consists of the hepatitis D RNA genome, hepatitis D antigen (HDAg), and a lipoprotein envelope containing HBV surface antigen (HBsAg) proteins.[2] Thus, HDV requires HBV in addition to cellular RNA polymerases for replication and cannot infect individuals without the presence of HBsAg, which is required for cell entry, virion assembly and export. Since the widespread availability of the hepatitis B vaccine with worldwide implementation of vaccination programs, a concomitant decrease in HDV alongside HBV would be expected. However, the prevalence of HDV seems to be increasing and may be attributed to the higher prevalence of HDV infection in human immunodeficiency virus (HIV) coinfected individuals and intravenous drug users.[3,4] The global burden of disease is estimated to be 62 million to 72 million, affecting nearly 1% of the general population.[4]

Clinical Presentation

Infection with hepatitis D can occur under 2 circumstances (**Fig. 1**). Coinfection occurs when an individual is exposed to both hepatitis B and D viruses simultaneously with a similar presentation to acute HBV infection and potential risk of acute liver failure (ALF). Superinfection occurs when an individual with established chronic hepatitis B infection (defined by the presence of HBsAg) is exposed to an acute hepatitis D infection. Although superinfection with HDV is more likely to develop into chronic infection, 95% of individuals with HBV-HDV coinfection ultimately have viral clearance.[5] Chronic HDV infection is the most aggressive form of viral hepatitis with greater rates of hepatocellular carcinoma and more rapid progression to cirrhosis compared with HBV monoinfection.[6–9]

Screening for HDV is recommended for individuals with chronic HBV (HBsAg positivity) and presence of 1 or more of the following risk factors[10]:

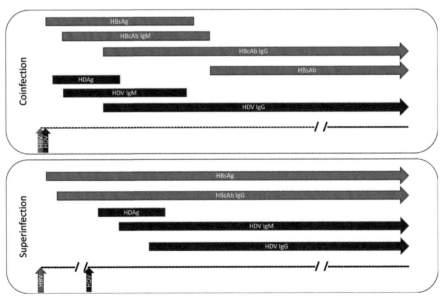

Fig. 1. Typical pattern of HBV and HDV serologies in HDV infection. Coinfection leads to clearance of both viruses in 95% of patients. Superinfection in a patient with preexisting chronic HBV infection most often leads to chronic HDV infection. HBcAb, hepatitis B core antibody; HBsAb, hepatitis B surface antibody; IgG, immunoglobulin G; IgM, immunoglobulin M.

- Individuals with HIV or hepatitis C virus (HCV) coinfection
- Current or past intravenous drug users
- Men who have sex with men
- Individuals with high-risk sexual behavior
- Immigrants from high-prevalence areas[11]
  - Africa (central and West Africa)
  - Asia (central and northern Asia, Vietnam, Mongolia, Pakistan, Japan, and Chinese Taipei)
  - Pacific Islands (Kiribati, Nauru)
  - Middle East (all countries)
  - Eastern Europe (eastern Mediterranean regions, Turkey)
  - South America (Amazon basin)
  - Greenland
- Individuals with high transaminase levels despite low or undetectable HBV DNA levels

Diagnosis

HDV infection is diagnosed with serum-based tests (**Table 1**). HDV antigen is typically only detected in the blood during the early acute phase of infection and is not a reliable test for diagnosis.[12] Acute HDV infection leads to both innate and adaptive immune responses with production of HDV immunoglobulin M (IgM) and immunoglobulin G (IgG), respectively. HDV IgM is detectable 1 to 3 weeks after exposure and remains positive in chronic active infection with levels reflective of disease activity.[13] HDV IgG is a marker of either current active or prior resolved infection. Thus, HDV IgG is checked first for chronic HDV screening, and HDV RNA is used to confirm active infection and to follow response to therapy. Because there remains ongoing work to standardize and improve HDV RNA assays, HDV IgM can be tested in patients with high clinical suspicion of HDV infection but an undetected RNA level.[14]

Table 1
Serologies in hepatitis B virus and hepatitis D virus infection

	HBsAg	Anti-HBc IgM	Anti-HBc IgG	HBV DNA	HDAg	Anti-HDV IgM	Anti-HDV IgG	HDV RNA
Acute HBV infection	+	+	+[a]	+	−	−	−	−
Chronic HBV infection	+	−	+	+	−	−	−	−
Acute HBV-HDV coinfection	+	+	+[a]	+	±[b]	+	+[a]	+
Acute HBV-HDV superinfection	+	−	+	+	±[b]	+	+[a]	+
Chronic HBV-HDV infection	+	−	+	+	±[b]	+[c]	+	+
Resolved HBV and HDV[d]	−	−	+	−	−	−	+	−

Abbreviations: anti-HBc, hepatitis B core antibody; HDAg, hepatitis D antigen; anti-HDV, hepatitis D antibody; IgG, immunoglobulin G; IgM, immunoglobulin M.
[a] May not be present yet in early infection.
[b] Present transiently, often not detected.
[c] Typically remains persistently increased.
[d] Occurs rarely in superinfection, more common in coinfection.

Noninvasive markers for fibrosis, including the FIB-4 score, have not been reliable in patients with chronic HDV infection.[15] The greater degree of inflammation in HDV compared with HBV monoinfection likely alters elastography measurement. A recent study showed that vibration-controlled transient elastography may have reasonable accuracy to detect cirrhosis[16] but remains to be validated and has not yet been studied for grading lesser degrees of fibrosis. Thus, liver biopsy is typically still required for accurate grading of inflammation and staging of fibrosis.

Treatment

Interferon alfa (IFN-α) is currently the only available treatment for chronic HDV infection. The goal of HDV therapy is to achieve viral suppression with sustained clearance of HDV after treatment completion. Thus far, no study has been able to achieve this in the majority of patients treated.[17] The Hep-Net International Delta Hepatitis Intervention Trial (HIDIT), a large multicenter initiative, treated patients with peginterferon α-2a and/or adefovir for 48 weeks of therapy. Six months after treatment completion, 28% of patients treated with interferon alone had continued undetectable HDV RNA with no additional benefit derived in those who also received adefovir and no response in individuals treated with adefovir alone.[18] In the follow-up study, HIDIT-II, treating with peginterferon α-2a with or without tenofovir, only 23% of patients had undetectable HDV RNA 24 weeks after completing a 96-week course of therapy with interferon and no additional benefit from concomitant tenofovir therapy.[19]

The international societies, including the American Association for the Study of Liver Diseases (AASLD), European Association for the Study of the Liver (EASL), and Asian Pacific Association for the Study of the Liver (APASL), do not provide specific guidelines on indications for chronic HDV treatment.[10,20,21] The decision to treat with interferon must be balanced between the suspected degree of inflammation and fibrosis and whether the trajectory of disease warrants the potential side effects from interferon therapy and expected low response rates. Although the presence of HDV typically suppresses HBV replication,[22] treatment with a nucleoside/nucleotide analogue (entecavir or tenofovir) is generally recommended for co-infected patients with HBV DNA levels greater than 2000 IU/mL and all patients with cirrhosis regardless of HBV replication status (**Table 2**).

The ability to achieve sustained virologic response (SVR) in the treatment of HDV remains uncertain given the high rates of late relapse. Follow-up of the HIDIT-I study participants at a median time of 4.5 years found detectable HDV RNA levels in half of the patients who had met the initial SVR definition with undetectable HDV RNA 24 weeks after treatment.[23] Likelihood of response may be predicted by HDV RNA and HBsAg

Table 2
Treatment recommendations in chronic hepatitis B virus and hepatitis D virus coinfection

HDV RNA	ALT	HBV DNA	Cirrhosis	Treatment
+	+	<2000 IU/mL	No	IFN alone
+	+	>2000 IU/mL	No	IFN + NA
+	+	<2000 IU/mL	Yes	IFN + NA
+	+	>2000 IU/mL	Yes	IFN + NA

IFN treatment for 48 weeks: Peg-IFN-α-2a (Pegasys) 180 μg weekly; Peg-IFN-α-2b (PegIntron) 1.5 μg/kg weekly.
NA treatment: entecavir (Baraclude) 0.5 to 1 mg daily; tenofovir dipovoxil fumarate (Viread) 300 mg daily; tenofovir alafenamide (Vemlidy) 25 mg daily.
Abbreviations: ALT, alanine transaminase; NA, nucleotide or nucleoside analogue.

kinetics during treatment.[24] Earlier decline of HDV RNA levels by more than 2 log copies per milliliter and HBsAg level less than 1000 IU/mL by week 24 of therapy indicate a higher likelihood of virologic response after treatment completion.[25,26] Because of the high rates of relapse, ongoing surveillance for HDV RNA is needed, particularly in the setting of increased transaminase levels after completion of prior therapy. However, loss of HBsAg after treatment of HDV with IFN is considered a marker of cure for both HBV and HDV.

In patients with chronic HDV infection who are decompensated and unable to tolerate IFN because of its side effects, liver transplant may be considered. As with all patients with cirrhosis, ongoing screening is needed for esophageal varices and hepatocellular carcinoma. For patients who undergo liver transplant, hepatitis B immune globulin is administered similar to patients with HBV monoinfection, which results in clearance of HBsAg and HDV RNA.[27]

Given the paucity of treatment options, high relapse rates, and poor side effect profile, there remains a need and ongoing investigation for a treatment option that may be more efficacious. Novel treatments with promising early data under investigation include myrcludex, an entry inhibitor that blocks both HDV and HBV hepatocyte entry; the prenylation inhibitor lonafarnib, which inhibits farnesyltransferase, a key enzyme required for HDV replication; and pegylated interferon lambda, a type 3 interferon.[28]

HEPATITIS E

Hepatitis E virus (HEV) is the most common cause of acute viral hepatitis worldwide. The original hepatitis E outbreak likely occurred in New Delhi in 1955, involving 29,000 individuals based on analysis of stored serum. The virus was initially isolated from the stool of Soviet soldiers experiencing hepatitis outbreaks during the military conflict in Afghanistan during the 1980s. HEV was subsequently named in 1990 to distinguish it from hepatitis A virus, an additional source of waterborne hepatitis epidemics at the time.[29] There are 4 known HEV genotypes. Infections with genotypes 1 and 2 are limited to humans and cause disease via consumption of contaminated water. HEV genotypes 3 and 4 cause zoonotic infections, with human disease attributed to consumption of raw or undercooked meat, particularly pork and wild game.[30] Thus, HEV endemic outbreaks are related to genotypes 1 and 2 typically in Asia, Africa, and Mexico, and sporadic cases caused by genotype 3 and 4 have been observed in nations worldwide.

Clinical Presentation

Clinical presentation in acute HEV infection depends on the exposed person's risk factors. Most healthy individuals are either asymptomatic or have a self-limited course of acute hepatitis with nonspecific symptoms and spontaneous resolution after 4 to 6 weeks.[31] More severe clinical courses are observed in infants, pregnant women, and individuals with excessive alcohol consumption or other chronic preexisting liver diseases.[30,32] Mortality from acute HEV genotype 1 and 2 infections in developing countries has been largely attributed to ALF in pregnant women.[33] In addition, HEV has been recognized as a cause of acute-on-chronic liver failure worldwide.[34]

Chronic HEV, defined by chronic hepatitis with increased aminotransferase levels and persistent detection of HEV RNA for 6 months after exposure, is rare in immunocompetent individuals but has been increasingly recognized with genotype 3 HEV infections in immunocompromised hosts, particularly in those with solid organ transplants (SOTs), stem cell transplants (SCTs), or HIV. This condition is likely caused by the impaired and/or insufficient immune T-cell response with an inability to control the virus in the immunocompromised state.[35] An estimated 60% of SOT recipients infected with HEV do not clear the virus and develop chronic infection with increased risk of rapid progression to cirrhosis.[36] Unlike immunocompetent individuals, HEV infection in immunocompromised patients typically presents with lower transaminase and bilirubin levels and minimal symptoms. Both acute and chronic HEV have been associated with numerous extrahepatic manifestations (**Table 3**), which may be the only sign or symptom at presentation.[37–41]

Table 3
Hepatitis E infection in immunocompetent and immunocompromised individuals

	Immunocompetent	Immunocompromised
Presentation		
Symptoms	Self-limited, nonspecific symptoms	Typically asymptomatic
ALT Level	High >1000 IU/L	Moderate 100–300 IU/L
Extrahepatic Manifestations	Neurologic: Guillain-Barré syndrome, radiculoneuropathy, amyotrophy, encephalitis Renal: membranous and membranoproliferative glomerulonephritis, IgA nephropathy Hematologic: aplastic anemia, autoimmune hemolytic anemia, cryoglobulinemia, thrombocytopenia Pancreatic: pancreatitis Rheumatologic: polyarthritis Cardiac: myocarditis Endocrine: thyroiditis	
Diagnosis		
Serologies	HEV IgM and/or HEV RNA	HEV RNA
Liver Biopsy	Varies: mixed inflammatory infiltrate, interface hepatitis, cholestasis, apoptotic bodies	Varies: minimal inflammation, mild acute cellular rejection
Differential Diagnoses	Acute viral hepatitis (HAV, HBV, HCV, HEV, CMV, EBV) Autoimmune hepatitis Drug-induced liver injury	Acute cellular rejection (liver transplant patients) Graft-versus-host disease (SOT or SCT patients) Drug-induced liver injury Chronic viral hepatitis (HBV, HCV, HDV) EBV and CMV hepatitis (reactivation)
Treatment	None Consider treatment if extrahepatic manifestations or high risk; ie, pregnancy, chronic liver disease	Reduction of immunosuppression (avoidance of calcineurin inhibitors) Ribavirin 600 mg for 3 mo, dose adjusted for weight and renal function
Prevention	Universal access to clean drinking water Avoidance of undercooked pork, wild game, and shellfish Screening of blood donors and/or products Vaccination (currently not available in most countries)	

Abbreviations: CMV, cytomegalovirus; EBV, Epstein-Barr virus; HAV, hepatitis A virus; HCV, hepatitis C virus; IgA, immunoglobulin A; SOT, solid organ transplant; SCT, stem cell transplant.

Diagnosis

After initial exposure and an incubation period of 2 to 8 weeks, HEV RNA may be detectable in the stool and serum for 1 to 2 weeks after onset of symptoms. The diagnostic window is narrow because patients typically present after the peak viremic period has concluded. Anti-HEV IgM is produced early after infection, coinciding with peak alanine transaminase levels, and may last 4 to 6 months. Anti-HEV IgG is first present at low titers and increases incrementally over time. Thus, patients who present early may only have detectable HEV RNA, whereas many patients do not present until the early viremic period has already subsided.[42] In immunocompetent hosts, diagnosis of acute HEV infection may require anti-HEV IgM or HEV RNA.

In immunocompromised hosts, levels of anti-HEV immunoglobulin are lower and frequently undetectable, so diagnosis often requires testing for HEV RNA by polymerase chain reaction (PCR) for confirmation. The World Health Organization has developed an international standard for nucleic acid amplification techniques to improve HEV RNA detection and quantification.[43] To increase diagnostic rates of HEV, use of at least 2 of the 3 markers mentioned earlier is suggested to increase yield, particularly because accuracy and reliability of anti-HEV immunoglobulin assays differ widely in laboratories and among the particular individuals being tested.[42,44] Although there are distinct HEV genotypes, the body's immune response and production of anti-HEV IgG antibodies are cross-reactive to all 4 known genotypes.[45]

Liver biopsy in acute HEV infection may show a wide range of features, including mixed inflammatory infiltrate, interface hepatitis, cholestasis, and apoptotic bodies, which may have similar overlapping features with other viral hepatitis, autoimmune hepatitis, or drug-induced liver injury.[46] Because most cases of acute HEV are self-limited in immunocompetent hosts, liver biopsy is often not necessary. By contrast, liver biopsy is often obtained before chronic HEV infection is suspected in immunosuppressed hosts because unexplained increase in transaminase levels is the typical presentation with no other clinical symptoms. In patients with known infection, liver biopsy may be beneficial for staging of fibrosis given the potential risk for accelerated progression to cirrhosis. HEV RNA may be detected in the liver biopsy specimen and histopathology ranges from minimal inflammation to clinical features suggestive of mild acute cellular rejection.[47] Given the nonspecific findings on histologic examination, HEV RNA should be tested in transplant recipients if a liver biopsy shows chronic hepatitis of uncertain cause or a nondiagnostic biopsy in the setting of persistently abnormal liver chemistries.[48]

Treatment of Chronic Hepatitis E Virus Infection

The initial step in management of chronic HEV is reduction of immunosuppression, if possible, particularly using medications with an effect on T cells (ie, calcineurin inhibitors and mammalian target of rapamycin inhibitors), which has been shown to be a sufficient strategy to allow clearance of the virus in one-third of patients.[49] The optimal immunosuppressive regimen still requires further studies, with current recommendations to minimize immunosuppression as much as possible and favoring use of mycophenolate rather than calcineurin or mammalian target of rapamycin inhibitors.[50] Interferon has been used for treatment of hepatitis B and C, so it has similarly been investigated in use for treatment of chronic HEV.[51] However, its long list of potential side effects, including the potential for graft rejection, makes it a poor treatment option. Ribavirin is used and tolerated well for treatment of chronic HEV in SOT recipients at a median dose of 600 mg daily (8 mg/kg) for 3 months and longer treatment courses for 6 to 12 months in those with partial response or relapse after treatment.[52] There is currently 1 licensed vaccine for hepatitis E (HEV 239, Hecolin) available in China, which is derived from a 26-KDa protein coded by ORF2 of HEV1.[53]

HUMAN HERPESVIRUSES

There are 8 viruses in the Herpesviridae family that can cause disease in humans, including viral hepatitis (**Table 4**). Initial infections with these viruses are typically self-limited. The viruses then become latent infections with the ability to reactivate when there is an immunocompromised or immunosuppressed state.

Herpes Simplex Virus

Herpes simplex virus type 1 (HSV-1) and type 2 (HSV-2) are common infections that cause both oral and genital vesicular lesions. Although immunocompetent individuals can develop disseminated HSV with hepatic involvement, it is more common in immunocompromised states, including pregnancy, HIV infection, and use of

Table 4
Human herpesviruses

	Alternate Name	Immunocompetent Host	Immunocompromised Hosts[c]	Liver Histology
HHV-1	HSV-1	Oral and genital ulcers	ALF, encephalitis	Hepatocyte necrosis, intranuclear inclusions, multinucleated giant cells
HHV-2	HSV-2	Oral and genital ulcers	ALF, encephalitis	Hepatocyte necrosis, intranuclear inclusions, multinucleated giant cells
HHV-3	VZV	Chickenpox, shingles	ALF, encephalitis	Hepatocyte necrosis, intranuclear inclusions, multinucleated giant cells
HHV-4	EBV	Infectious mononucleosis[a]	Hepatitis, PTLD, lymphoma	Sinusoidal lymphocytic infiltration
HHV-5	CMV	Mononucleosislike syndrome[a]	Multisystemic organ involvement[b]	Mononuclear portal and sinusoidal infiltration, owl's eye nuclear inclusions
HHV-6		Roseola	Rare	Nonspecific
HHV-7		Pityriasis rosea	Rare	Nonspecific
HHV-8	KSHV	Fever, rash, lymphadenopathy	Kaposi sarcoma, Castleman disease	Proliferation of spindle-shaped cells

Abbreviations: CMV, cytomegalovirus; EBV, Epstein-Barr virus; HHV, human herpesvirus; HSV, herpes simplex virus; KSHV, Kaposi sarcoma–associated herpes virus; PTLD, posttransplant lymphoproliferative disease; VZV, varicella zoster virus.
   [a] Mononucleosis syndrome is the classic triad of fever, pharyngitis, and lymphadenopathy.
   [b] Hepatitis, pneumonitis, colitis, myocarditis, retinitis, encephalitis, cytopenias.
   [c] Mild hepatitis may occur with all HHV infections but severe hepatitis and ALF typically only occur in immunocompromised hosts.

immunosuppressant medications. HSV hepatitis, more commonly caused by HSV-2, is less likely to manifest with characteristic mucocutaneous vesicular lesions and typically presents with fever and ALF leading to death or liver transplant in most cases.[54] Diagnosis should be made with HSV DNA by PCR rather than serologies (HSV IgG or IgM) because of the latter's inaccuracies in acute hepatitis.[55] Liver biopsy may be needed for definitive diagnosis and shows hepatocellular necrosis with intranuclear inclusions and immunostaining for HSV. However, immediate initiation of empiric treatment with intravenous acyclovir is recommended given the severity and potentially rapid progression of disease, including death if treatment is delayed.[54]

Varicella Zoster Virus

Varicella zoster virus (VZV) is commonly known for causing chickenpox in children at the time of initial infection, and later becoming latent in the dorsal root ganglia with reactivation causing shingles in adults. Transmission occurs via aerosolized nasopharyngeal secretions or direct contact with fluid from vesicular lesions. VZV-associated hepatitis has been rarely reported in the literature but can present similarly to HSV hepatitis.[56] Liver biopsy typically looks similar to HSV hepatitis, although diagnosis is made by checking serum VZV PCR. Similar to HSV, treatment with acyclovir is recommended. In immunocompromised hosts, varicella zoster immune globulin may be considered if known exposure occurs.[57] An inactivated zoster vaccine (Shingrix) is now available and recommended for posttransplant and other immunocompromised patients.[58]

Epstein-Barr Virus

Epstein-Barr virus (EBV) is a common infection that causes infectious mononucleosis with fevers, pharyngitis, and lymphadenopathy. More than 90% of the population has evidence of prior exposure by 20 years of age.[59] Unlike the other herpesviruses, mild hepatitis with hepatomegaly and increased transaminase level typically occurs with EBV infection. However, ALF caused by EBV is less common, accounting for 1 in 500 cases of the Acute Liver Failure Study Group and may occur in young and immunocompetent individuals, unlike the other herpesviruses that typically only lead to ALF in the immunocompromised host.[60] After primary infection, the virus becomes latent in the memory B cells.[61] EBV PCR and in situ hybridization of liver tissue can be used to identify the presence of virus, although confirmation of EBV-related hepatitis also requires the appropriate clinical features, including increased transaminase levels with serologies (viral capsid IgG/IgM and Epstein-Barr nuclear antigen antibody and EBV DNA).[62] Virtually all cases of EBV hepatitis are self-limited, but rare cases of severe hepatitis or ALF may require liver transplant.

EBV infection after liver transplant has been associated with posttransplant lymphoproliferative disorder (PTLD), particularly in cases that occur in the first 18 months after transplant.[63] Risk factors for PTLD within the first year of transplant include primary EBV infection, use of antilymphocyte antibodies, younger age at transplant, and transplant of the intestine, lung, or heart. Risk factors for PTLD after the first year of transplant include longer duration of immunosuppression and older age at transplant.[64] Symptoms of PTLD are similar to other lymphoproliferative disorders, including malaise, fevers, weight loss, and lymphadenopathy. Diagnosis requires biopsy of the affected organ, which is typically an excisional biopsy of an enlarged lymph node. Treatment of PTLD first requires the reduction of immunosuppression, but use of anti-CD20 (anti–cluster of differentiation 20) monoclonal antibodies (ie, rituximab) or other therapies may be needed in more refractory cases.[64]

Cytomegalovirus

Cytomegalovirus (CMV) infection may be asymptomatic or lead to a mononucleosis-like syndrome, with an estimated 64% of adults having evidence of prior CMV infection by 50 years of age.[65] Mild transaminase level increases are common and may persist for months after infection.[66] In solid organ transplant recipients, CMV infection is associated with increased death and graft loss, particularly within the first year of transplant.[67] In these cases, CMV hepatitis may be difficult to differentiate from graft rejection. CMV may also lead to a multisystemic disease with end-organ involvement including cytopenias, pneumonitis, colitis, retinitis, myocarditis, and encephalitis. Although CMV IgM may be checked as a marker of acute infection in immunocompetent individuals, serologies are not reliable in immunocompromised hosts. CMV PCR or immunostaining of liver tissue is needed for diagnosis. Preemptive antiviral therapy with valganciclovir has been recommended for SOT recipients at risk, particularly those with no evidence of prior CMV exposure (ie, CMV IgG is negative) who receive allografts from CMV IgG-positive donors.[68] Oral valganciclovir or intravenous ganciclovir may be used to treat CMV hepatitis depending on the severity of illness.

Human Herpes Viruses 6 and 7

Human herpesvirus 6 (HHV-6) and 7 (HHV-7) are typically subclinical infections that may present as roseola or pityriasis rosea, respectively. Reactivation in transplant recipients has been reported to cause hepatitis, graft rejection, and liver failure alongside extrahepatic manifestations including colitis, pneumonitis, encephalitis, and bone marrow suppression.[69] Tissue biopsy with viral PCR is available but not standardized, and positive results do not necessarily confirm causation of clinical disease.[70]

Kaposi Sarcoma–Associated Herpesvirus

Human herpesvirus 8 (HHV-8), also called Kaposi sarcoma–associated herpesvirus, is a known cause of Kaposi sarcoma, lymphoma, and multicentric Castleman disease. Although Kaposi sarcoma is more commonly reported in association with acquired immunodeficiency syndrome, there have also been reported cases in transplant recipients, particularly in liver transplant recipients, who may have graft involvement with hepatitis.[70] Reduction of immunosuppression, including conversion to mammalian target of rapamycin inhibitors, leads to response in most patients, whereas chemotherapy is reserved for those with severe disease with visceral involvement.[71]

MISCELLANEOUS VIRUSES

Additional viruses have been reported to cause a range of clinical presentations, from mild to severe acute hepatitis and ALF, including:[72]

- Adenoviridae
- Arenaviridae: Lassa virus
- Coronaviridae: severe acute respiratory syndrome virus
- Filoviridae: Ebola virus
- Flaviviridae: Dengue virus, West Nile virus, yellow fever virus, Zika virus
- Orthomyxoviridae: influenza virus
- Paramyxoviridae: measles morbillivirus
- Parvoviridae: parvovirus B19
- Picornaviridae: Coxsackie virus, echovirus, poliovirus
- Retroviridae: HIV
- Togaviridae: chikungunya virus

SUMMARY

Both HDV and HEV are causes of disease worldwide and diagnosis requires high clinical suspicion to test for disease presence. HDV remains difficult to treat with the current available therapies and typically leads to chronic disease after superinfection with an accelerated course to cirrhosis or related complications. HEV leading to chronic hepatitis is more common in immunocompromised hosts. Although the hepatotropic viruses (HAV, HBV, HCV, HDV, HEV) may cause disease in all exposed individuals, the nonhepatotropic viruses (ie, HSV-1, HSV-2, VZV, EBV, CMV) typically have self-limited courses that may include a mild hepatitis caused by the immune system's response to the virus at the time of primary infection. For immunocompromised hosts, the risk of clinical disease from the nonhepatotropic viruses is typically at the time of reactivation, with the potential for significant morbidity and mortality.

DISCLOSURE

A. Cheung has nothing to disclose. P. Kwo has received grant support from Eiger.

REFERENCES

1. Rizzetto M, Canese MG, Aricò S, et al. Immunofluorescence detection of new antigen-antibody system (delta/anti-delta) associated to hepatitis B virus in liver and in serum of HBsAg carriers. Gut 1977;18(12):997–1003.
2. Heller T, Koh C, Glenn JS. Hepatitis D. In: Sanyal A, Boyer T, Lindor K, et al, editors. Zakim and Boyer's hepatology: a textbook of liver disease. 7th edition. Philadelphia: Elsevier; 2018. p. 501–11.
3. Lin HH, Lee SS, Yu ML, et al. Changing hepatitis D virus epidemiology in a hepatitis B virus endemic area with a national vaccination program. Hepatology 2015; 61(6):1870–9.
4. Chen HY, Shen D, Ji D, et al. Prevalence and burden of hepatitis D virus infection in the global population: a systematic review and meta-analysis. Gut 2019;68: 512–21.
5. Caredda F, Rossi E, d'Arminio Monforte A, et al. Hepatitis B virus-associated coinfection and superinfection with delta agent: indistinguishable disease with different outcome. J Infect Dis 1985;151(5):925–8.
6. Fattovich G, Boscaro S, Noventa F, et al. Influence of hepatitis delta virus infection on progression to cirrhosis in chronic hepatitis type B. J Infect Dis 1987;155(5): 931–5.
7. Romeo R, Del Ninno E, Rumi M, et al. A 28-year study of the course of hepatitis Delta infection: a risk factor for cirrhosis and hepatocellular carcinoma. Gastroenterology 2009;136(5):1629–38.
8. Ji J, Sundquist K, Sundquist J. A population-based study of hepatitis D virus as potential risk factor for hepatocellular carcinoma. J Natl Cancer Inst 2012; 104(10):790–2.
9. Mahale P, Aka P, Chen X, et al. Hepatitis D virus infection, cirrhosis and hepatocellular carcinoma in the Gambia. J Viral Hepat 2019;26(6):738–49.
10. Terrault NA, Lok ASF, McMahon BJ, et al. Update on prevention, diagnosis, and treatment of chronic hepatitis B: AASLD 2018 Hepatitis B guidance. Clin Liver Dis (Hoboken) 2018;12(1):33–4.
11. World Health Organization. Hepatitis D (fact sheet). 2019. Available at: https://www.who.int/en/news-room/fact-sheets/detail/hepatitis-d. Accessed November 22, 2019.

12. Aragona M, Macagno S, Caredda F, et al. Serological response to the hepatitis delta virus in hepatitis D. Lancet 1987;1(8531):478–80.

13. Wranke A, Heidrich B, Ernst S, et al. Anti-HDV IgM as a marker of disease activity in hepatitis delta. PLoS One 2014;9(7):e101002.

14. Le Gal F, Brichler S, Sahli R, et al. First international external quality assessment for hepatitis delta virus RNA quantification in plasma. Hepatology 2016;64(5): 1483–94.

15. Takyar V, Surana P, Kleiner DE, et al. Noninvasive markers for staging fibrosis in chronic delta hepatitis. Aliment Pharmacol Ther 2017;45(1):127–38.

16. Da BL, Surana P, Takyar V, et al. Vibration-controlled transient elastography for the detection of cirrhosis in chronic Hepatitis D infection. J Viral Hepat 2020; 27(4):428–36.

17. Hughes SA, Wedemeyer H, Harrison PM. Hepatitis delta virus. Lancet 2011; 378(9785):73–85.

18. Wedemeyer H, Yurdaydin C, Dalekos GN, et al. Peginterferon plus adefovir versus either drug alone for hepatitis delta. N Engl J Med 2011;364(4):322–31.

19. Wedemeyer H, Yurdaydin C, Hardtke S, et al. Peginterferon alfa-2a plus tenofovir disoproxil fumarate for hepatitis D (HIDIT-II): a randomised, placebo controlled, phase 2 trial. Lancet Infect Dis 2019;19(3):275–86.

20. European Association for the Study of the Liver. EASL 2017 clinical practice guidelines on the management of hepatitis B virus infection. J Hepatol 2017; 67(2):370–98.

21. Sarin SK, Kumar M, Lau GK, et al. Asian-Pacific clinical practice guidelines on the management of hepatitis B: a 2015 update. Hepatol Int 2016;10(1):1–98.

22. Zachou K, Yurdaydin C, Drebber U, et al. Quantitative HBsAg and HDV-RNA levels in chronic delta hepatitis. Liver Int 2010;30(3):430–7.

23. Heidrich B, Yurdaydin C, Kabaçam G, et al. Late HDV RNA relapse after peginterferon alpha-based therapy of chronic hepatitis delta. Hepatology 2014;60(1): 87–97.

24. Guedj J, Rotman Y, Cotler SJ, et al. Understanding early serum hepatitis D virus and hepatitis B surface antigen kinetics during pegylated interferon-alpha therapy via mathematical modeling. Hepatology 2014;60(6):1902–10.

25. Keskin O, Wedemeyer H, Tüzün A, et al. Association between level of Hepatitis D virus RNA at week 24 of pegylated interferon therapy and outcome. Clin Gastroenterol Hepatol 2015;13(13):2342–9.e1-2.

26. Niro GA, Smedile A, Fontana R, et al. HBsAg kinetics in chronic hepatitis D during interferon therapy: on-treatment prediction of response. Aliment Pharmacol Ther 2016;44(6):620–8.

27. Samuel D, Zignego AL, Reynes M, et al. Long-term clinical and virological outcome after liver transplantation for cirrhosis caused by chronic delta hepatitis. Hepatology 1995;21(2):333–9.

28. Yurdaydin C, Abbas Z, Buti M, et al. Treating chronic hepatitis delta: the need for surrogate markers of treatment efficacy. J Hepatol 2019;70(5):1008–15.

29. Reyes GR, Huang CC, Yarbough PO, et al. Hepatitis E virus. Comparison of 'new and Old World' isolates. J Hepatol 1991;13(Suppl 4):S155–61.

30. Kamar N, Bendall R, Legrand-Abravanel F, et al. Hepatitis E. Lancet 2012; 379(9835):2477–88.

31. Scobie L, Dalton HR. Hepatitis E: source and route of infection, clinical manifestations and new developments. J Viral Hepat 2013;20(1):1–11.

32. Kumar Acharya S, Kumar Sharma P, Singh R, et al. Hepatitis E virus (HEV) infection in patients with cirrhosis is associated with rapid decompensation and death. J Hepatol 2007;46(3):387–94.
33. Navaneethan U, Al Mohajer M, Shata MT. Hepatitis E and pregnancy: understanding the pathogenesis. Liver Int 2008;28(9):1190–9.
34. Sarin SK, Choudhury A, Sharma MK, et al. Acute-on-chronic liver failure: consensus recommendations of the Asian Pacific association for the study of the liver (APASL): an update. Hepatol Int 2019;13(4):353–90.
35. Suneetha PV, Pischke S, Schlaphoff V, et al. Hepatitis E virus (HEV)-specific T-cell responses are associated with control of HEV infection. Hepatology 2012;55(3): 695–708.
36. Kamar N, Garrouste C, Haagsma EB, et al. Factors associated with chronic hepatitis in patients with hepatitis E virus infection who have received solid organ transplants. Gastroenterology 2011;140(5):1481–9.
37. Fernandes B, Dias E, Mascarenhas-Saraiva M, et al. Rheumatologic manifestations of hepatic diseases. Ann Gastroenterol 2019;32(4):352–60.
38. Kamar N, Marion O, Abravanel F, et al. Extrahepatic manifestations of hepatitis E virus. Liver Int 2016;36(4):467–72.
39. Haffar S, Bazerbachi F, Garg S, et al. Frequency and prognosis of acute pancreatitis associated with acute hepatitis E: a systematic review. Pancreatology 2015; 15(4):321–6.
40. Cheung MC, Maguire J, Carey I, et al. Review of the neurological manifestations of hepatitis E infection. Ann Hepatol 2012;11(5):618–22.
41. Kamar N, Weclawiak H, Guilbeau-Frugier C, et al. Hepatitis E virus and the kidney in solid-organ transplant patients. Transplantation 2012;93(6):617–23.
42. Huang S, Zhang X, Jiang H, et al. Profile of acute infectious markers in sporadic hepatitis E. PLoS One 2010;5(10):e13560.
43. Baylis SA, Wallace P, McCulloch E, et al. Standardization of nucleic acid tests: the approach of the World Health Organization. J Clin Microbiol 2019;57(1) [pii: e01056-18].
44. Norder H, Karlsson M, Mellgren Å, et al. Diagnostic performance of five assays for anti-hepatitis E virus IgG and IgM in a large cohort study. J Clin Microbiol 2016;54(3):549–55.
45. Emerson SU, Clemente-Casares P, Moiduddin N, et al. Putative neutralization epitopes and broad cross-genotype neutralization of Hepatitis E virus confirmed by a quantitative cell-culture assay. J Gen Virol 2006;87(Pt 3):697–704.
46. Malcolm P, Dalton H, Hussaini HS, et al. The histology of acute autochthonous hepatitis E virus infection. Histopathology 2007;51(2):190–4.
47. Protzer U, Böhm F, Longerich T, et al. Molecular detection of hepatitis E virus (HEV) in liver biopsies after liver transplantation. Mod Pathol 2015;28(4):523–32.
48. Te H, Doucette K. Viral hepatitis: guidelines by the American society of transplantation infectious disease community of practice. Clin Transplant 2019;33(9): e13514.
49. Unzueta A, Rakela J. Hepatitis E infection in liver transplant recipients. Liver Transpl 2014;20(1):15–24.
50. Behrendt P, Steinmann E, Manns MP, et al. The impact of hepatitis E in the liver transplant setting. J Hepatol 2014;61(6):1418–29.
51. Haagsma EB, Riezebos-Brilman A, van den Berg AP, et al. Treatment of chronic hepatitis E in liver transplant recipients with pegylated interferon alpha-2b. Liver Transpl 2010;16(4):474–7.

52. Kamar N, Izopet J, Tripon S, et al. Ribavirin for chronic hepatitis E virus infection in transplant recipients. N Engl J Med 2014;370(12):1111–20.
53. Li SW, Zhao Q, Wu T, et al. The development of a recombinant hepatitis E vaccine HEV 239. Hum Vaccin Immunother 2015;11(4):908–14.
54. Norvell JP, Blei AT, Jovanovic BD, et al. Herpes simplex virus hepatitis: an analysis of the published literature and institutional cases. Liver Transpl 2007; 13(10):1428–34.
55. Levitsky J, Duddempudi AT, Lakeman FD, et al. Detection and diagnosis of herpes simplex virus infection in adults with acute liver failure. Liver Transpl 2008; 14(10):1498–504.
56. Patti ME, Selvaggi KJ, Kroboth FJ. Varicella hepatitis in the immunocompromised adult: a case report and review of the literature. Am J Med 1990;88(1):77–80.
57. Kusne S, Pappo O, Manez R, et al. Varicella-zoster virus hepatitis and a suggested management plan for prevention of VZV infection in adult liver transplant recipients. Transplantation 1995;60(6):619–21.
58. Danziger-Isakov L, Kumar D, Practice AICo. Vaccination of solid organ transplant candidates and recipients: guidelines from the American society of transplantation infectious diseases community of practice. Clin Transplant 2019;33(9): e13563.
59. Kofteridis DP, Koulentaki M, Valachis A, et al. Epstein Barr virus hepatitis. Eur J Intern Med 2011;22(1):73–6.
60. Mellinger JL, Rossaro L, Naugler WE, et al. Epstein-Barr virus (EBV) related acute liver failure: a case series from the US Acute Liver Failure Study Group. Dig Dis Sci 2014;59(7):1630–7.
61. Babcock GJ, Decker LL, Volk M, et al. EBV persistence in memory B cells in vivo. Immunity 1998;9(3):395–404.
62. Suh N, Liapis H, Misdraji J, et al. Epstein-Barr virus hepatitis: diagnostic value of in situ hybridization, polymerase chain reaction, and immunohistochemistry on liver biopsy from immunocompetent patients. Am J Surg Pathol 2007;31(9): 1403–9.
63. Kremers WK, Devarbhavi HC, Wiesner RH, et al. Post-transplant lymphoproliferative disorders following liver transplantation: incidence, risk factors and survival. Am J Transplant 2006;6(5 Pt 1):1017–24.
64. Allen UD, Preiksaitis JK, Practice AIDCo. Post-transplant lymphoproliferative disorders, epstein-barr virus infection, and disease in solid organ transplantation: guidelines from the American Society of Transplantation Infectious Diseases Community of Practice. Clin Transplant 2019;33(9):e13652.
65. Bate SL, Dollard SC, Cannon MJ. Cytomegalovirus seroprevalence in the United States: the national health and nutrition examination surveys, 1988-2004. Clin Infect Dis 2010;50(11):1439–47.
66. Cohen JI, Corey GR. Cytomegalovirus infection in the normal host. Medicine (Baltimore) 1985;64(2):100–14.
67. Bosch W, Heckman MG, Diehl NN, et al. Association of cytomegalovirus infection and disease with death and graft loss after liver transplant in high-risk recipients. Am J Transplant 2011;11(10):2181–9.
68. Kotton CN, Kumar D, Caliendo AM, et al. The third international consensus guidelines on the management of cytomegalovirus in solid-organ transplantation. Transplantation 2018;102(6):900–31.
69. Abdel Massih RC, Razonable RR. Human herpesvirus 6 infections after liver transplantation. World J Gastroenterol 2009;15(21):2561–9.

70. Pellett Madan R, Hand J, Practice AIDCo. Human herpesvirus 6, 7, and 8 in solid organ transplantation: guidelines from the American society of transplantation infectious diseases community of practice. Clin Transplant 2019;33(9):e13518.

71. Delyon J, Rabate C, Euvrard S, et al. Management of Kaposi sarcoma after solid organ transplantation: a European retrospective study. J Am Acad Dermatol 2019;81(2):448–55.

72. Mrzljak A, Tabain I, Premac H, et al. The role of emerging and neglected viruses in the etiology of hepatitis. Curr Infect Dis Rep 2019;21(12):51.

Cholangiocarcinoma
Diagnosis and Management

Adam P. Buckholz, MD, Robert S. Brown Jr, MD, MPH*

KEYWORDS

- Cholangiocarcinoma • Diagnosis • Management • Transplant • Resection
- Chemotherapy • ERCP

KEY POINTS

- Cholangiocarcinoma is relatively rare but highly lethal so requires a high index of suspicion in order to detect disease at an early stage.
- Diagnosis requires a combination of imaging with magnetic resonance cholangiopancreatography, laboratory testing, and endoscopic retrograde cholangiopancreatography.
- Primary sclerosing cholangitis is a strong risk factor, and patients should be enrolled in surveillance programs with imaging and laboratory testing.
- Surgical resection and transplantation are potentially curative; unfortunately, high recurrence rates persist with 5-year survival rates of 50% to 70%.
- Systemic chemotherapy, locoregional therapy, and radiation provide marginal benefit but should be offered to patients without surgical resection options.

INTRODUCTION

Cholangiocarcinoma (CCA) is a biliary tract epithelial malignancy and the second most common primary hepatic cancer. Defined as a cancer with cholangiocyte origin, CCA is otherwise quite heterogeneous in location, histology, and clinical course, providing diagnostic and management challenges even for experts. Despite recent advances, CCA still has a high mortality with poor prognosis, especially in advanced disease.

In this review, CCA is considered a distinct entity from primary gallbladder or ampulla of Vater cancer. Although the localization can be challenging, CCA is subdivided by anatomic location within the biliary tract. Tumors proximal to the main intrahepatic ducts are termed intrahepatic cholangiocarcinoma (iCCA), extrahepatic tumors (eCCA) proximal to the cystic duct are perihilar cholangiocarcinoma (pCCA),

Division of Gastroenterology and Hepatology, NewYork–Presbyterian/Weill Cornell Medical College, 1305 York Avenue, 4th Floor, New York, NY 10021, USA
* Corresponding author.
E-mail address: rsb2005@med.cornell.edu

Clin Liver Dis 24 (2020) 421–436
https://doi.org/10.1016/j.cld.2020.04.005
1089-3261/20/© 2020 Elsevier Inc. All rights reserved.

liver.theclinics.com

and distal to the cystic duct are distal cholangiocarcinoma (dCCA) (**Fig. 1**).[1] Frequency of occurrence by the various subtypes differs by risk factors. Location impacts surgical options and outcomes and treatment choice in unresectable disease. pCCA is the most common subtype, accounting for approximately 50% to 60% of cases, with dCCA another 25% of cases, and iCCA 20% of cases.[2] CCA can be further subdivided by histologic subtype, but almost all are sclerosing-type carcinomas.[2]

The incidence of iCCA appears to be increasing, whereas that of eCCA is decreasing.[3] Some of this is likely due to improved diagnostic techniques and more accurate classification; for example, 1 study found that many hepatic lesions previously described as Cancer of Unknown Primary were likely in fact CCA.[4] However, increased burden of chronic viral hepatitis and nonalcoholic fatty liver disease likely accounts for some of the documented increase in iCCA.[5] There are several known risk factors helpful to understand when considering a diagnosis of CCA. Some of these risk factors are unlikely to be encountered in a western setting, such as the endemic liver fluke of Northern Thailand, which increases risk by up to 100-fold,[6] or the inherited choledochal cystic Caroli disease (lifetime CCA risk 10%–30%).[7] More common risk factors with lower disease hazard include obesity, viral hepatitis, and cholelithiasis, especially for iCCA. Likewise, advanced liver disease and cirrhosis appear to be independent risk factors.[8] Alcohol appears to have a moderate (odds ratio 2.4)[9] increase in risk of CCA, whereas the contribution of tobacco use is controversial. Primary sclerosing cholangitis (PSC) is a well-established risk factor and is discussed further elsewhere.

DIAGNOSIS

There are 3 distinct but interrelated circumstances that should prompt consideration for CCA: a patient with asymptomatic cholestatic elevation of liver enzymes, a patient with symptoms or imaging findings concerning for hepatobiliary malignancy (**Fig. 2**), or a patient with known ulcerative colitis (UC) or PSC (**Fig. 3**).

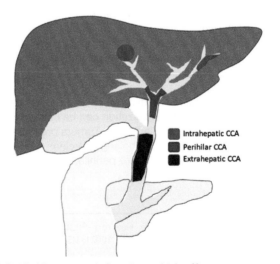

Intrahepatic CCA
Perihilar CCA
Extrahepatic CCA

Fig. 1. CCA is subdivided by anatomic location, which affects management and prognosis. dCCA is distal to the cystic duct, pCCA is from proximal to the cystic duct to the hilum and main hepatic ducts, whereas CCA involving the small proximal ducts within the liver is intrahepatic.

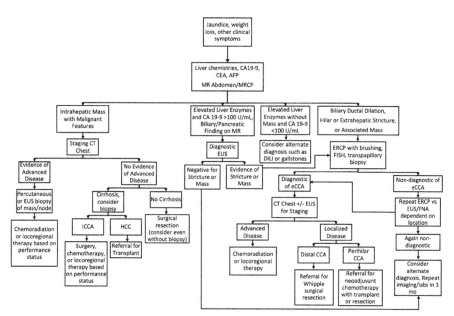

Fig. 2. Diagnosis and management of suspected CCA in patients without PSC. AFP, alpha feto protein; DILI, drug induced liver injury.

Elevated Liver Panel

The typical laboratory pattern for CCA is a cholestatic liver injury, with alkaline phosphatase greater than twice normal with elevated gamma-glutamyl transferase and often bilirubin. Persistent biliary obstruction from tumor or iCCA can also result in elevated transaminases and prolongation of the international normalized ratio. Unfortunately, none of these tests have high specificity for CCA, and the differential diagnosis for this laboratory pattern is broad (**Table 1**). CCA incidence increases with age, most commonly presenting between 50 and 70; there is a slight male predominance, and people of Asian descent are at higher risk.[10] Although rare, its lethality demands a high level of suspicion.

Patients should be questioned for a history of gallstone disease, inflammatory bowel disease, or hepatitis. Substance abuse, travel, and family histories (for example, Lynch syndrome) should be taken. Symptoms such as weight loss, malaise, dark urine, clay-colored stools, or pruritis are nonspecific but suggest biliary obstruction with possible associated malignancy. Nonetheless, CCA is often clinically silent until an advanced stage, and cholangitis is a rare presentation.[11] Laboratory analyses should include Carbohydrate antigen 19-9 (CA 19-9), a tumor antigen with sensitivity for CCA of 50% to 70% at levels greater than 100 U/mL.[12] Its utility is limited due to false positives in the setting of cholangitis or other benign biliary disease. Likewise, 7% to 10% of patients do not express Lewis antigen and will not have an elevated CA 19-9. Other markers such as carcinoembryonic antigen (CEA), matrix metalloproteinase-7, and cytokeratin-19 fragment have been shown to be elevated in CCA[13] but suffer from a combination of low sensitivity, specificity, or availability in clinical practice. Some data suggest that combining all 4 markers could provide sensitivity and specificity greater than 90%,[14] but this is not guideline based and does not obviate eventual invasive testing. Immunoglobulin G4 elevations could suggest autoimmune

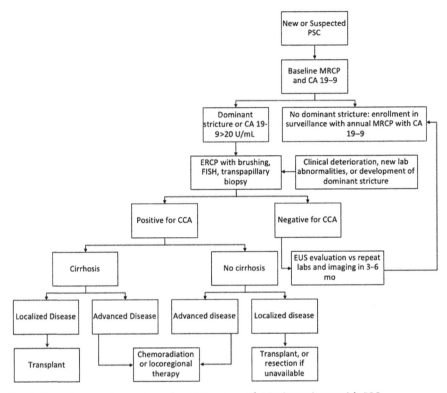

Fig. 3. Surveillance, diagnosis, and management of CCA in patients with PSC.

cholangiopathy, but is likewise nonspecific as elevations have been seen in CCA.[15] For this reason, unexplained elevation in liver enzymes should prompt further evaluation with imaging.

In the patient presenting with symptoms or cholestatic liver enzyme elevation, the best test is a magnetic resonance/magnetic resonance cholangiopancreatography (MR/MRCP), which offers sensitivity of 88% and specificity of 75% to 85%. Addition of contrast increases sensitivity by 10%, so a contrast-enhanced study should be

Table 1
Differential diagnosis for common presenting symptoms and findings in cholangiocarcinoma

Cholestatic Liver Enzyme Elevation	Biliary Dilation or Stricture	Intrahepatic Mass
• Gallstone disease	• Choledocholithiasis	• HCC
• Non-CCA malignant obstruction	• PSC	• Hepatic adenoma
• Drug-induced liver injury	• Ampulla of Vater carcinoma	• Focal nodular hyperplasia
• Primary biliary cholangitis	• Pancreatic cancer	• Hepatic hemangioma
• PSC	• Secondary sclerosing cholangitis	• Metastatic disease
• AIDS cholangiopathy	• Extrinsic gallstone compression (Mirizzi syndrome)	
• Cholestasis of pregnancy		
• Cholangitis		
• Autoimmune cholangiopathy		

performed in the absence of contraindications, such as renal failure or allergy.[16] Patients with renal failure should have a noncontrast MRCP rather than ultrasound. Findings of a mass, ductal dilation, stricture, contrast enhancement, and ductal wall thickening or irregularity should prompt invasive evaluation and tissue sampling.

Patients with Abnormal Liver Imaging

All patients who present with a biliary dilatation or a mass on imaging concerning for CCA should have an MRCP, ideally with contrast, as well as the laboratory workup above if not already performed. In a patient presenting with an intrahepatic mass, care must be taken to differentiate iCCA from other causes (see **Table 1**). Contrast-enhanced imaging characteristics help with this differentiation. Unlike the washout seen with hepatocellular carcinoma (HCC), iCCA tends to have progressive uptake in both the arterial and the venous contrast phases[17]; however, the classic heterogeneous uptake was only seen 70% of the time in 1 series,[18] and mixed tumors with both HCC and CCA can occur. MR can occasionally help with differentiation, but is not always definitive. Despite best efforts, CCA, especially intrahepatic, can still be mistaken for HCC, with 1 study reporting 1.5% of explants for presumed HCC actually representing early CCA.[19] Tumors less than 2 cm are less likely to have classic washout appearance to help delineate iCCA from HCC.[20] Any imaging assessment of an intrahepatic lesion concerning for iCCA should include a computed tomographic (CT) scan of the chest to assess for metastatic disease. The role of PET-CT is likely confined to metastatic disease.[21] If there is no evidence of distant metastasis and the lesion is concerning for iCCA, referral for surgical resection without biopsy is appropriate. In cirrhosis, a biopsy with endoscopic ultrasound (EUS) or percutaneously may be necessary for determination of transplant candidacy, despite a known risk of needle tract seeding. All patients with imaging findings concerning for iCCA should be referred early to a multidisciplinary team at a specialized center.

Perihilar or Extrahepatic Mass

Perihilar tumors less commonly present as a defined mass and more often appear nodular or infiltrating on cross-sectional imaging. CT is fairly accurate for detection of portal vein (sensitivity and specificity 89% and 92%) and hepatic artery (83% and 93%) involvement, whereas less accurate for lymph node detection (61% and 88%).[22] Still, MR/MRCP has become an essential and preferred evaluation tool for pCCA because of its ability to better characterize the biliary tree and extent of intrabiliary lesion.[16] Further anatomic subdivision of pCCA is by the Bismuth-Corlette classification.

In patients with imaging or symptoms concerning for pCCA, endoscopic retrograde cholangiopancreatography (ERCP) has become the test of choice for obtaining a tissue diagnosis. Multiple studies have shown low yield to cytology brushings alone.[23] Fluorescence in situ hybridization (FISH) increases the diagnostic yield of brushings[24] to approximately 35% or better.[25] Transpapillary biopsy in combination with FISH and brushing increases overall sensitivity to 82%,[26] whereas a recent study suggested improved diagnostic yield for combining FISH with single-operator cholangiography from 64.5% to 71.5% over transpapillary biopsy.[27] Intraductal ultrasound can be used as an adjunct for visual confirmation of difficult-to-characterize lesions. In expert hands, sensitivity has reached 93%, although its inability to collect tissue for cytology or detect regional adenopathy limits practical use.[28]

The use of EUS before or at the time of ERCP is somewhat controversial. Noninvasive EUS is likely helpful and has high sensitivity (90%–100%) for detecting an extrahepatic lesion, with increasing sensitivity in more distal tumors.[29] In addition, it likely has a role in determining resectability of a tumor; in 1 series, EUS had 53% sensitivity and 97% specificity for unresectability[29] in part due to its excellent performance at identifying and sampling regional lymph nodes.[30] Fine needle aspiration (FNA) of the primary tumor also increases diagnostic yield. A recent metaanalysis including 294 patients with concern for malignant stricture noted improved diagnostic sensitivity of EUS-FNA over ERCP with transpapillary biopsy (75 vs 49%), albeit both had low negative predictive values.[31] EUS-FNA should be used in patients with an indeterminate initial ERCP; sensitivity in this setting ranges from 43% to 86%.[32] In 1 study, following an indeterminate ERCP with transpapillary biopsy with stepwise repeat, ERCP for intrinsic lesions or EUS-FNA for extrinsic lesions increased overall diagnostic yield to greater than 96%.[32] EUS-FNA does, however, raise concern for tumor seeding and should be avoided in patients who are possible transplant candidates. This concern is primarily in pCCA rather than dCCA, because the duodenal bulb is part of the surgical resection in the latter case. Although some studies have suggested that seeding is probably a clinically rare event,[33] it remains a contraindication for transplant at some centers, most notably the Mayo Clinic.[34] Overall strategy depends on tumor location, characteristics, and center expertise.

Patients with Primary Sclerosing Cholangitis

PSC is a chronic, inflammatory cholangiopathy characterized by progressive cholestasis, fibrosis, and stricturing.[35] It is strongly associated with inflammatory bowel disease, especially UC. Patients with PSC are twice as likely to develop cancer as the general population, and PSC is a known risk factor for multiple cancers, including CCA, colorectal, primary gallbladder, and HCC.[36] Unfortunately, it remains unclear which patients with UC will develop PSC and which of those will develop CCA.[37,38]

When referred a patient to rule out PSC or with a diagnosis of PSC, the clinician must have an immediate concern about the implications of CCA. Burden of CCA in this population is up to 1500 times the general population,[39] and despite this knowledge, most CCA is unresectable at diagnosis.[1] CCA is the largest cause of mortality in patients with PSC,[36] and the lifetime risk is approximately 10% to 15%, with annual incidence approximately 1%.[40] Early studies noted that approximately 50% of CCA is diagnosed within a year of PSC diagnosis,[41] and recent work suggests that the risk persists and is increased with longer disease course.[42] The fact that patients with PSC are often diagnosed with CCA early in their course suggests that many patients are diagnosed with PSC only after development of a dominant, malignant, stricture.

In newly diagnosed or suspected PSC, imaging with MRCP and laboratory testing including liver chemistries and a CA 19-9 are appropriate initial steps. These tests serve the dual purpose of identifying any possible malignant stricture and serving as a baseline in the case of laboratory, symptom, or imaging changes in the future. Most patients with PSC will at 1 time have a dominant stricture; although only about 25% of these will prove malignant,[43] ERCP with brushing/biopsy as discussed above is generally recommended to rule out CCA.

Definitive surveillance guidelines for this population have proven elusive.[39] As previously reported, the 1% annual incidence of CCA in PSC is roughly the same as HCC in cirrhosis, which could serve to justify a surveillance program.[44] At the moment, expert consensus supports annual or semiannual CA 19-9 with either abdominal ultrasound or preferably MRCP.[45] Because of the high rate of elevated CA 19-9 in benign PSC as well as elevation in other diseases, such as cholangitis,[46] care must be taken not to rely solely on laboratory data. A new dominant stricture or CA 19-9 greater than 20 U/mL should prompt ERCP with brush cytology, FISH, and biopsy. In patients with PSC, FISH has a high false positive rate[47] but still provides useful diagnostic information. A recent study of surveillance for all hepatobiliary cancer in PSC found that patients enrolled in surveillance programs had lower all-cause mortality and that CCA was diagnosed with smaller lesions and less nodal involvement; surveilled patients received more liver transplants (LT) and had higher survival even in the absence of transplantation.[48] Despite this, the most recent consensus guidelines out of the United Kingdom fail to recommend routine surveillance.[49]

No medication or supplement, including ursodeoxycholic acid[50] or curcumin,[51] has been consistently shown to decrease risk of CCA. Patients are likely to ask about such options, but at this time the evidence is insufficient to advise their use. With curcumin, promising in vitro data suggested possible antitumorigenicity, but a resultant small clinical trial failed to show any change in cholestatic markers.[52] Smoking and alcohol avoidance is recommended, even in the absence of cirrhosis.

MANAGEMENT OPTIONS

The primary management strategies for CCA include surgical resection, LT, systemic chemotherapy, and locoregional therapy. Multidisciplinary expert involvement is critical to quickly identify those patients for whom potentially curative resection or transplant is available.

Surgical Resection

Surgery is the only potentially curative management of CCA. Typically, resection is reserved for patients without retroperitoneal or periceliac node involvement, no main portal vein or hepatic artery invasion, no invasion of adjacent organs, and no distant metastasis. There are other individualized factors that can limit resection candidacy beyond the scope of this review. Only approximately half of patients with iCCA present with tumors that are considered candidates for resection, and recurrence rates are high with 5-year survival ranging from 40% to 60% even with R0 resection.[53] Likewise, metastatic disease not seen on imaging can be discovered during attempted surgical resection. Some experts recommend preresection diagnostic laparoscopy,[54] but this is controversial. Portal lymphadenectomy may be needed for some patients. Vascular involvement, large tumor size, lymphadenopathy, and positive resection margin are among the factors predicting recurrence.[55] Surgery for more distal tumors is likewise complex. Whipple procedures are generally performed for dCCA; even with R0 resection (negative microscopic margins), 5-year survival is approximately 27%.[56] Surgical options for pCCA are related to Bismuth classification, but often involve lobectomy, bile duct resection, lymphadenectomy,[57] and hepaticojejunostomy.[58] Overall, recurrence rates (70%–80%) and 5-year survival (30%–50%)[59] have improved for resection of pCCA likely because of improved patient selection[60] and improved surgical technique.[61] Those treated with neoadjuvant therapy who become surgically resectable likely have similar outcomes to those with primary resectable disease.[62]

Because of the high recurrence rates, adjuvant chemoradiotherapy is often used. Previous retrospective or nonrandomized studies demonstrated mixed results with a possible trend toward survival benefit especially in those with R1 or lymph node–positive resection.[63] Randomized phase 3 data from the PROTIGE[64] and BILCAP[65] trials have conflicting results, exacerbated by heterogeneous study populations. PROTIGE randomized 196 patients with biliary cancer (including primary gallbladder) and R0 or R1 resections to receiving gemcitabine and oxaliplatin; there was no difference in relapse-free survival or mortality with a median follow-up of 46.5 months, including in subgroup analysis of iCCA and eCCA. In BILCAP, 447 patients were randomized to postoperative capecitabine or observation with median follow-up of 51 months. There was no overall survival (OS) improvement by the intention-to-treat analysis, but sensitivity and per-protocol analyses suggested a benefit. Even though both BILCAP and PROTIGE were technically negative studies, their trends toward significance may lead to increased usage of adjuvant capecitabine or gemcitabine.

Liver Transplantation

CCA was long considered a contraindication to transplantation (LT), but has been reevaluated as an option in selected patients with pCCA because of high recurrence and mortality rates after surgical resection. In an early study evaluating surgical options for CCA, LT was associated with the lowest rate of recurrence, albeit with high overall rates in part because of the high number of stage IV patients included.[58] However, in the absence of posttransplant adjuvant therapy such as radiation, recurrence rates are untenable for both pCCA[66] and iCCA[67]; 1 study reported recurrence of approximately 50% within 1 year.[68] For context, in HCC within Milan criteria, 1-year recurrence-free survival for LT surpasses 80%.[69] Fortunately, the addition of neoadjuvant chemoradiation for patients with unresectable pCCA has allowed transplantation to become a viable option again,[70] with 5-year recurrence-free survival of 65%.[71] In response, the Mayo Clinic Protocol for patient selection and neoadjuvant chemoradiation therapy has been adopted by the United Network of Organ Sharing and allows allocation of transplant exception points for pCCA similar to that of HCC after review by the National Liver Review Board.[72] To date, no randomized controlled trial has evaluated transplantation versus resection for pCCA. Similar rates of success for LT in iCCA have been difficult to achieve; guidelines recommend against LT in this population.[5] Recent data, largely from explants with unintentionally discovered iCCA, have renewed interest in LT for early iCCA,[73] but overall recurrence rates remain higher even for pathologically early iCCA.[19] A prospective trial is currently underway (NCT02878473).[74]

In PSC, CCA is often detected at a more advanced stage and with more underlying liver disease, complicating surgical management. Diffuse, difficult-to-discern disease could make a resection specimen clear of disease, while dysplasia persists elsewhere.[75] Randomized data are lacking, but several small studies have evaluated orthotopic liver transplantation for dysplasia or CCA in PSC, sometimes with the addition of radiotherapy[76] or chemotherapy.[77] In addition, coincident Whipple procedure is often performed.

Treatment of Locally Advanced or Unresectable Disease

In patients without surgically resectable disease, palliative chemotherapy or locoregional therapy can be offered. Since the ABC-02 trial, the mainstay of therapy has been gemcitabine in combination with cisplatin, offering a mean OS of 11.7 months compared with 8 months with gemcitabine alone.[78] Almost all patients eventually fail this therapy, and no standard second-line regimen exists. Second-line therapies with gemcitabine or combining 5-fluorouracil with either oxaliplatin or irinotecan have shown additional OS of approximately 13 months in retrospective studies.[79,80] A recent randomized study of supportive care or 5-fluorouracil plus oxaliplatin for any advanced biliary cancer demonstrated improved (25.9 vs 11.4%) 12-month OS with chemotherapy.[81] Tyrosine kinase inhibitors against vascular endothelial growth factor-2 have shown disappointing results in small studies.[82] Some patients will require ERCP with stenting to normalize serum bilirubin before chemotherapy.

Most mortality in CCA is due to local progression and obstruction rather than distant metastasis,[83] so patients without resection options should be considered for locoregional disease control.

Palliative stenting improves biliary drainage and quality of life at the expense of increased cholangitis occurrence; endoscopically placed self-expanding metal stents are generally thought to be superior to plastic stents or percutaneous stents for this purpose.[84,85] Endoscopic radiofrequency ablation[86] in combination with stenting may improve survival in pCCA and eCCA and likely improves stent patency.[87] Similarly, photodynamic therapy[88] may reduce stent blockage and has some mortality benefit. Lack of head-to-head comparison with other methodologies or high-quality studies precludes these therapies being guideline based; an individualized approach is needed with pCCA and dCCA, and they are not effective for iCCA.[89]

Vascular therapies, including transarterial chemoembolization (TACE), hepatic artery infusion (HAI) of chemotherapy, and yttrium-90 (^{90}Y) radioembolization, have been used for disease control and occasional conversion to resectability, especially for iCCA. Of these, the most evidence exists for ^{90}Y therapy, which uses catheter-delivered radiolabeled microspheres.[90] Response rates in iCCA vary from 5% to 36% with median survival increases of approximately 9 to 22 months.[91] Small studies have suggested prolonged benefit when combined with systemic chemotherapy.[92] Recently, a French multicenter single-arm prospective study (MISPHEC)[93] treated 41 patients with locally advanced disease with cisplatin, gemcitabine, and ^{90}Y. They noted a 39% response rate, with 20% of enrolled patients able to subsequently undergo R0 resection and progression-free survival (PFS) of 14 months. Given the efficacy and relatively minimal toxicity of ^{90}Y, it is considered second-line therapy by some experts.[57] Potential hepatotoxicity means it is currently not recommended for patients with cirrhosis. Randomized trial data comparing TACE, HAI, and ^{90}Y are lacking but potentially forthcoming.[94]

Radiation therapy with external beam radiation or stereotactic body radiotherapy (SBRT) is often offered for unresectable tumors. Survival data are mixed, but it appears that there is some benefit to high-dose radiotherapy.[95] SBRT may offer similar marginal disease control, with 1 study finding a PFS of 10 months among patients with either iCCA or pCCA.[96] A recent systematic review noted that although most studies of SBRT are not robust, efficacy appears to approach that of chemotherapy alone for survival and disease control.[97]

The recent proliferation of tumor genomic testing and new technologies, such as immunotherapy, likely will impact management of unresectable disease in the coming years. The heterogeneity of CCA makes standardization difficult, but some tumors demonstrate programmed cell death protein-1 ligand and mismatch repair protein deficiency, representing possible targets for immunotherapy.[98] Early phase studies of immunotherapy in unresectable patients have shown some promise,[99] and multiple clinical trials are currently enrolling.[100] It is reasonable to consider tumor genomics and enrollment in clinical trials for patients with advanced CCA and good performance status.

SUMMARY

CCA is a heterogeneous and highly lethal cancer that lacks reliable disease markers and often presents with symptoms late in its course and in an unresectable state. Patients with known PSC should be enrolled in a surveillance program early in their course. In any patient with symptoms or biochemical evidence of cholestasis, laboratory testing with CA 19-9 and imaging with abdominal ultrasound or preferably MRCP should be performed. CT exposes patients to radiation without added diagnostic efficacy, whereas CEA and other tumor markers can be collected but with probable minimal clinical benefit. Imaging is especially crucial to delineate between other causes of cholestasis or obstruction, localizing CCA as intrahepatic, perihilar, or distal, and guiding management.

A suspicious lesion on MR generally demands invasive testing for tissue confirmation. A possible exception would be a patient with cirrhosis whom is a transplant candidate. ERCP with brush cytology, FISH, and transpapillary biopsy is generally preferred for tissue acquisition. EUS is useful for more distal tumors, lymph node evaluation or sampling, and in the setting of a negative ERCP. Other tools, such as intraductal ultrasound, cholangioscopy, or percutaneous biopsy, have utility in specific settings.

Most important in the diagnosis and staging of CCA is deciding on resection and transplant candidacy, because these are the only potentially curative therapies. Patients with advanced liver disease are not candidates for resection. Transplantation is available for select patients with local perihilar disease undergoing neoadjuvant chemoradiation per the Mayo Clinic Protocol and offers acceptable cure rates. Without resectable disease, prognosis is generally dismal. For patients with good performance status, systemic chemotherapy with gemcitabine/cisplatin and locoregional therapy provides some survival benefit and occasionally can shrink tumors enough to offer surgical resection. The choice of locoregional therapy depends on patient characteristics, presence of distant metastases, location of CCA, and center expertise. For patients with poor performance status, palliative stenting is a viable option to provide some symptom control.

Further advances in this field are necessary. Ongoing topics of research include noninvasive markers of disease, head-to-head comparison of adjuvant therapies, better delineation of appropriate transplant candidates, targeted systemic therapy such as immunotherapy, and improved surveillance methods for patients with PSC.

DISCLOSURE

Dr A.P. Buckholz and Dr R.S. Brown have nothing to disclose.

REFERENCES

1. Rizvi S, Gores GJ. Pathogenesis, diagnosis, and management of cholangiocarcinoma. Gastroenterology 2013. https://doi.org/10.1053/j.gastro.2013.10.013.
2. Nakeeb A, Pitt HA, Sohn TA, et al. Cholangiocarcinoma: a spectrum of intrahepatic, perihilar, and distal tumors. Ann Surg 1996. https://doi.org/10.1097/00000658-199610000-00005.
3. Everhart JE, Ruhl CE. Burden of digestive diseases in the United States part III: liver, biliary tract, and pancreas. Gastroenterology 2009. https://doi.org/10.1053/j.gastro.2009.02.038.
4. Glitza IC, Varadhachary GR. Carcinoma of Unknown primary (CUP). In: Cancer Consult: expertise for clinical practice. 2014. https://doi.org/10.1002/9781118589199.ch127.
5. Bridgewater J, Galle PR, Khan SA, et al. Guidelines for the diagnosis and management of intrahepatic cholangiocarcinoma. J Hepatol 2014. https://doi.org/10.1016/j.jhep.2014.01.021.
6. Sripa B, Pairojkul C. Cholangiocarcinoma: lessons from Thailand. Curr Opin Gastroenterol 2008. https://doi.org/10.1097/MOG.0b013e3282fbf9b3.

7. Söreide K, Körner H, Havnen J, et al. Bile duct cysts in adults. Br J Surg 2004. https://doi.org/10.1002/bjs.4815.

8. Tyson GL, El-Serag HB. Risk factors for cholangiocarcinoma. Hepatology 2011. https://doi.org/10.1002/hep.24351.

9. Palmer WC, Patel T. Are common factors involved in the pathogenesis of primary liver cancers? A meta-analysis of risk factors for intrahepatic cholangiocarcinoma. J Hepatol 2012. https://doi.org/10.1016/j.jhep.2012.02.022.

10. Shaib Y, El-Serag H. The epidemiology of cholangiocarcinoma. Semin Liver Dis 2004;24(02):115–25.

11. Rassi ZE, Partensky C, Scoazec JY, et al. Peripheral cholangiocarcinoma: presentation, diagnosis, pathology and management. Eur J Surg Oncol 1999;25(4): 375–80.

12. Patel AH, Harnois DM, Klee GG, et al. The utility of CA 19-9 in the diagnoses of cholangiocarcinoma in patients without primary sclerosing cholangitis. Am J Gastroenterol 2000. https://doi.org/10.1016/S0002-9270(99)00744-3.

13. Grunnet M, Mau-Sørensen M. Serum tumor markers in bile duct cancer–a review. Biomarkers 2014;19(6):437–43.

14. Lumachi F, Lo Re G, Tozzoli R, et al. Measurement of serum carcinoembryonic antigen, carbohydrate antigen 19-9, cytokeratin-19 fragment and matrix metalloproteinase-7 for detecting cholangiocarcinoma: a preliminary case-control study. Anticancer Res 2014;34(11):6663–7. Available at: http://www.ncbi.nlm.nih.gov/pubmed/25368272. Accessed November 17, 2019.

15. Oseini AM, Chaiteerakij R, Shire AM, et al. Utility of serum immunoglobulin G4 in distinguishing immunoglobulin G4-associated cholangitis from cholangiocarcinoma. Hepatology 2011;54(3):940–8.

16. Charatcharoenwitthaya P, Enders FB, Halling KC, et al. Utility of serum tumor markers, imaging, and biliary cytology for detecting cholangiocarcinoma in primary sclerosing cholangitis. Hepatology 2008. https://doi.org/10.1002/hep.22441.

17. Iavarone M, Piscaglia F, Vavassori S, et al. Contrast enhanced CT-scan to diagnose intrahepatic cholangiocarcinoma in patients with cirrhosis. J Hepatol 2013. https://doi.org/10.1016/j.jhep.2013.02.013.

18. Kim SH, Lee CH, Kim BH, et al. Typical and atypical imaging findings of intrahepatic cholangiocarcinoma using gadolinium ethoxybenzyl diethylenetriamine pentaacetic acid-enhanced magnetic resonance imaging. J Comput Assist Tomogr 2012. https://doi.org/10.1097/RCT.0b013e3182706562.

19. Lee DD, Croome KP, Musto KR, et al. Liver transplantation for intrahepatic cholangiocarcinoma. Liver Transpl 2018. https://doi.org/10.1002/lt.25052.

20. Huang B, Wu L, Lu XY, et al. Small intrahepatic cholangiocarcinoma and hepatocellular carcinoma in cirrhotic livers may share similar enhancement patterns at multiphase dynamic MR imaging. Radiology 2016. https://doi.org/10.1148/radiol.2016151205.

21. Anderson CD, Rice MH, Pinson CW, et al. Fluorodeoxyglucose PET imaging in the evaluation of gallbladder carcinoma and cholangiocarcinoma. J Gastrointest Surg 2004. https://doi.org/10.1016/j.gassur.2003.10.003.

22. Ruys AT, Van Beem BE, Engelbrecht MRW, et al. Radiological staging in patients with hilar cholangiocarcinoma: a systematic review and meta-analysis. Br J Radiol 2012. https://doi.org/10.1259/bjr/88405305.

23. Korc P, Sherman S. ERCP tissue sampling. Gastrointest Endosc 2016. https://doi.org/10.1016/j.gie.2016.04.039.

24. Kipp BR, Stadheim LM, Halling SA, et al. A comparison of routine cytology and fluorescence in situ hybridization for the detection of malignant bile duct strictures. Am J Gastroenterol 2004. https://doi.org/10.1111/j.1572-0241.2004.30281.x.

25. Smoczynski M, Jablonska A, Matyskiel A, et al. Routine brush cytology and fluorescence in situ hybridization for assessment of pancreatobiliary strictures. Gastrointest Endosc 2012. https://doi.org/10.1016/j.gie.2011.08.040.

26. Nanda A, Brown JM, Berger SH, et al. Triple modality testing by endoscopic retrograde cholangiopancreatography for the diagnosis of cholangiocarcinoma. Therap Adv Gastroenterol 2015. https://doi.org/10.1177/1756283X14564674.

27. Kaura K, Sawas T, Bazerbachi F, et al. Cholangioscopy biopsies improve detection of cholangiocarcinoma when combined with cytology and FISH, but not in patients with PSC. Dig Dis Sci 2019. https://doi.org/10.1007/s10620-019-05866-2.

28. Meister T, Heinzow HS, Woestmeyer C, et al. Intraductal ultrasound substantiates diagnostics of bile duct strictures of uncertain etiology. World J Gastroenterol 2013. https://doi.org/10.3748/wjg.v19.i6.874.

29. Mohamadnejad M, Dewitt JM, Sherman S, et al. Role of EUS for preoperative evaluation of cholangiocarcinoma: a large single-center experience. Gastrointest Endosc 2011. https://doi.org/10.1016/j.gie.2010.08.050.

30. Gleeson FC, Rajan E, Levy MJ, et al. EUS-guided FNA of regional lymph nodes in patients with unresectable hilar cholangiocarcinoma. Gastrointest Endosc 2008. https://doi.org/10.1016/j.gie.2007.07.018.

31. De Moura DTH, De Moura EGH, Bernardo WM, et al. Endoscopic retrograde cholangiopancreatography versus endoscopic ultrasound for tissue diagnosis of malignant biliary stricture: systematic review and meta-analysis. Endosc Ultrasound 2018. https://doi.org/10.4103/2303-9027.193597.

32. Lee YN, Moon JH, Choi HJ, et al. Diagnostic approach using ERCP-guided transpapillary forceps biopsy or EUS-guided fine-needle aspiration biopsy according to the nature of stricture segment for patients with suspected malignant biliary stricture. Cancer Med 2017. https://doi.org/10.1002/cam4.1034.

33. Chafic AH El, Dewitt J, LeBlanc JK, et al. Impact of preoperative endoscopic ultrasound-guided fine needle aspiration on postoperative recurrence and survival in cholangiocarcinoma patients. Endoscopy 2013. https://doi.org/10.1055/s-0033-1344760.

34. Levy MJ, Heimbach JK, Gores GJ. Endoscopic ultrasound staging of cholangiocarcinoma. Curr Opin Gastroenterol 2012. https://doi.org/10.1097/MOG.0b013e32835005bc.

35. Lazaridis KN, Strazzabosco M, Larusso NF. The cholangiopathies: disorders of biliary epithelia. Gastroenterology 2004. https://doi.org/10.1053/j.gastro.2004.08.006.

36. Boonstra K, Weersma RK, van Erpecum KJ, et al. Population-based epidemiology, malignancy risk, and outcome of primary sclerosing cholangitis. Hepatology 2013. https://doi.org/10.1002/hep.26565.

37. Wiesner RH, Grambsch PM, Dickson ER, et al. Primary sclerosing cholangitis: natural history, prognostic factors and survival analysis. Hepatology 1989. https://doi.org/10.1002/hep.1840100406.

38. Takakura WR, Tabibian JH, Bowlus CL. The evolution of natural history of primary sclerosing cholangitis. Curr Opin Gastroenterol 2017. https://doi.org/10.1097/MOG.0000000000000341.

39. Burak K, Angulo P, Pasha TM, et al. Incidence and risk factors for cholangiocarcinoma in primary sclerosing cholangitis. Am J Gastroenterol 2004. https://doi.org/10.1111/j.1572-0241.2004.04067.x.

40. Claessen MMH, Vleggaar FP, Tytgat KMAJ, et al. High lifetime risk of cancer in primary sclerosing cholangitis. J Hepatol 2009. https://doi.org/10.1016/j.jhep.2008.08.013.

41. Fevery J, Verslype C, Lai G, et al. Incidence, diagnosis, and therapy of cholangiocarcinoma in patients with primary sclerosing cholangitis. Dig Dis Sci 2007. https://doi.org/10.1007/s10620-006-9681-4.

42. Gulamhusein AF, Eaton JE, Tabibian JH, et al. Duration of inflammatory bowel disease is associated with increased risk of cholangiocarcinoma in patients with primary sclerosing cholangitis and IBD. Am J Gastroenterol 2016. https://doi.org/10.1038/ajg.2016.55.

43. Chapman MH, Webster GJM, Bannoo S, et al. Cholangiocarcinoma and dominant strictures in patients with primary sclerosing cholangitis: a 25-year single-centre experience. Eur J Gastroenterol Hepatol 2012. https://doi.org/10.1097/MEG.0b013e3283554bbf.

44. Razumilava N, Gores GJ. Surveillance for cholangiocarcinoma in patients with primary sclerosing cholangitis: effective and justified? Clin Liver Dis 2016. https://doi.org/10.1002/cld.567.

45. Razumilava N, Gores GJ, Lindor KD. Cancer surveillance in patients with primary sclerosing cholangitis. Hepatology 2011. https://doi.org/10.1002/hep.24570.

46. Wannhoff A, Gotthardt DN. Recent developments in the research on biomarkers of cholangiocarcinoma in primary sclerosing cholangitis. Clin Res Hepatol Gastroenterol 2019;43(3):236–43.

47. Bangarulingam SY, Bjornsson E, Enders F, et al. Long-term outcomes of positive fluorescence in situ hybridization tests in primary sclerosing cholangitis. Hepatology 2010. https://doi.org/10.1002/hep.23277.

48. Ali AH, Tabibian JH, Nasser-Ghodsi N, et al. Surveillance for hepatobiliary cancers in patients with primary sclerosing cholangitis. Hepatology 2018. https://doi.org/10.1002/hep.29730.

49. Chapman MH, Thorburn D, Hirschfield GM, et al. British Society of Gastroenterology and UK-PSC guidelines for the diagnosis and management of primary sclerosing cholangitis. Gut 2019;68(8):1356–78.

50. Eaton JE, Silveira MG, Pardi DS, et al. High-dose ursodeoxycholic acid is associated with the development of colorectal neoplasia in patients with ulcerative colitis and primary sclerosing cholangitis. Am J Gastroenterol 2011. https://doi.org/10.1038/ajg.2011.156.

51. Hu RW, Carey EJ, Lindor KD, et al. Curcumin in hepatobiliary disease: pharmacotherapeutic properties and emerging potential clinical applications. Ann Hepatol 2017. https://doi.org/10.5604/01.3001.0010.5273.

52. Eaton JE, Nelson KM, Gossard AA, et al. Efficacy and safety of curcumin in primary sclerosing cholangitis: an open label pilot study. Scand J Gastroenterol 2019. https://doi.org/10.1080/00365521.2019.1611917.

53. Choi S-B, Kim K-S, Choi J-Y, et al. The prognosis and survival outcome of intrahepatic cholangiocarcinoma following surgical resection: association of lymph node metastasis and lymph node dissection with survival. Ann Surg Oncol 2009;16(11):3048–56.

54. Weber SM, Jarnagin WR, Klimstra D, et al. Intrahepatic cholangiocarcinoma: resectability, recurrence pattern, and outcomes. J Am Coll Surg 2001;193(4): 384–91.

55. Mavros MN, Economopoulos KP, Alexiou VG, et al. Treatment and prognosis for patients with intrahepatic cholangiocarcinoma. JAMA Surg 2014;149(6):565.

56. DeOliveira ML, Cunningham SC, Cameron JL, et al. Cholangiocarcinoma: thirty-one-year experience with 564 patients at a single institution. Ann Surg 2007. https://doi.org/10.1097/01.sla.0000251366.62632.d3.

57. Valle JW, Borbath I, Khan SA, et al. Biliary cancer: ESMO clinical practice guide-lines for diagnosis, treatment and follow-up. Ann Oncol 2016. https://doi.org/10.1093/annonc/mdw324.

58. Neuhaus P, Jonas S, Bechstein WO, et al. Extended resections for hilar cholan-giocarcinoma. Ann Surg 1999. https://doi.org/10.1097/00000658-199912000-00010.

59. Groot Koerkamp B, Wiggers JK, Allen PJ, et al. Recurrence rate and pattern of perihilar cholangiocarcinoma after curative intent resection. J Am Coll Surg 2015;221(6):1041–9.

60. Nakeeb A, Tran KQ, Black MJ, et al. Improved survival in resected biliary malig-nancies. Surgery 2002. https://doi.org/10.1067/msy.2002.127555.

61. Nagino M, Ebata T, Yokoyama Y, et al. Evolution of surgical treatment for perihilar cholangiocarcinoma: a single-center 34-year review of 574 consecutive resec-tions. Ann Surg 2013;258(1):129–40.

62. Le Roy B, Gelli M, Pittau G, et al. Neoadjuvant chemotherapy for initially unre-sectable intrahepatic cholangiocarcinoma. Br J Surg 2018. https://doi.org/10.1002/bjs.10641.

63. Horgan AM, Amir E, Walter T, et al. Adjuvant therapy in the treatment of biliary tract cancer: a systematic review and meta-analysis. J Clin Oncol 2012; 30(16):1934–40.

64. Edeline J, Benabdelghani M, Bertaut A, et al. Gemcitabine and oxaliplatin chemotherapy or surveillance in resected biliary tract cancer (Prodige 12-accord 18-Unicancer GI): a randomized phase III study. J Clin Oncol 2019. https://doi.org/10.1200/JCO.18.00050.

65. Primrose JN, Fox RP, Palmer DH, et al. Capecitabine compared with observation in resected biliary tract cancer (BILCAP): a randomised, controlled, multicentre, phase 3 study. Lancet Oncol 2019. https://doi.org/10.1016/S1470-2045(18)30915-X.

66. Ghali P, Marotta PJ, Yoshida EM, et al. Liver transplantation for incidental chol-angiocarcinoma: analysis of the Canadian experience. Liver Transpl 2005. https://doi.org/10.1002/lt.20512.

67. Sotiropoulos GC, Kaiser GM, Lang H, et al. Liver transplantation as a primary indication for intrahepatic cholangiocarcinoma: a single-center experience. Transplant Proc 2008. https://doi.org/10.1016/j.transproceed.2008.08.053.

68. Fu BS, Zhang T, Li H, et al. The role of liver transplantation for intrahepatic chol-angiocarcinoma: a single-center experience. Eur Surg Res 2011. https://doi.org/10.1159/000332827.

69. Doyle MBM, Vachharajani N, Maynard E, et al. Liver transplantation for hepato-cellular carcinoma: long-term results suggest excellent outcomes. J Am Coll Surg 2012. https://doi.org/10.1016/j.jamcollsurg.2012.02.022.

70. Sudan D, DeRoover A, Chinnakotla S, et al. Radiochemotherapy and transplan-tation allow long-term survival for nonresectable hilar cholangiocarcinoma. Am J Transplant 2002. https://doi.org/10.1034/j.1600-6143.2002.20812.x.

71. Darwish Murad S, Kim WR, Harnois DM, et al. Efficacy of neoadjuvant chemo-radiation, followed by liver transplantation, for perihilar cholangiocarcinoma at 12 US centers. Gastroenterology 2012. https://doi.org/10.1053/j.gastro.2012.04.008.

72. Gores GJ, Gish RG, Sudan D, et al. Model for End-Stage Liver Disease (MELD) exception for cholangiocarcinoma or biliary dysplasia. Liver Transpl 2006. https://doi.org/10.1002/lt.20965.

73. Sapisochin G, Facciuto M, Rubbia-Brandt L, et al. Liver transplantation for "very early" intrahepatic cholangiocarcinoma: international retrospective study supporting a prospective assessment. Hepatology 2016. https://doi.org/10.1002/hep.28744.

74. Sapisochin G. Liver transplantation for early intrahepatic cholangiocarcinoma (LT for iCCA). Available at: https://clinicaltrials.gov/ct2/show/NCT02878473.

75. Bergquist A, Glaumann H, Persson B, et al. Risk factors and clinical presentation of hepatobiliary carcinoma in patients with primary sclerosing cholangitis: a case-control study. Hepatology 1998. https://doi.org/10.1002/hep.510270201.

76. Wu YM, Johlin FC, Rayhill SC, et al. Long-term, tumor-free survival after radio-therapy combining hepatectomy-Whipple en bloc and orthotopic liver transplantation for early-stage hilar cholangiocarcinoma. Zhonghua Wai Ke Za Zhi 2009. https://doi.org/10.1002/lt.21287.

77. Nikeghbalian S, Shamsaeefar A, Eshraghian A, et al. Liver transplantation and Whipple surgery combined with chemoradiotherapy for treatment of hilar cholangiocarcinoma in patients with primary sclerosing cholangitis. Liver Transpl 2015. https://doi.org/10.1002/lt.24095.

78. Valle J, Wasan H, Palmer DH, et al. Cisplatin plus gemcitabine versus gemcitabine for biliary tract cancer for the ABC-02 Trial Investigators*. N Engl J Med 2010. https://doi.org/10.1056/NEJMoa0908721.

79. Brieau B, Dahan L, De Rycke Y, et al. Second-line chemotherapy for advanced biliary tract cancer after failure of the gemcitabine-platinum combination: a large multicenter study by the Association des Gastro-Entérologues Oncologues. Cancer 2015. https://doi.org/10.1002/cncr.29471.

80. Lowery MA, Goff LW, Keenan BP, et al. Second-line chemotherapy in advanced biliary cancers: a retrospective, multicenter analysis of outcomes. Cancer 2019. https://doi.org/10.1002/cncr.32463.

81. Lamarca A, Palmer DH, Wasan HS, et al. ABC-06 | A randomised phase III, multi-centre, open-label study of active symptom control (ASC) alone or ASC with oxaliplatin/5-FU chemotherapy (ASC+mFOLFOX) for patients (pts) with locally advanced/metastatic biliary tract cancers (ABC) previously-treated with cisplatin/gemcitabine (CisGem) chemotherapy. J Clin Oncol 2019; 37(15_suppl):4003.

82. Goyal L, Zheng H, Yurgelun MB, et al. A phase 2 and biomarker study of cabozantinib in patients with advanced cholangiocarcinoma. Cancer 2017;123(11): 1979–88.

83. Patel T. Cholangiocarcinoma—controversies and challenges. Nat Rev Gastroenterol Hepatol 2011;8(4):189–200.

84. Almadi MA, Barkun A, Martel M. Plastic vs. self-expandable metal stents for palliation in malignant biliary obstruction: a series of meta-analyses. Am J Gastroenterol 2017;112(2):260–73.

85. Dumonceau J-M, Tringali A, Papanikolaou I, et al. Endoscopic biliary stenting: indications, choice of stents, and results: European Society of Gastrointestinal

Endoscopy (ESGE) clinical guideline–updated October 2017. Endoscopy 2018; 50(09):910–30.

86. Sharaiha RZ, Natov N, Glockenberg KS, et al. Comparison of metal stenting with radiofrequency ablation versus stenting alone for treating malignant biliary strictures: is there an added benefit? Dig Dis Sci 2014;59(12):3099–102.

87. Yang J, Wang J, Zhou H, et al. Efficacy and safety of endoscopic radiofrequency ablation for unresectable extrahepatic cholangiocarcinoma: a randomized trial. Endoscopy 2018;50(08):751–60.

88. Moole H, Tathireddy H, Dharmapuri S, et al. Success of photodynamic therapy in palliating patients with nonresectable cholangiocarcinoma: a systematic review and meta-analysis. World J Gastroenterol 2017;23(7):1278.

89. Khan SA, Davidson BR, Goldin RD, et al. Guidelines for the diagnosis and treatment of cholangiocarcinoma: an update. Gut 2012;61(12):1657–69.

90. Gangi A, Shah J, Hatfield N, et al. Intrahepatic cholangiocarcinoma treated with transarterial yttrium-90 glass microsphere radioembolization: results of a single institution retrospective study. J Vasc Interv Radiol 2018. https://doi.org/10.1016/j.jvir.2018.04.001.

91. Saxena A, Bester L, Chua TC, et al. Yttrium-90 radiotherapy for unresectable intrahepatic cholangiocarcinoma: a preliminary assessment of this novel treatment option. Ann Surg Oncol 2010. https://doi.org/10.1245/s10434-009-0777-x.

92. Edeline J, Du F Le, Rayar M, et al. Glass microspheres 90Y selective internal radiation therapy and chemotherapy as first-line treatment of intrahepatic cholangiocarcinoma. Clin Nucl Med 2015. https://doi.org/10.1097/RLU.0000000000000904.

93. Edeline J, Touchefeu Y, Guiu B, et al. Radioembolization plus chemotherapy for first-line treatment of locally advanced intrahepatic cholangiocarcinoma. JAMA Oncol 2019. https://doi.org/10.1001/jamaoncol.2019.3702.

94. Kloeckner R, Ruckes C, Kronfeld K, et al. Selective internal radiotherapy (SIRT) versus transarterial chemoembolization (TACE) for the treatment of intrahepatic cholangiocellular carcinoma (CCC): study protocol for a randomized controlled trial. Trials 2014;15(1):311.

95. Tao R, Krishnan S, Bhosale PR, et al. Ablative radiotherapy doses lead to a substantial prolongation of survival in patients with inoperable intrahepatic cholangiocarcinoma: a retrospective dose response analysis. J Clin Oncol 2016;34(3):219–26.

96. Mahadevan A, Dagoglu N, Mancias J, et al. Stereotactic body radiotherapy (SBRT) for intrahepatic and hilar cholangiocarcinoma. J Cancer 2015;6(11):1099–104.

97. Frakulli R, Buwenge M, Macchia G, et al. Stereotactic body radiation therapy in cholangiocarcinoma: a systematic review. Br J Radiol 2019;92(1097):20180688.

98. Gani F, Nagarajan N, Kim Y, et al. Program death 1 immune checkpoint and tumor microenvironment: implications for patients with intrahepatic cholangiocarcinoma. Ann Surg Oncol 2016. https://doi.org/10.1245/s10434-016-5101-y.

99. Bang Y-J, Ueno M, Malka D, et al. Pembrolizumab (PEMBRO) for advanced biliary adenocarcinoma: results from the KEYNOTE-028 (KN028) and KEYNOTE-158 (KN158) basket studies. J Clin Oncol 2019;37(15_suppl):4079.

100. Chen W, Li G, Hu Z, et al. Significant response to anti-PD-1 based immunotherapy plus lenvatinib for recurrent intrahepatic cholangiocarcinoma with bone metastasis. Medicine (Baltimore) 2019;98(45):e17832.

Thrombocytopenia in Chronic Liver Disease
New Management Strategies

Kathy M. Nilles, MD[a], Steven L. Flamm, MD[b],*

KEYWORDS

- Thrombocytopenia • Thrombopoietin • TPO receptor agonists • Cirrhosis
- Advanced liver disease • Invasive procedures • Low platelets

KEY POINTS

- Thrombocytopenia is common in advanced liver disease and can pose management difficulties in patients who require invasive procedures.
- One mechanism of thrombocytopenia in advanced liver disease is decreased hepatocyte production of thrombopoietin.
- Although platelet transfusions are the current standard of care to address preprocedure thrombocytopenia, disadvantages include patient risks, costs, and logistical difficulties.
- Two novel thrombopoietin receptor agonists, avatrombopag and lusutrombopag, were approved in the United States to augment platelet counts before elective procedures in patients with thrombocytopenia caused by advanced liver disease.
- These agents are effective and generally safe in carefully selected patient populations, including those with lower Model for End-stage Liver Disease and Child-Turcotte-Pugh scores.

INTRODUCTION

Chronic liver disease caused by cirrhosis is frequently complicated by thrombocytopenia, particularly when portal hypertension is present. Coagulopathy manifested by increases in prothrombin time (PT) and International Normalized Ratio (INR), in the absence of vitamin K deficiency, are other laboratory signs indicating hepatic synthetic dysfunction. Many patients show both thrombocytopenia and coagulopathy. Consequently, these patients are often assumed to be at higher risk of bleeding complications from invasive procedures, including gastrointestinal endoscopy. Moreover,

[a] Division of Gastroenterology and Hepatology, MedStar Georgetown Transplant Institute, Georgetown University School of Medicine, 3800 Reservoir Road NW, 2-PHC, Washington, DC 20007, USA; [b] Division of Gastroenterology and Hepatology, Comprehensive Transplant Center, Northwestern University Feinberg School of Medicine, 676 North St Clair Street, Arkes Suite 1900, Chicago, IL 60611, USA
* Corresponding author.
E-mail address: S-flamm@northwestern.edu

Clin Liver Dis 24 (2020) 437–451
https://doi.org/10.1016/j.cld.2020.04.009
1089-3261/20/© 2020 Elsevier Inc. All rights reserved.

liver.theclinics.com

this patient population is more ill than the general population, and thus more likely to need invasive procedures in general. Invasive procedures are especially common in patients with cirrhosis and complications of portal hypertension, including those undergoing liver transplant evaluation.

Thrombocytopenia may be the first laboratory sign heralding the presence of liver dysfunction. The severity of thrombocytopenia correlates to both severity of liver disease as well as to long-term outcomes.[1] Thrombocytopenia is categorized as mild (platelet count >75,000/μL), moderate (50,000–75,000/μL), and severe (<50,000/μL).[2] It is also common. As many as 76% of patients with cirrhosis have mild thrombocytopenia, and an additional 13% may have more significant degrees of thrombocytopenia.[1]

MECHANISMS OF THROMBOCYTOPENIA IN LIVER DISEASE

The thrombocytopenia observed in liver disease is often multifactorial.[2,3] The most commonly taught mechanism is the sequestration of platelets by the spleen as a result of portal hypertension. Thrombocytopenia in patients with liver disease is such a specific marker of portal hypertension that it is an indication for screening endoscopy for gastroesophageal varices according to the Baveno VI guidelines.[4] However, other causes of thrombocytopenia exist (**Box 1**).

In the setting of hepatic dysfunction, platelets are also underproduced. The growth factor thrombopoietin (TPO), discovered in 1994, is the main regulator of platelet production.[3] TPO acts to prevent platelet apoptosis and increases both the size and number of platelets, as well as their differentiation via binding to its receptor on platelet and megakaryocyte membranes.[2,5] TPO is primarily produced by hepatocytes, and its production is reduced in patients with hepatic dysfunction.[6] In addition, attenuation in platelet response to TPO has been observed in liver disease,[7] and restoration of functioning hepatocytes via liver transplant has been shown to increase both TPO levels and circulating platelets levels.[8] In addition to reduction of TPO, platelets may also be underproduced in liver disease because of concurrent bone marrow suppression from alcohol abuse, untreated hepatitis C virus (HCV), other infections, medications, and nutritional deficiencies.

Increased destruction of existing platelets is a third mechanism of thrombocytopenia in liver disease. These mechanisms include immune-mediated destruction by autoantibodies as well as direct splenic destruction. In addition, dilutional thrombocytopenia is a less common phenomenon in patients with liver disease but can occur with massive blood transfusions or large amounts of crystalloid or colloid for volume resuscitation.

Box 1
Mechanisms of thrombocytopenia in liver disease

Decreased platelet production
• Reduction in thrombopoietin production in hepatic dysfunction
• Marrow suppression (alcohol, hepatitis C virus, nutritional deficiencies, medications)

Removal of circulating platelets
• Hypersplenism/sequestration caused by portal hypertension
• Immune-mediated destruction (autoantibodies)
• Direct splenic destruction

Dilutional
• Intravascular volume resuscitation with crystalloid or colloid
• Massive blood transfusions

The platelet counts measured on routine blood counts are a quantitative measure only, and the numerical value provides no information about platelet function. Platelet dysfunction, even with normal platelet counts, may occur in the setting of chronic kidney disease with uremia, and use of medications that inhibit platelets, such as aspirin, clopidogrel, nonsteroidal antiinflammatory drugs, and serotonin agents. Infections, and sepsis in particular, as well as nutritional deficiencies can also impair platelet function. In addition, in liver disease, bile salts, apolipoprotein E, and fibrinogen degradation products also can inhibit platelet function.[9] The impairment in platelet function directly correlates with the degree of liver dysfunction as measured by the Child-Turcotte-Pugh (CTP) score.[10]

Despite the thrombocytopenia and coagulopathy, patients with liver disease show an increased risk of thromboembolism, particularly in the mesenteric and portal venous circulations. Decreased hepatic synthesis of the anticoagulants antithrombin III and protein C, increases in the procoagulant factor VIII, and decreased fibrinolysis all contribute to a prothrombotic state.[11] When these are combined with reduced velocity of blood flow through the portal circulation from cirrhosis and portal hypertension, portal and/or mesenteric vein thrombosis may occur.

This thrombotic tendency is not measured on routine laboratory testing and this makes it difficult to accurately estimate the bleeding risks in patients with liver disease. Measures of platelet count, PT, and partial thromboplastin time (PTT) are only a partial reflection of the overall hemostatic balance in liver disease.[11,12] Discrepancies exist in perception of bleeding risk, with some data suggesting thrombin generation is adequate for clotting as long as platelets are at least $56,000/\mu L$,[13] whereas other studies have shown higher procedure bleeding risk caused by thrombocytopenia.[14,15] To obviate this issue, some centers use thromboelastography (TEG) or rotational thromboelastometry (ROTEM) to help characterize specific degradations in clot formation and dissolution and thus clarify whether a patient has tendencies toward bleeding versus clotting. TEG is commonly used during liver transplant[16] and increasingly used in inpatient settings to help guide transfusions.

AVAILABLE THROMBOPOIETIN AGONISTS

The cloning of TPO in 1994 generated interest in the use of TPO receptor agonists to treat thrombocytopenia.[3] The original agents mimicked the structure of TPO but caused severe cross reactivity and subsequent inhibition of endogenous TPO, resulting in a paradoxic reduction in platelet counts.[2,3] Newer agents are structurally dissimilar to TPO and thus avoid this cross reactivity.

The original TPO receptor agonist was romiplastin (Nplate, Romiplate). Only small studies exist in patients with liver disease, and currently it is limited to use for hematological disorders.[17–19] A second agent, eltrombopag (Promacta, Revolade), was used to address thrombocytopenia in patients with liver disease. However, both romiplastin and eltrombopag carry significant safety concerns, including formation of portal venous thrombosis (PVT),[20–22] and additionally, eltrombopag has risks of hepatotoxicity. Thus, neither agent is currently recommended for use in patients with thrombocytopenia caused by liver disease.

The interest in platelet count augmentation with TPO receptor agonists increased once again with the development of newer oral agents with high efficacy and fewer safety concerns. In 2018, 2 oral agents, avatrombopag (Doptelet), and lusutrombopag (Mulpleta), were both approved by the US Food and Drug Administration (FDA) for use in patients with thrombocytopenia caused by liver disease undergoing elective procedures.

Avatrombopag was studied in the ADAPT-1 and ADAPT-2 studies.[23,24] These studies were randomized, double-blind, placebo-controlled, multicenter, global phase III clinical trials. In both trials, avatrombopag at dosages of 40 or 60 mg/d (based on initial platelet counts <40,000/μL or ≥40,000/μL but <50,000/μL) for 5 days, or placebo, was administered to 231 (ADAPT-1) and 204 (ADAPT-2) patients with thrombocytopenia caused by advanced liver disease who were undergoing scheduled outpatient procedures. The study drug was taken orally once daily for a total of 5 days. The platelet counts were measured again at the procedure date, as well as 1 week and 5 weeks after the procedure.

The procedures varied in bleeding risk but were deemed lower risk in 61% of the patients, and no higher-risk (intracranial/intraspinal) procedures were included. In addition, because of the potential PVT risk observed with earlier TPO receptor agonists, patients were carefully selected to reduce this risk. Patients with known prior PVT or advanced hepatocellular carcinoma (HCC), prior thrombosis, current mesenteric or PVT, or decreased portal vein velocities were excluded.

Avatrombopag increased the platelet count by a mean of 31,000 to 32,000/μL at the higher dosage of 60 mg/d, versus a change of 800 to 3000/μL for placebo groups. At the lower dosage of 40 mg/d, for patients with slightly higher baseline counts, the mean platelet count increased by 37,000 to 45,000/μL in both trials, compared with 1000 to 6000/μL in the placebo group. Overall, 65% of patients in the lower platelet count group, and 87% in the higher baseline platelet group, reached the primary end point of platelet count greater than 50,000/μL and no bleeding events before the procedure, compared with placebo rates of 22% to 23%. Platelet counts began to increase by day 4, peaked between 10 and 13 days, and gradually returned to baseline over the next month.

The drug showed an excellent safety profile. With the exclusion criteria listed earlier, PVT risks were overall low, occurring in 1 patient on 40 mg, discovered on day 18 and not thought to be related to the study drug. The overall thromboembolic rate was not different than placebo.[23,24]

Lusutrombopag had been used in the correction of thrombocytopenia caused by liver disease in patients in Asia for a few years before approval in the United States, mostly in procedures done by interventional radiology.[25-30] However, the FDA approval for lusutrombopag use in the United States came after the completion of the phase III L-PLUS-1 and L-PLUS-2 trials.[31,32]

In these randomized, double-blind, placebo-controlled studies, patients with liver disease and thrombocytopenia undergoing procedures necessitating platelet correction were administered 3 mg/d of oral lusutrombopag or placebo before their elective procedures. These procedures were performed 9 to 14 days after the first dose. The L-PLUS-1 trial included 97 patients and the L-PLUS-2 included 215 patients. Unlike the ADAPT trials, the L-PLUS-1 and L-PLUS-2 trials included platelet monitoring at days 5 to 8, and, if the platelet count surpassed the 50,000/μL target by days 5 to 7, the drug could be stopped early. In addition, screening ultrasonography scans were used to detect PVT before and after study drug dosing.

In the L-PLUS-1 trial, 79% of patients receiving lusutrombopag achieved platelet counts of greater than 50,000/μL, compared with 12.5% in the placebo group. In the L-PLUS-2 trial, 70% of patients who received lusutrombopag achieved the target platelet count and showed an increase greater than 20,000/μL, compared with 14% in the placebo group. The mean increase in platelet count was approximately 45,000/μL compared with 11,000/μL in the placebo group. Similar to avatrombopag, lusutrombopag did not have an increased risk of PVT. One patient receiving lusutrombopag developed a PVT not thought to be related to the study drug, but the overall thrombosis rates between the study drug and placebo were similar.

These studies showed the safety and efficacy of oral TPO receptor agonists to augment platelet counts with sustained duration, allowing completion of procedures, in patients who were not at increased risk of PVT formation.

INDIVIDUALIZED APPROACHES TO THROMBOCYTOPENIA

In the elective procedure setting, significant variation is observed in the approach to thrombocytopenia management. Although society guidelines are available, these reflect recommendations in the general population and are not specific to thrombocytopenia or coagulopathy in patients with advanced liver disease. As discussed earlier, bleeding and thrombosis in liver disease are not accurately reflected in the routine laboratory abnormalities observed in advanced liver disease, making estimation of bleeding risk in these patients less straightforward than in those with thrombocytopenia from a hematological abnormality.

Many components contribute to the variation in the approach to thrombocytopenia,[33] summarized in **Table 1**. Factors that are specific to each patient include the degree of thrombocytopenia, in conjunction with coexistent coagulopathy (PT/INR or PTT increases), as well as use of medications that could increase bleeding risks (such as aspirin, nonsteroidal antiinflammatory drugs, clopidogrel, low-molecular-weight heparin, warfarin, and newer oral anticoagulants). The presence and degree of uremia in patients with kidney disease may also affect platelet function. Thus, severe thrombocytopenia in a patient with coexistent kidney disease with uremia is likely clinically different than the same platelet count in a patient without kidney disease.

In addition, a prior history of bleeding (particularly procedurally related), the severity of prior bleeding, the precise platelet count, the procedure, and other circumstances in which the bleeding occurred are also relevant. Spontaneous or unprovoked bleeding, such as severe bleeding from routine polypectomy, may be viewed with more concern than bleeding from higher-risk procedures, such as severe bleeding from biliary sphincterotomy. Prior response to platelet transfusions may also be relevant. Attempts to transfuse platelets preprocedure may be inadvisable in patients who

Table 1 Factors influencing platelet count preferences		
Patient Specific	**Provider Specific**	**Procedure Specific**
• Severity of thrombocytopenia	• Institutional protocols	• Procedure bleeding risk in general population
• Concurrent coagulopathy	• Local practice patterns	• Severity of bleeding outcomes (likelihood of catastrophic outcome vs minor manageable outcome)
• Medications (antiplatelet agents, anticoagulants)	• Population socioeconomics and medical-legal culture	
• Prior bleeding history and degree of thrombocytopenia at prior bleeding	• Degree of risk aversion, including concerns about litigation or recent poor outcome	• Location/facility type: stand-alone endoscopy center or tertiary center with emergency room, interventional radiology, and surgery readily available
• Known platelet refractoriness	• Prior training methods	
	• Degree of experience and comfort with the procedure	

have historically responded poorly, and procedure-specific modifications may be undertaken in patients with known platelet transfusion refractoriness.

Provider-specific factors also occur. The clinical experience of the provider, training patterns, personality, and degree of risk aversion all contribute to stylistic differences in baseline platelet count preferences before a particular procedure.

Practice locale and patient population may also affect practice patterns. Providers who frequently perform procedures for patients with advanced liver disease may have less aversion to procedures and have lower thresholds for concern with lower platelet counts in these patients, compared with those who rarely care for such patients. Institutional culture and formally designed protocols, patient socioeconomic status, and associated regional medicolegal culture may also influence practice patterns. Facility factors are relevant; some practitioners, particularly in stand-alone procedure facilities, may prefer to avoid higher-risk procedures in patients with severe thrombocytopenia and instead perform them at hospital-based facilities, where emergency department, interventional radiology, laboratory and blood bank services, and surgical backup are immediately available. In such centers, that same provider may tolerate a greater degree of bleeding risk (including lower platelet counts) than in an isolated facility requiring ambulance transport if a complication occurred.

In addition, another consideration is the severity of bleeding; consequences may be vastly different depending on the location within the body, as well as available methods to treat the bleeding. For example, intracranial bleeding could be catastrophic with long-term sequelae, whereas biliary sphincterotomy bleeding is often self-limited and overall less likely to have long-term consequences. Treatment options are also a factor. For example, a severe polypectomy bleed where interventional radiology is not readily available for embolization may result in emergent partial colectomy to control bleeding. Thus, all of these considerations are important in any specific provider's approach to an elective procedure in patients with advanced liver disease and severe thrombocytopenia.

In addition, and most importantly, the risk stratification of the procedure is critical in influencing whether platelet counts must be augmented in patients with severe thrombocytopenia. Patients with advanced liver disease often require many different types of procedure (**Table 2**). Within gastroenterology, the American Society of Gastrointestinal Endoscopy (ASGE) guidelines designate procedures as higher or lower risk.[34] Procedures in which bleeding is lower risk include paracentesis and routine esophagogastroduodenoscopy (EGD) or colonoscopy with biopsy, as well as polypectomy of smaller polyps, endoscopic variceal ligation, push or balloon enteroscopy, and capsule endoscopy. More advanced procedures at lower risk of bleeding include Barrett esophageal ablation, argon plasma coagulation, endoscopic ultrasonography (EUS) without fine-needle aspiration (FNA), and endoscopic retrograde cholangiopancreatography (ERCP) without sphincterotomy. Transjugular liver biopsy is also considered by some clinicians to be low risk, but opinions on this vary widely.

Moderate-risk procedures in terms of bleeding include percutaneous liver biopsy, colonoscopy with polypectomy of larger polyps, ERCP with sphincterotomy, placement of percutaneous gastrostomy or jejunostomy tubes, cystogastrostomy, ampullectomy, endoscopic mucosal resection or submucosal dissection, and pneumatic dilation of esophageal or other strictures. Many other procedures outside gastroenterology and hepatology are low or moderate risk, such as bronchoscopy, cardiac catheterization, bone marrow biopsy, and lumbar puncture. Those procedures deemed at the highest bleeding risk are generally intracranial or intraspinal procedures.

In general, the provider who is performing a procedure determines the specific platelet threshold for a specific procedure. This decision is individualized but may

Table 2		
Commonly performed procedures in patients with liver disease		
Bleeding Risk Suggested Platelet Target	Gastroenterology/Hepatology	Other Procedures/Specialists
Low >20,000/μL	Paracentesis Small polypectomy Diagnostic EGD or colonoscopy Mucosal biopsies Push enteroscopy Capsule endoscopy EUS without FNA Enteral stent deployment Argon plasma coagulation Barrett esophagus ablation ERCP without balloon dilation ERCP without stent Prophylactic variceal banding	Transjugular liver biopsy Bone marrow biopsy Central line placement Bronchoscopy, without biopsy Thoracentesis Percutaneous biliary interventions TIPS placement
Moderate >50,000/μL	Percutaneous liver biopsy Large polypectomy CystogastrostomyAmpullectomy Endoscopic mucosal resection or submucosal dissection Pneumatic or bougie dilation ERCP with sphincterotomy Endoscopic tumor ablation Percutaneous gastrostomy/ jejunostomy tube EUS with FNA Endoscopic hemostasis	Cardiac catheterization Percutaneous organ biopsy Lumbar puncture Locoregional therapy for HCC Surgery (noncranial, nonspine)
High >100,000/μL	—	Intracranial Intraspinal

Abbreviations: EGD, esophagogastroduodenoscopy; ERCP, endoscopic retrograde cholangiopancreatography; EUS, endoscopic ultrasonography; FNA, fine-needle aspiration; TIPS, transvenous intrahepatic portosystemic shunt.

be made in collaboration with the referring provider. Providers in specialties outside of gastroenterology and hepatology who perform procedures on patients with advanced liver disease and severe thrombocytopenia determine the thrombocytopenia management strategy.

PROCEDURE-SPECIFIC PLATELET RECOMMENDATIONS

Despite the aforementioned variations in practice, certain procedures have established recommendations for platelet goals. Guidelines from the ASGE for gastrointestinal endoscopy procedures[35] suggest routine laboratory monitoring before procedures in patients who may have a higher risk of bleeding, which generally includes patients with advanced liver disease.[34] Although higher-risk procedures may be safest if platelets are augmented to at least 50,000/μL, lower-risk procedures such as diagnostic upper endoscopy may be safely performed at platelet counts of 20,000/μL.[36]

The American Association for the Study of Liver Disease (AASLD) guidelines for paracentesis[37] do not recommend augmenting platelets before performing this procedure because of low bleeding risks even in patients with severe thrombocytopenia.[38] In contrast, liver biopsy is considered a higher-risk procedure, with nonsevere bleeding occurring in 1 in 500 cases.[39] Most hepatologists and interventional radiologists performing percutaneous liver biopsies prefer to correct thrombocytopenia to levels of at least 50,000/μL before the procedure.

Providers outside of gastroenterology and hepatology performing procedures in patients with advanced liver disease often prefer platelet counts of at least 50,000/μL. This level is supported by guidelines,[40–43] even if not directly studied in advanced liver disease. However, in 2019, the Society of Interventional Radiology released updated guidelines on this topic.[44,45] Procedures are now categorized as low or high risk. Recommendations for low-risk procedures include a platelet threshold of 20,000/μL, and, for higher-risk procedures, at least 50,000/μL. Lower-risk procedures relevant to patients with advanced liver disease include paracentesis, thoracentesis, lumbar puncture, and transvenous liver biopsy. Higher-risk procedures performed by interventional radiologists include biliary and portal vein interventions, percutaneous liver and other solid organ biopsies, arterial interventions (including locoregional therapy for HCC), and placement of transvenous intrahepatic portosystemic shunt (TIPS). These updated guidelines will likely result in the evolution of practice patterns of correction of thrombocytopenia in the future.

MANAGEMENT OF THROMBOCYTOPENIA

Two major strategies exist to address periprocedure thrombocytopenia. These strategies include modification of the procedure technique, setting, or personnel, or augmentation of the patient's platelet count via platelet transfusion or use of the TPO receptor agonists.

Procedural Modifications

Rather than correcting thrombocytopenia, postponement of the intended procedure may be justified in some cases. For example, biopsies are generally considered low risk, but they may be forsaken in patients who have salmon-colored esophageal mucosa suggestive of Barrett esophagus with no visible lesion, in the setting of esophageal varices. Deferral of elective procedures until after liver transplant is also an option for some patients.

In addition, if a procedure is necessary, providers who are less comfortable can refer the patient to another provider. Further, a provider may choose to perform a procedure in a hospital-based setting instead of an outpatient facility if there is increased risk.

In cases where the procedure must be performed (such as ERCP for choledocholithiasis and cholangitis), the endoscopist may alter the procedure technique to minimize bleeding risks, such as avoiding sphincterotomy. Even hemostatic techniques are influenced by thrombocytopenia and coagulopathy; electrocautery methods may be avoided in favor or mechanical options, such as hemostatic clips.

Platelet Transfusions

Frequently, elective procedures must be performed in patients with advanced liver disease and severe thrombocytopenia. In these settings, transfusion of platelets is the standard of care and the most rapid method to correct thrombocytopenia.

In the general patient population, 1 unit of platelets increases the total platelet count by approximately 30,000/μL, within the first few minutes of completion. One unit of platelets can be administered in 20 to 30 minutes.[40] However, in patients with advanced liver disease, platelet transfusions are less effective in increasing the platelet count; the average increase in platelet count is only 12,000/μL. Despite this, studies of rotational thromboelastometry in patients with liver disease have shown that, even though the increase in platelet counts may be blunted, clot firmness is still augmented.[46]

Issues with platelet transfusions are summarized in **Box 2**. Although platelet transfusion is generally considered safe and efficacious, adverse events are common.[40] Febrile, allergic, or hypersensitivity reactions are observed, and, in some cases, patients must be pretreated with diphenhydramine, acetaminophen, and/or prednisone. Transfusion-related acute lung injury and transfusion-associated circulatory overload can also occur; however, this is likely more common in the inpatient setting when patients require a large number of transfusions, and less likely in an outpatient setting when fewer units are transfused.

Additional medical risks of platelet transfusions include transfusion-related graft-versus-host disease; bacterial, viral, or parasitic infections; and hemolysis.[40] In addition, in patients who have required multiple blood product transfusions, alloimmunization can occur, whereby recipients form antibodies against donor platelets. Alloimmunization is difficult to prevent in the setting of frequent transfusions. It may contribute to the refractoriness seen in some patients who fail to achieve an adequate increase in platelet counts after platelet transfusion. For patients with significant alloimmunization, matched platelets can be sought. Although effective, the strategy of matching platelets can cause significant delays related to availability. In patients who are liver transplant candidates, alloimmunity can create significant difficulty

---

Box 2
Platelet transfusion issues

Medical safety issues
- Febrile reactions
- Allergic or hypersensitivity reactions
- Transfusion-related lung injury or cardiac overload
- Graft-versus-host disease
- Hemolysis (minor ABO incompatibilities)
- Infections (viral, bacterial, and parasitic)
- Alloimmunization/platelet refractoriness

Failure of platelet counts to increase to desired target
- Additional units must be ordered/administered
- Procedure is canceled, delayed, or modified to address thrombocytopenia

Cost issues
- Actual platelet doses
- Pretreatment of patients with prior sensitivity
- Monitoring during/after transfusion
- Any necessary treatment of reactions
- Lost productivity for patient/caregiver, transportation, and parking costs

Logistical issues
- Patients must come to a transfusion center or hospital setting for monitoring
- Availability of platelets must be timed, including matched platelets
- Scheduling issues (holidays/center closures, patient scheduling)
- Storage and shelf life of platelets (doses may be discarded, and so forth)

with appropriate response to platelets intraoperatively. Thus, particularly in patients who are liver transplant candidates or undergoing other major surgeries in which large amounts of blood products may be required, repeated platelet transfusions are best avoided when possible.

In addition, transfusion of platelets is associated with high costs and logistical issues. One study estimated that the cost of platelet transfusion in patients undergoing percutaneous liver biopsy was more than $7000.[47] In addition, platelet transfusions are usually administered in either a transfusion center or hospital center to allow for adequate monitoring; this may pose logistical difficulties if patients must travel to the center. Logistical issues may result in missed days of work or school for the patient or caregivers, as well as nonadherence to transfusion strategies if transportation is burdensome. Additional logistical issues include availability of platelets (particularly if matched platelets are necessary), scheduling of transfusions in coordination with the scheduled procedure, and the storage and shelf life of platelets. However, despite these issues, platelet transfusion remains the mainstay of managing thrombocytopenia before invasive procedures in the inpatient and outpatient settings.

Correction of Thrombocytopenia via Thrombopoietin Receptor Agonists

TPO receptor agonists are a useful alternative to outpatient platelet transfusions in appropriate settings. With these agents, platelet counts remain increased for a longer duration than platelet transfusions, and thus allow a longer window to complete, reschedule, or even repeat the procedure. After 5 doses of avatrombopag, platelet counts increase, and return to baseline over the next month.[23] With lusutrombopag, platelet counts may remain more than 50,000/µL for up to 3 weeks.[31,48,49]

TPO receptor agonists are inappropriate in certain populations. The products were not studied in pediatric populations or in pregnant and lactating women. There are also few data in patients with significant kidney disease. However, in patients with creatinine clearance more than 30 mL/min, no dose adjustments are needed. Both approved drugs undergo hepatic metabolism. Lusutrombopag was only studied in cirrhotic patients with CTP class A and B, whereas avatrombopag was studied in CTP A, B, and C, but only in patients with Model for End-stage Liver Disease (MELD) scores less than 23. In these specific populations, neither drug needs to be dose reduced. However, in patients with more severe liver disease, dosing is not specified, and caution or complete avoidance is suggested.

No antidotes are available in the setting of overdose of TPO receptor agonists and neither drug can be removed by hemodialysis. Furthermore, rapid increases in platelet count with older TPO receptor agonists were associated with the formation of PVT.[49,50] Patients at higher risk of PVT have a relative, but not necessarily absolute, contraindication, to use of the newer agents. These patients include those with advanced hepatocellular carcinoma, Budd-Chiari syndrome, sinusoidal obstructive syndrome, and those with inherited hypercoagulable states. The presence of slow portal vein flow (<10 cm/s) and/or prior platelet transfusions within 7 days were also exclusion criteria in the pivotal studies, and thus patients meeting these conditions should ideally avoid these agents. Absolute contraindications to use of TPO receptor agonists include patients with prior PVT or current thrombosis of the portal or mesenteric vessels.

Usage of TPO receptor agonists must be timed correctly before the planned date of the elective procedure. Because of potential delays related to insurance, it is recommended to prescribe the medication several weeks in advance of the procedure.

The dosing of TPO receptor agonists is based on baseline platelet count, and timing is based on the date of the procedure. Avatrombopag comes in 20-mg tablets. The dosage of 60 mg/d is used for patients with platelet counts less than 40,000/μL, whereas the 40 mg dose is used if platelet counts are greater than or equal to 40,000 to 49,000/μL. Both regimens are dosed once daily for 5 days. After the last dose, the procedure is recommended to be performed 5 to 8 days later. Thus, if day 1 is designated as the first dose, the procedure can be performed on day 10 to 13. Lusutrombopag has 1 dosing schedule of 3 mg/d for 7 days for patients with any platelet count less than 50,000/μL. The procedure should be performed in a 7-day window beginning 1 day after the drug is finished. Assuming day 1 represents the first dose of lusutrombopag, the procedure is ideally performed on day 9 to 15.

Platelet counts should be obtained on the day of the procedure or the day preceding to ensure they are at or greater than the desired target range[49,50]; if they are not, platelet transfusion may still be necessary. There are no recommendations on checking the platelet count during the course of therapy.

Ideally, the procedure should not be deferred after the patient has started the medication, and, if the procedure is delayed outside the recommended window, platelet counts must be rechecked. Prescribing a second course or extending the course of the dose to accommodate procedure schedule delays was not studied. Thus, it is ideal to confirm the procedure date with the patient, the proceduralist, and the location earlier than usual to ensure that rescheduling is unnecessary, that the patient obtained the medication, and that the patients is completely clear on when to start the medication.

FUTURE STUDIES

Avatrombopag and lusutrombopag are still new, and postmarketing data will be important to help clinicians refine the use of these agents. At present, none of the American gastroenterology and hepatology societies have incorporated these agents into their guidelines. Many questions remain unanswered. These questions include the appropriate dosing for patients with thrombocytopenia who have platelet goals lower or higher than 50,000/μL. Furthermore, monitoring of the platelet count during the course of therapy is not delineated by current prescribing guidelines. It is also unclear whether additional doses are safe and result in longer duration of increased platelets counts, or whether repeated courses of the drugs are safe and effective. Although small studies suggest overall safety with repeated dosing,[25,27] the appropriate safety period between a first and second course has yet to be determined.

In addition, whether or not patients should be monitored for PVT is unclear. It may be prudent to obtain baseline portal vein imaging with MRI or Doppler ultrasonography to avoid prescribing these agents in patients with unidentified PVT.

In addition, use of TPO receptor agonists in patients with platelet counts 50,000/μL or higher in need of neurosurgical procedures that require platelet counts of greater than 100,000/μL is also unstudied.

Another potential area of study is the effect of TPO receptor agonists on the clotting and dissolution parameters measured by TEG and ROTEM. If thrombocytopenia is corrected but the TEG parameters suggest that the patient remains at increased risk for bleeding based on platelet dysfunction, platelet transfusion may still be necessary. In the clinical trials, the absence of bleeding was used as a surrogate marker for adequate platelet function.

Although these novel agents are exciting, caution must be exercised. These issues will be important to revisit in the next few years as more experience with the TPO receptor agonists is gained.

SUMMARY

Patients with underlying advanced liver disease develop thrombocytopenia from a variety of mechanisms, and may or may not be at higher risk of bleeding from invasive procedures than those with normal platelet counts. In patients who need procedures for which target platelet counts more than 50,000/μL are recommended, the TPO receptor agonists, avatrombopag and lusutrombopag, are a convenient alternative method to platelet transfusion to augment platelet counts. These oral agents can be taken at home before the planned, elective procedure and thus may avoid the routine use of platelet transfusions normally administered for this purpose. In addition, unlike the rapid decline in platelet counts observed after platelet transfusion, these agents provide a more sustained increase in platelet counts, thus allowing a longer window of opportunity to safely perform the procedure. Avatrombopag and lusutrombopag are overall safe, without the increased risks of PVT concerns of first-generation agents, at least in the setting of selection of patients at lowest risk for this complication. In specific populations of patients with advanced liver disease and severe thrombocytopenia for whom an elective procedure is planned, a TPO agonist may be optimal. However, for certain patients, these agents may be inappropriate, so judicious use is indicated.

DISCLOSURE

K.M. Nilles has nothing to disclose. S.L. Flamm is a consultant for Shionogi.

REFERENCES

1. Giannini EG. Review article: thrombocytopenia in chronic liver disease and pharmacologic treatment options. Aliment Pharmacol Ther 2006;23(8):1055–65.
2. Afdhal N, McHutchison J, Brown R, et al. Thrombocytopenia associated with chronic liver disease. J Hepatol 2008;48(6):1000–7.
3. Maan R, de Knegt RJ, Veldt BJ. Management of thrombocytopenia in chronic liver disease: focus on pharmacotherapeutic strategies. Drugs 2015;75(17):1981–92.
4. de Franchis R, Baveno VIF. Expanding consensus in portal hypertension: report of the Baveno VI Consensus Workshop: stratifying risk and individualizing care for portal hypertension. J Hepatol 2015;63(3):743–52.
5. Kaushansky K. Thrombopoietin. N Engl J Med 1998;339(11):746–54.
6. Peck-Radosavljevic M, Zacherl J, Meng YG, et al. Is inadequate thrombopoietin production a major cause of thrombocytopenia in cirrhosis of the liver? J Hepatol 1997;27(1):127–31.
7. Peck-Radosavljevic M, Wichlas M, Pidlich J, et al. Blunted thrombopoietin response to interferon alfa-induced thrombocytopenia during treatment for hepatitis C. Hepatology 1998;28(5):1424–9.
8. Peck-Radosavljevic M, Wichlas M, Zacherl J, et al. Thrombopoietin induces rapid resolution of thrombocytopenia after orthotopic liver transplantation through increased platelet production. Blood 2000;95(3):795–801.
9. Witters P, Freson K, Verslype C, et al. Review article: blood platelet number and function in chronic liver disease and cirrhosis. Aliment Pharmacol Ther 2008; 27(11):1017–29.
10. Tapper EB, Robson SC, Malik R. Coagulopathy in cirrhosis - the role of the platelet in hemostasis. J Hepatol 2013;59(4):889–90.
11. Tripodi A, Mannucci PM. The coagulopathy of chronic liver disease. N Engl J Med 2011;365(2):147–56.

12. Intagliata NM, Argo CK, Stine JG, et al. Concepts and controversies in haemostasis and thrombosis associated with liver disease: proceedings of the 7th international coagulation in liver disease conference. Thromb Haemost 2018;118(8): 1491–506.

13. Tripodi A, Primignani M, Chantarangkul V, et al. Thrombin generation in patients with cirrhosis: the role of platelets. Hepatology 2006;44(2):440–5.

14. Sharma M, Yong C, Majure D, et al. Safety of cardiac catheterization in patients with end-stage liver disease awaiting liver transplantation. Am J Cardiol 2009; 103(5):742–6.

15. Giannini EG, Greco A, Marenco S, et al. Incidence of bleeding following invasive procedures in patients with thrombocytopenia and advanced liver disease. Clin Gastroenterol Hepatol 2010;8(10):899–902 [quiz: e109].

16. Stravitz RT. Potential applications of thromboelastography in patients with acute and chronic liver disease. Gastroenterol Hepatol (N Y) 2012;8(8):513–20.

17. Moussa MM, Mowafy N. Preoperative use of romiplostim in thrombocytopenic patients with chronic hepatitis C and liver cirrhosis. J Gastroenterol Hepatol 2013; 28(2):335–41.

18. Voican CS, Naveau S, Perlemuter G. Successful antiviral therapy for hepatitis C virus-induced cirrhosis after an increase in the platelet count with romiplostim: two case reports. Eur J Gastroenterol Hepatol 2012;24(12):1455–8.

19. Al-Samkari H, Marshall AL, Goodarzi K, et al. Romiplostim for the management of perioperative thrombocytopenia. Br J Haematol 2018;182(1):106–13.

20. Afdhal NH, Giannini EG, Tayyab G, et al. Eltrombopag before procedures in patients with cirrhosis and thrombocytopenia. N Engl J Med 2012;367(8):716–24.

21. Afdhal NH, Dusheiko GM, Giannini EG, et al. Eltrombopag increases platelet numbers in thrombocytopenic patients with HCV infection and cirrhosis, allowing for effective antiviral therapy. Gastroenterology 2014;146(2):442–452 e441.

22. Dultz G, Kronenberger B, Azizi A, et al. Portal vein thrombosis as complication of romiplostim treatment in a cirrhotic patient with hepatitis C-associated immune thrombocytopenic purpura. J Hepatol 2011;55(1):229–32.

23. Terrault N, Chen YC, Izumi N, et al. Avatrombopag before procedures reduces need for platelet transfusion in patients with chronic liver disease and thrombocytopenia. Gastroenterology 2018;155(3):705–18.

24. Terrault NA, Hassanein T, Howell CD, et al. Phase II study of avatrombopag in thrombocytopenic patients with cirrhosis undergoing an elective procedure. J Hepatol 2014;61(6):1253–9.

25. Sato S, Miyake T, Kataoka M, et al. Efficacy of repeated lusutrombopag administration for thrombocytopenia in a patient scheduled for invasive hepatocellular carcinoma treatment. Intern Med 2017;56(21):2887–90.

26. Sakamaki A, Watanabe T, Abe S, et al. Lusutrombopag increases hematocytes in a compensated liver cirrhosis patient. Clin J Gastroenterol 2017;10(3):261–4.

27. Kotani S, Kohge N, Tsukano K, et al. Avoidance of platelet transfusion with readministration of lusutrombopag before radiofrequency ablation in hepatocellular carcinoma: a case report. Nihon Shokakibyo Gakkai Zasshi 2017;114(10): 1853–9.

28. Fujita M, Abe K, Hayashi M, et al. Two cases of liver cirrhosis treated with lusutrombopag before partial splenic embolization. Fukushima J Med Sci 2017; 63(3):165–71.

29. Kim ES. Lusutrombopag: first global approval. Drugs 2016;76(1):155–8.

30. Tateishi R, Seike M, Kudo M, et al. A randomized controlled trial of lusutrombopag in Japanese patients with chronic liver disease undergoing radiofrequency ablation. J Gastroenterol 2018;54(2):171–81.

31. Hidaka H, Kurosaki M, Tanaka H, et al. Lusutrombopag reduces need for platelet transfusion in patients with thrombocytopenia undergoing invasive procedures. Clin Gastroenterol Hepatol 2018;17(6):1192–200.

32. Peck-Radosavljevic M, Simon K, Iacobellis A, et al. Lusutrombopag for the treatment of thrombocytopenia in patients with chronic liver disease undergoing invasive procedures (L-PLUS 2). Hepatology 2019;70(4):1336–48.

33. Nilles KM, Caldwell SH, Flamm SL. Thrombocytopenia and procedural prophylaxis in the era of thrombopoietin receptor agonists. Hepatol Commun 2019; 3(11):1423–34.

34. Committee ASoP, Pasha SF, Acosta R, et al. Routine laboratory testing before endoscopic procedures. Gastrointest Endosc 2014;80(1):28–33.

35. Committee ASoP, Acosta RD, Abraham NS, et al. The management of antithrombotic agents for patients undergoing GI endoscopy. Gastrointest Endosc 2016; 83(1):3–16.

36. Committee ASoP, Ben-Menachem T, Decker GA, et al. Adverse events of upper GI endoscopy. Gastrointest Endosc 2012;76(4):707–18.

37. Runyon BA, Aasld. Introduction to the revised American Association for the Study of Liver Diseases Practice Guideline management of adult patients with ascites due to cirrhosis 2012. Hepatology 2013;57(4):1651–3.

38. Grabau CM, Crago SF, Hoff LK, et al. Performance standards for therapeutic abdominal paracentesis. Hepatology 2004;40(2):484–8.

39. Rockey DC, Caldwell SH, Goodman ZD, et al. American association for the study of liver D. Liver biopsy. Hepatology 2009;49(3):1017–44.

40. Schiffer CA, Bohlke K, Delaney M, et al. Platelet transfusion for patients with cancer: American society of clinical Oncology clinical practice guideline update. J Clin Oncol 2018;36(3):283–99.

41. Patel IJ, Davidson JC, Nikolic B, et al. Consensus guidelines for periprocedural management of coagulation status and hemostasis risk in percutaneous image-guided interventions. J Vasc Interv Radiol 2012;23(6):727–36.

42. Kaufman RM, Djulbegovic B, Gernsheimer T, et al. Platelet transfusion: a clinical practice guideline from the AABB. Ann Intern Med 2015;162(3):205–13.

43. Szczepiorkowski ZM, Dunbar NM. Transfusion guidelines: when to transfuse. Hematology Am Soc Hematol Educ Program 2013;2013:638–44.

44. Davidson JC, Rahim S, Hanks SE, et al. Society of Interventional Radiology Consensus Guidelines for the periprocedural management of thrombotic and bleeding risk in patients undergoing percutaneous image-guided interventions-Part I: review of anticoagulation agents and clinical considerations: endorsed by the Canadian Association for Interventional Radiology and the Cardiovascular and Interventional Radiological Society of Europe. J Vasc Interv Radiol 2019; 30(8):1155–67.

45. Patel IJ, Rahim S, Davidson JC, et al. Society of interventional radiology consensus guidelines for the periprocedural management of thrombotic and bleeding risk in patients undergoing percutaneous image-guided interventions-part II: recommendations: Endorsed by the Canadian Association for Interventional Radiology and the Cardiovascular and Interventional Radiological Society of Europe. J Vasc Interv Radiol 2019;30(8):1168–84.e1.

46. Tripodi A, Primignani M, Chantarangkul V, et al. Global hemostasis tests in patients with cirrhosis before and after prophylactic platelet transfusion. Liver Int 2013;33(3):362–7.
47. Basu PNT, Farhat S, Shah NJ, et al. Single use of romiplostim thrombopoietin analogue in severe thrombocytopenia for outpatient percutaneous liver biopsy in patients with chronic liver disease–a randomized double blinded prospective trial. J Hepatol 2012;56(Supplement 2):S38.
48. Afdhal N, Duggal A, Ochiai T, et al. Lusutrombopag for treatment of thrombocytopenia in patients with chronic liver disease who are undergoing non-emergency invasive procedures: results from an international phase 3, randomized, double-blind, placebo-controlled study (L-PLUS-2). Hepatology 2017;66(6):1254A.
49. FDA prescribing information Mulpleta (lusutrombopag). Available at: https://www.accessdata.fda.gov/drugsatfda_docs/label/2018/210923s000lbl.pdf. Accessed November 1, 2018.
50. FDA prescribing information doptelet (avatrombopag). 2018. Available at: https://www.accessdata.fda.gov/drugsatfda_docs/label/2018/210238s000lbl.pdf. Accessed November 1, 2018.

Budd-Chiari Syndrome
An Uncommon Cause of Chronic Liver Disease that Cannot Be Missed

Lamia Y.K. Haque, MD, MPH[a], Joseph K. Lim, MD[b],*

KEYWORDS

- Splanchnic thrombosis • Hepatic venous outflow tract obstruction • Thrombophilia
- Anticoagulation • Angioplasty • Portal shunt
- Transjugular intrahepatic portosystemic shunt • Transplantation

KEY POINTS

- Budd-Chiari syndrome, or hepatic venous outflow tract obstruction, is a rare entity with variable presentation but high mortality that requires a high index of suspicion.
- Primary Budd-Chiari syndrome often results from the combined effect of multiple thrombophilic risk factors and, therefore, necessitates a thorough work-up to identify all possible underlying conditions in order to address them.
- Lifelong anticoagulation is recommended in the absence of contraindications.
- Management of Budd-Chiari syndrome requires a multidisciplinary, individualized, step-wise approach, consisting of prompt anticoagulation, management of complications of portal hypertension, treatment of any underlying risk factors, and sequential use of endovascular therapy, portosystemic shunting, or liver transplantation, depending on a patient's clinical course.
- Patients with Budd-Chiari syndrome are at increased risk of developing hepatocellular carcinoma; however, the development of regenerative nodules makes a radiographic diagnosis of hepatocellular carcinoma challenging.

INTRODUCTION

Budd-Chiari syndrome (BCS), or hepatic venous (HV) outflow tract obstruction, was first described in the medical literature in the 1800s by George Budd[1] and Hans Chiari.[2] Whereas Budd reported the presence of membranous material within the HV, Chiari described the presence of HV thrombosis.[1,2] At present, BCS refers to obstruction of the HV outflow tract that can occur in various locations, including small HVs, large HVs, and the inferior vena cava (IVC) up to the level of the right atrium.[3–5] HV

[a] Section of Digestive Diseases, Yale University School of Medicine, 333 Cedar Street, LMP 1080, New Haven, CT 06520, USA; [b] Section of Digestive Diseases, Yale Liver Center, Yale University School of Medicine, 333 Cedar Street, LMP 1080, New Haven, CT 06520, USA
* Corresponding author.
E-mail address: joseph.lim@yale.edu

Clin Liver Dis 24 (2020) 453–481
https://doi.org/10.1016/j.cld.2020.04.012
1089-3261/20/© 2020 Elsevier Inc. All rights reserved.

liver.theclinics.com

outflow tract obstruction due to sinusoidal obstruction or pericardial pathology generally has been excluded from this definition.[4] Whereas primary BCS refers to the presence of venous thrombosis, secondary BCS occurs due to mechanical obstruction from malignancy, abscess, cysts, large hepatic nodules, surgical manipulation, and blunt abdominal trauma.[3,4] Primary BCS, which is the main focus of this review, often is a result of multiple risk factors, most commonly inherited and acquired thrombophilic states.[3] Due to the rare nature of this disease, it is imperative to maintain a high index of suspicion in the appropriate clinical scenario, particularly in younger adult patients with new-onset ascites, hepatomegaly, or caudate lobe enlargement.[6,7] Although high-quality evidence in the form of randomized controlled trials to guide management is lacking, progress has been made in the management of BCS using an individualized, stepwise, multidisciplinary approach, consisting of anticoagulation and other pharmacotherapy, endovascular interventions, transjugular intrahepatic portosystemic shunts (TIPSs), surgical shunts, and liver transplantation.[3,4,6,8–11]

EPIDEMIOLOGY

A recent meta-analysis pooling data from several large studies across Europe and Asia found the yearly incidence of BCS to be 1 per million, with rates varying between 0.168 per million and 4.09 per million, and the pooled prevalence 11 per million, ranging between 2.4 per million and 33.1 per million, depending on geographic location.[12] The epidemiology of BCS is characterized by significant regional variation. A nationwide analysis of French data revealed a prevalence of 4.04 per million,[13] and another recent study from centers in Italy reported an incidence of 2.2 per million and 2 per million in women and men, respectively.[14] The incidence and prevalence of BCS based on a Swedish study were 0.8 per million per year and 1.4 per million, respectively.[15] A study from Nepal reported that 17% of patients treated at a liver unit over 3 years had BCS.[16] A Japanese study revealed a similar prevalence of 2.4 per million,[17] whereas a more recent population-based study from South Korea reported an incidence and prevalence of 0.87 per million per year and 5.29 per million, respectively.[18] BCS is more common in China, where the overall incidence and prevalence are 0.88 per million per year and 7.69 million per year, respectively, with significant variation by province.[19,20]

Although the risk of venous thromboembolism as a whole increases with age,[21] BCS usually occurs in patients in their third, fourth, or fifth decade of life. Two European studies reported a mean age of 40 years, whereas a Japanese study reported mean ages of 46.5 years and 36.4 years in women and men, respectively.[13,15,17] BCS is extremely rare in children. A retrospective analysis of records between 2001 and 2015 at King's College Hospital in the United Kingdom yielded only 7 pediatric cases of primary BCS.[22] Risk factors in this population included polycythemia vera, paroxysmal nocturnal hemoglobinuria (PNH), and antiphospholipid antibody syndrome.[22]

CLASSIFICATION

BCS can result from HV obstruction at various levels, including small intrahepatic veins, large intrahepatic veins, and the IVC.[7] Causes of primary BCS include HV thrombosis, IVC thrombosis, and membranous obstruction.[23] In an Indian study, HV thrombosis was present in 59.1% of patients with BCS,[23] which contrasts with older reports that described IVC obstruction cava as the most common mechanism.[24] A French study revealed a similar distribution of thrombus location in which pure HV thrombosis was present in 76.6% of cases whereas combined HV and IVC thrombosis occurred in 37% of cases.[13] Concomitant portal vein (PV) thrombosis also can occur with BCS and has been reported in 3.2% to 15% of cases.[3,13] Patterns of venous obstruction leading to BCS in East Asian nations, such as China, Japan, and Nepal, are distinct in that involvement of the hepatic vena cava as well as a more indolent course are more common than in European populations.[17,19,25–27] A large case series from China reported that 63% of consecutive patients with BCS had a combination of HV and IVC obstruction, with membranous obstruction present in 61% of cases.[28]

DIAGNOSIS AND CLINICAL FEATURES

The clinical presentation of BCS varies significantly between patients and may correlate with the acuity and severity of venous obstruction, ranging from the complete absence of symptoms[29] to rapidly progressive acute liver failure.[30] Distinctions, therefore, have been made between fulminant, acute, subacute, and chronic presentations of BCS.[7,31] In fulminant BCS, hepatic encephalopathy occurs within days to weeks of developing jaundice. Acute BCS is characterized by acute-onset ascites and hepatic necrosis in the absence of venous collaterals, whereas subacute disease is associated with a more subtle clinical presentation due to the development of portal and hepatic collateral circulation.[31] Chronic BCS may manifest as cirrhosis and portal hypertension.[31]

The most commonly reported symptoms overall include abdominal fullness, abdominal discomfort, lower extremity swelling, jaundice, fever, malaise, and altered mental status.[15,17,23,32] Physical examination findings include ascites, hepatosplenomegaly, jaundice, edema, lower extremity ulcers, and dilated subcutaneous veins, particularly along the trunk or lower extremities.[17,33,34] A study of patients with BCS in India reported that 42% presented with chronic BCS, 41% presented with acute BCS, 8% had fulminant disease, and 6% were asymptomatic.[23] In an Egyptian study, 79.8% of patients presented with chronic BCS, 19.1% presented with acute BCS, and 1.1% had fulminant disease.[35] The lack of symptoms in some patients may be due to the presence of large spontaneous intrahepatic portosystemic shunts.[29] Whereas patients in Western nations tend to present with acute HV thrombosis in the presence of at least 1 hypercoagulable risk factor, many patients in China present with chronic occlusion of the hepatic vena cava manifesting as long-standing lower extremity swelling and abdominal wall varices.[25] A summary of symptoms and signs associated with BCS is presented in **Table 1**.

Laboratory abnormalities in BCS vary based on the acuity of the obstruction and can include elevated transaminases, elevated alkaline phosphatase, elevated bilirubin, elevated international normalized ratio (INR), or low serum albumin.[3] In some cases, laboratory parameters may be within normal range.[3] Ascitic fluid analysis usually

Table 1 Clinical features of Budd-Chiari syndrome	
Symptoms	**Physical Examination Findings**
Abdominal discomfort	Ascites
Abdominal fullness	Jaundice
Hematemesis	Fever
Melena	Hepatosplenomegaly
Malaise	Lower extremity edema
Leg swelling	Dilated subcutaneous trunk veins
Varicose veins	Hepatic encephalopathy

reveals a serum-ascites albumin gradient of 1.1 g/dL or greater; however, ascitic protein levels can vary.[3]

Diagnosis of BCS is confirmed with imaging. Relevant imaging modalities include Doppler ultrasound, computed tomography (CT), magnetic resonance imaging (MRI), and hepatic venography. Doppler ultrasound is cost effective, avoids radiation, and provides information regarding the blood flow pattern within the splanchnic vessels.[36] Limitations of ultrasound include the ability to characterize focal lesions in the hepatic parenchyma as well as difficulty in identifying collaterals.[36] In addition to better outlining the hepatic vasculature and collaterals, CT imaging provides information regarding liver morphology as well as patterns of parenchymal enhancement and perfusion.[36] MRI may be useful in distinguishing between acute and chronic forms of BCS based on the presence of ascites, degree of signal intensity within the HV or IVC, spleen size, and presence of collaterals.[37,38]

Typical findings on imaging include obstruction of the HVs, occlusion of IVC, hypertrophy of the caudate lobe, heterogeneous liver parenchymal enhancement, and presence of vascular collaterals or nodules.[39,40] Additional elements may include thrombi, narrowing, or weblike structures within the IVC or ascites.[41] Whereas acute BCS is characterized by hepatomegaly, ascites, and lack of enhancement of HVs, chronic BCS is associated with liver atrophy, enlargement of the caudate lobe, vascular collaterals, and regenerative nodules.[42] Because the caudate lobe drains independently into the IVC, it appears to have normal perfusion on imaging in acute BCS and hypertrophies over time.[7,43] Vascular collaterals may be identified by a spiderweb vascular pattern on hepatic venography.[43]

Histologic features in acute BCS include congestion, hemorrhage, necrosis, fibrosis, scarring, and the presence of regenerative nodules.[32,44] A study in which imaging findings in patients with BCS were correlated with histology on explanted livers revealed radiographic evidence of decreased portal perfusion in a majority of patients and increased arterial perfusion in a minority of patients.[45] Histologic findings were consistent with nodular regenerative hyperplasia and obstructive portal venopathy in all patients, although those with increased arterial perfusion on imaging had greater large regenerative nodules on pathology.[45] Although liver biopsy rarely is indicated for large vessel disease, it is pursued more commonly in cases involving isolated small vessel involvement due to lesser certainty regarding diagnosis.[46] Various patterns of fibrosis in BCS have been described and the presence of PV disease may play a role in whether a patient eventually develops venocentric cirrhosis or nodular regenerative hyperplasia.[47] Findings on liver biopsy do not necessarily correlate with clinical outcome.[48]

ETIOLOGY, PATHOGENESIS, AND RISK FACTORS

The etiology of venous thromboembolism often is multifactorial and this is particularly relevant in BCS given its rarity.[21,49,50] In 1 case series, 84% of patients with BCS had at least 1 risk factor for thrombosis, and 46% of patients had more than 1.[51] Patients with more extensive thrombosis of the splanchnic vasculature beyond isolated HV thrombosis, such as those with combined HV-PV thrombosis, are even more likely to have multiple risk factors.[52] A summary of risk factors is outlined in **Box 1**. Patients with BCS are likely to have impairments in mechanisms of fibrinolysis.[53] Hemodynamic analyses in patients with primary BCS and severe portal hypertension reveal that unlike patients with cirrhosis who develop vasodilation and hyperdynamic circulation, patients with BCS tend to have normal hemodynamics without vasodilation.[54] Despite this, patients with BCS have increases in plasma volume, renin activity, aldosterone, and norepinephrine levels.[54]

Box 1
Etiologies and risk factors for Budd-Chiari syndrome

Myeloproliferative disorders
  Polycythemia vera
  Essential thrombocytosis
  Myelofibrosis

Inherited thrombophilia
  Factor V Leiden
  Prothrombin gene mutation
  Protein C deficiency

Acquired thrombotic states
  Antiphospholipid syndrome
  Behçet disease
  PNH
  Sarcoidosis
  Sjögren disease
  Systemic lupus erythematosus
  Inflammatory bowel disease
  Celiac enteropathy
  Nephrotic syndrome
  Malignancy and tumors
  Sepsis
  Obesity
  Pregnancy
  Oral contraceptive therapy

Myeloproliferative Disorders

Myeloproliferative disorders are a result of clonal transformation of hematopoietic stem cells leading to increased production of mature blood cells.[55] Myeloproliferative disorders associated with BCS include polycythemia vera, essential thrombocytosis, and myelofibrosis in which the Janus kinase 2 (JAK2) V617F somatic mutation commonly is found.[8,56–59] The mechanism by which myeloproliferative disorders lead to hypercoagulability may be due to the effects of active protein C resistance as well as reduction in free protein S levels.[60] Patients with myeloproliferative disorders and BCS are more likely to have younger age, female sex, inherited thrombophilia, and the JAK2 V617F mutation than patients who develop thromboses in other locations.[61] Routine testing for JAK2 V617F mutations in patients with chronic, latent, or idiopathic BCS can uncover a myeloproliferative disorder that otherwise would be unidentified.[62]

A study of 115 consecutive cases of BCS in Algeria revealed that 27% of patients had multiple risk factors, the most common being myeloproliferative disorders, which occurred in 34%.[63] In an Italian cohort, the JAK2 V617F mutation was identified in 40% of patients with BCS.[58] Myeloproliferative disorders were identified in 38% of individuals in a Swedish study and 49% of patients in European case series.[15,51] Myeloproliferative disorders are much less common in East Asian patients with BCS. In several studies from China, only approximately 5% of patients were reported to have a JAK2 V617F mutation–positive myeloproliferative neoplasm.[28,64] The JAK2 46/1 haplotype has been associated with BCS.[65]

Other less common mutations that have been associated with myeloproliferative disorders involve the calreticulin (CALR) gene and thrombopoietin receptor (MPL) gene.[61,66] Testing for CALR gene mutations is recommended in patients who have

BCS in context of suspected myeloproliferative disorder but are JAK2 V617F nega-tive.[67–71] A recent meta-analysis revealed that 17.2% of such patients had a mutation in CALR.[72]

The presence of massive splenomegaly and platelet count above 200×10^9 cells/L has been associated with underlying myeloproliferative neoplasms with high speci-ficity but low sensitivity.[73,74] Due to the high prevalence of myeloproliferative disorders among patients with BCS, routine testing is recommended.[7,75] In patients with myelo-proliferative disorder, the presence of splenomegaly, leukocytosis, and history of prior thrombosis also were associated with a greater likelihood of future recurrent thrombosis.[76]

Inherited Thrombophilia

A multicenter case-control study assessing the risk of BCS associated with various inherited thrombophilic disorders reported that patients with factor V Leiden mutation, prothrombin gene mutation, and protein C deficiency had higher relative risks of BCS of 11.3, 2.1, and 6.8, respectively, compared with population controls.[77] The risk of BCS was not elevated in patients with prothrombin gene mutation, antithrombin defi-ciency, or inherited protein S deficiency.[77,78] Factor V Leiden was reported in 30% of patients with BCS in another series and was found to co-occur often with additional risk factors for thrombosis.[79,80] The most common mutation found in an Egyptian cohort was factor V Leiden mutation.[35] A study of 53 patients with BCS in India revealed that factor V Leiden was the most prevalent risk factor and occurred in 26.4% of cases.[81] Other risk factors for BCS in this cohort included protein C defi-ciency, antiphospholipid syndrome, pregnancy, oral contraceptive therapy, and sur-gery. Prothrombin gene mutation was not detected.[81] In contrast, another study of 59 patients with BCS in India revealed that only 4 patients had factor V Leiden hetero-zygosity.[82] The G20210A prothrombin gene mutation also was absent in this series of patients.[82] A recent meta-analysis reported pooled prevalences of antithrombin, pro-tein C, and protein S deficiencies in BCS to be 2.3%, 3.8%, and 3%, respectively.[83]

Acquired Prothrombotic States

Several acquired thrombophilic states can contribute to the risk of BCS. Antiphospho-lipid syndrome is a condition in which autoantibodies, such as lupus anticoagulant and antiphospholipid antibodies, lead to a hypercoagulable state.[84] Antiphospholipid syn-drome is considered primary if it occurs in isolation or secondary if it occurs in the setting of other autoimmune conditions.[84] Both arterial and venous thromboses can occur in any area of the body, although the most common manifestations are stroke and lower extremity venous thromboembolism.[85] In a prospective study of 22 patients with BCS, 4 were noted to have antiphospholipid syndrome.[86]

Behçet disease is a clinical syndrome characterized by the presence of oral and genital ulcerations, ocular disease such as uveitis, and neurologic symptoms.[87] Among patients with Behçet disease, the development of BCS has been correlated with younger age and male sex.[88] A study comparing patients with BCS with and without Behçet disease revealed that patients in the latter group were more likely to be male and of North African descent.[89] Furthermore, patients with Behçet disease are more likely to have obstruction at the level of the IVC and have a more fulminant course.[88–90]

PNH is a known risk factor for BCS. It is caused by a mutation in the phosphatidy-linositol glycan class A gene, which leads to a deficiency in glycosylphosphatidylino-sitol and results in the absence of complement regulatory proteins CD55 and CD59 from affected hematopoietic stem cells.[91] This leads to a profoundly hypercoagulable state, and patients often develop complement-mediated intravascular hemolysis, bone marrow dysfunction, and venous thrombosis.[91,92] Analyses using data from a multicenter European study revealed that the majority of patients with BCS and PNH had additional bone marrow disorders, such as aplastic anemia or myelodysplastic syndrome, and some also had co-occurring myeloproliferative disease.[91] Studies of patients with BCS in China revealed a very small prevalence of PNH, with up to 1.6% of patients exhibiting deficiencies in CD55 and CD59.[93,94] PNH can be cured only through allogenic hematopoietic stem cell transplantation, and in 1 cohort of 163 patients with PNH and BCS, 6 underwent stem cell transplantation and 5 had a favorable post-transplant course.[91]

Hyperhomocysteinemia resulting from mutations in the methylenetetrahydrofolate reductase (MTHFR) gene also has been associated with BCS, although the literature is limited by small size and heterogeneity among studies.[95] A meta-analysis revealed that patients with BCS were more likely to have elevated plasma homocysteine levels and MTHFR C677T mutation homozygosity than healthy controls.[95]

Sepsis leads to hypercoagulability and thrombus formation through multiple mechanisms, including the effects of tissue factor emerging from monocytes and neutrophils as well as activation of platelets and the coagulation cascade.[96] An association between BCS involving the hepatic vena cava and bacteremia has been reported in a Nepalese cohort.[97] Intra-abdominal foci of infection, such as abscesses causing direct compression of the HV system, can lead to secondary BCS.[3]

Central obesity, characterized as large waist circumference, greater than 88 cm and 102 cm for women and men, respectively, has been associated with nontumorous noncirrhotic PV thrombosis, but the implications for the risk of BCS are unclear.[98] One possible mechanism for the elevated risk of splanchnic thrombosis in this group is the increased presence of systemic inflammation mediated via interleukin 6 secretion by visceral fat.[99] Chronic low-grade inflammation can activate prothrombotic cascades within vascular beds due to the effects of cytokines, tissue factor, platelet activation, and impaired fibrinolysis.[100]

Inflammatory bowel disease is associated with an increased risk of thrombosis that is provoked by intestinal inflammation leading to a systemic prothrombotic milieu due to the effects of tissue factor, thrombocytosis, and abnormalities in thrombolysis.[100] Although literature linking BCS to inflammatory bowel disease is limited, splanchnic thrombosis has been reported in this subgroup, and the overall risk of first venous thromboembolism is 2.8-times greater than in the general population.[100,101] Isolated cases of BCS also have been reported in patients with celiac disease and sarcoidosis.[102,103]

Malignancy is associated with a higher risk of venous thrombosis overall due to effects of procoagulant molecules, such as tissue factor, inflammatory cytokines, and proangiogenic factors.[104] Tumors directly obstructing the IVC or HV are rare and can lead to secondary BCS due to obstruction. One such case involved a patient with leiomyosarcoma of the IVC that led to acute BCS.[105] Another series reported cases of 4 patients with renal cell carcinoma who developed concomitant tumor thrombus leading to BCS.[106]

A systematic review and meta-analysis determined that the pooled prevalence of BCS attributed to pregnancy is 6.8%,[107] although associated with geographic variation, ranging from 5% in European nations, 7.1% in Asia, and 10.6% in Egypt.[107] Among 105 patients with BCS at a single center in India, 16 were diagnosed in the postpartum period and were attributed to pregnancy.[108] There is a paucity of studies confirming a link between pregnancy and BCS with careful evaluation of other risk factors, although it is possible that pregnancy may contribute to BCS in the presence of additional prothrombotic risk factors.[109]

Medications

Oral contraceptives have been implicated in some cases of BCS. The overall prevalence of BCS among patients taking oral contraceptives is low, suggesting the presence of additional risk factors in patients who develop BCS while on contraceptive therapy.[110] In a Swedish study, oral contraceptives were implicated in 30% of cases of BCS.[15] In an older French study, the relative risk of BCS was 2.37 in patients taking oral contraceptives compared with those who were not.[9] A case of a patient who developed BCS in the setting of tamoxifen exposure and underlying myeloproliferative disorder also has been reported. More evidence is needed, however, to clarify any causal link between tamoxifen and BCS.[111]

MANAGEMENT

Stepwise multidisciplinary management delivered in an individualized fashion with gradually increasing levels of invasiveness is the recommended approach to treatment of BCS, as outlined in **Fig. 1**.[8,112,113] The primary goals of therapy include improvement in signs and symptoms of portal hypertension, preservation of liver function, and recanalization of the vasculature if feasible.[114] A study in which outcomes among a cohort of 37 patients with BCS treated at a Belgian center compared with data from the European Network for Vascular Disorders of the Liver revealed that 7.21% were treated with anticoagulation alone, 4.21% underwent venous recanalization, 9.26% received portosystemic shunts, and 14.4% underwent liver transplantation.[115] The stepwise approach at this center consisted of anticoagulation for all patients except those receiving emergent liver transplantation and angioplasty for patients with focal HV thromboses as first-line therapies. If patients did not respond to first-line therapy, TIPS was offered if technically feasible, followed by liver transplantation if patients had progressive acute liver failure and/or TIPS failure.[115]

Initial Testing and Identification of Risk Factors

Addressing the underlying etiology of thrombosis is an important aspect of the initial work-up in patients with BCS. Obtaining a detailed history to assess for the presence of risk factors, such as oral contraceptive use, can be valuable. Comorbidities, such as pregnancy, postpartum state, inflammatory bowel disease, celiac disease, and malignancy, should be identified. Assessment for myeloproliferative disorders and hypercoagulable states can provide information on the expected clinical course, prognosis, and specific treatments to reduce the likelihood of progressive or recurrent disease.[112]

Genetic testing for JAK2 617F should be performed to assess for the presence of myeloproliferative disorder in patients with BCS.[116] If JAK2 617F testing is negative, testing for additional mutations, such as CALR or MPL, should be pursued.[68,69,71,112] In rare cases, bone marrow biopsy may be needed if genetic testing is negative but suspicion for myeloproliferative disease remains high.[112] Testing to identify other inherited or acquired thrombophilias includes assessment of activated protein C resistance, genetic testing for factor V Leiden with R605Q factor V mutation, assessment of antithrombin activity to identify antithrombin deficiency, assessment of protein C activity to identify protein C deficiency, assessment of free protein S levels to identify protein S deficiency, and assessment of antiphospholipid antibodies to identify antiphospholipid syndrome.[112] Flow cytometry to identify CD55 and CD59 deficiency can be used to assess for the presence of PNH.[112]

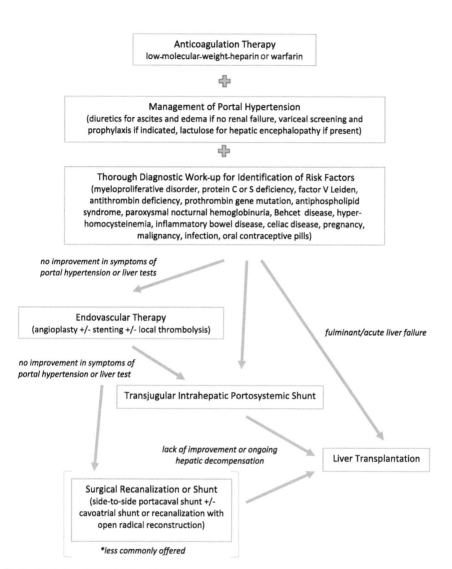

Fig. 1. Stepwise management of BCS.

Anticoagulation and Medical Therapy

Historically, anticoagulation with heparin and vitamin K antagonists have been recommended for patients with BCS, although studies delineating the optimal intensity of anticoagulation are lacking.[3,117] Beginning anticoagulation with low-molecular-weight heparin (LMWH) immediately upon diagnosis is recommended and dosing may be titrated to anti-Xa activity of 0.5 IU/mL to 0.8 IU/mL.[3,112] In a series of 43 consecutive patients treated with warfarin alone, with a goal INR range of 2 to 3, more than 60% experienced resolution of ascites and normalization of liver chemistries at a median follow-up of 23 months.[118] Low Child-Turcotte-Pugh (CTP) score was associated with a higher likelihood of response.[118]

Although not yet approved for patients with BCS, direct-acting oral anticoagulants (DOACs) have been used to treat selected patients with BCS and may represent an alternative for patients who have experienced recurrent thromboses on therapeutic levels of warfarin and/or LMWH.[117,119] A recent study comparing outcomes in patients with acute venous thromboembolism in atypical locations, such as the splanchnic veins, who were treated with DOACs versus those with deep venous thromboembolism of the extremities or pulmonary embolism treated with DOACs revealed similar rates of thrombus recurrence, and major bleeding was similar between groups.[120] This suggests that DOACs may be as effective in splanchnic thrombosis as they are in other thromboses; however, more studies are needed prior to standard use.

Systemic thrombolysis with recombinant tissue plasminogen activator has been used in rare cases with limited evidence describing its use.[121,122] The role of systemic thrombolysis as a primary therapy for BCS likely is limited to circumstances in which a high degree of clot burden prohibits alternative endovascular or surgical options.[122] Furthermore, systemic thrombolysis is unlikely to provide benefit in chronic BCS. In cases of acute thrombus formation provoked or exacerbated by endovascular instrumentation, locally delivered thrombolytics may increase the likelihood of vessel recanalization.[121]

Major bleeding can occur in patients with BCS due to the use of anticoagulation. In 1 study, 94 consecutive patients with BCS were evaluated for the incidence of major bleeding, defined as blood loss requiring hospitalization, need for transfusion of 2 or more units of red blood cells, intracranial or retroperitoneal bleeding, or bleeding that led to death, and the overall incidence was 22.8 per 100 patient-years.[123] Bleeding most commonly was related to invasive procedures for the treatment of BCS, portal hypertensive bleeding, nonportal hypertensive gastrointestinal bleeding, and genital bleeding.[123] The severity of BCS was associated with prognosis after a bleeding episode.[123]

In patients with concomitant myeloproliferative disorders, cytoreductive therapy may reduce the risk of recurrent thrombosis by addressing the underlying cause.[117,124] Hydroxyurea is a recommended first-line therapy in patients with underlying polycythemia vera and essential thrombocythemia.[117] For those with polycythemia vera who do not respond or are intolerant of hydroxyurea or for patients with myelofibrosis, ruxolitinib can be considered.[117] The involvement of hematology specialists is particularly important in guiding treatment of the underlying disease process in patients with myeloproliferative disorders.

Management of complications of portal hypertension, such as ascites, encephalopathy, renal insufficiency, and gastrointestinal bleeding, is an important aspect of initial therapy in patients with BCS.[112] Patients require screening for gastroesophageal varices and, if found, prophylaxis with nonselective β-blockers may be indicated. For patients with noncirrhotic portal hypertension who experience variceal bleeding, secondary prophylaxis includes β-blockers and endoscopic variceal band ligation.[125]

Percutaneous Angioplasty and Stenting

Endovascular approaches, such as angioplasty and stenting, have gained popularity over the past 2 decades.[126,127] The use of high-quality diagnostic imaging to help guide interventional approaches is encouraged.[128] Angioplasty often is pursued when short-length stenoses of the HV or IVC, including membranous obstruction, are suspected.[128–132] In a study of 60 patients with BCS due to HV thrombosis who underwent percutaneous intervention between 1995 and 2014, technical success was achieved in all patients.[133] HV angioplasty occurred in 18 patients and combined HV and IVC angioplasty was performed in 9 patients.[133] Another study of 143 patients with HV occlusion who were treated with angioplasty revealed vascular patency rates of 91.1%, 77.4%, and 74% as well as survival rates of 97.7%, 92.2%, and 90% at 1 year, 3 years and 6 years, respectively.[134] Another study revealed that endovascular recanalization via angioplasty resulted in a transplant-free survival rate of 94% at both 1 year and 5 years.[135] Balloon angioplasty also can be performed successfully in patients with combined obstruction of both the HV and IVC.[136] In 1 study, recanalization of both sites was achieved in 96% of patients.[136] Endovascular recanalization using balloon dilatation and stenting of accessory HVs also has been performed successfully in patients with extensive obstruction of HVs.[137,138]

Angioplasty may be combined with the placement of permanent or retrievable stents, particularly in cases involving IVC obstruction.[139,140] A study in which patients with BCS due to long-segment IVC obstruction of the IVC were treated with either permanent or retrievable stents removed within 1 month later revealed that primary stent patency may be superior in the latter group.[139] Periprocedural complications that were reported include inability to cannulate, pulmonary embolism, and cerebrovascular accident.[139] The approach to endovascular therapy in patients with thrombosis of the IVC varies based on the characteristics and distribution of the thrombus.[141,142] Modified approaches using local thrombolysis, thrombus aspiration, dilation, and stenting are used depending on the individual characteristics of the thrombus and can lead to favorable results.[141–143] In a study of 108 patients who underwent endovascular therapy with individualized technique, survival rates at 1 year, 5 years, and 10 years were 95%, 86%, and 81%, respectively.[142] Use of stenting in addition to angioplasty may be associated with higher rates of patency compared with angioplasty alone.[144] In 1 series in which patients with BCS underwent stenting of the HVC, IVC, or both structures, 90.9% of HV stents and 96.7% of IVC stents remained open at a mean follow-up of 45 months to 49 months.[145] Another study focusing on patients who underwent catheter aspiration of the thrombus with recanalization of the IVC using angioplasty with or without stenting revealed that patency rates at 1 year and 5 years were 93.6% and 83.2%, respectively.[146] A recently published randomized trial comparing 45 patients with BCS who received angioplasty alone versus 43 who received angioplasty and routine stent revealed that patients in the stenting group achieved superior stenosis-free vascular patency compared with angioplasty alone (98% vs 60%, respectively) within 27 months of follow-up.[147] Survival rates without re-stenosis at 3 years were 90% and 60.4%, respectively, in those with angioplasty plus stenting compared with angioplasty alone.[147]

Local thrombolysis using streptokinase or urokinase has been combined with angioplasty in rare cases with variable effect,[121,128,135,142,148] although it has been associated with a high rate of major bleeding. In a series of 12 patients treated with local thrombolytic therapy, 50% developed major procedure-related bleeding.[149] The presence of acute, extensive, multivessel splanchnic vein thrombosis was associated with the development of procedure-related bleeding.[149] Benefits from locally delivered thrombolysis may be limited to situations in which acute recurrent thrombi occur after endovascular procedures.[121]

An uncommon but well-recognized complication of percutaneous balloon angioplasty in patients with BCS is the development of pulmonary embolism.[150] The risk of pulmonary embolism increases in patients with large clot burdens affecting the IVC.[150] Pretreatment with warfarin with a goal INR between 2 and 3 prior to balloon angioplasty in order to facilitate stabilization and reduction of thrombus size prior to the procedure was effective in improving the symptoms of portal hypertension and reduced the incidence of pulmonary embolism in a series of 16 patients with a median follow-up of 40 months.[150] Continuation of anticoagulants after percutaneous intervention is recommended to reduce the likelihood of recurrent thrombosis and to preserve stent patency.[145,151,152] A recent study comparing warfarin to dabigatran found no significant difference in stent patency at 12 months.[153]

Transjugular Intrahepatic Portosystemic Shunt

Surgical shunts have become less common with the advent of TIPSs for BCS in the 1990s, which involves placement of a portosystemic shunt between the PV and HV through a percutaneous technique with the goal of reducing the HV pressure gradient to 12 mm Hg or less.[154–157] TIPS is performed in patients who do not respond to angioplasty with or without stenting.[158] The decision to pursue TIPS prior to percutaneous recanalization depends on anatomic considerations and the degree of venous obstruction.[159] A study of 15 patients with BCS who underwent TIPS revealed that although all patients with chronic BCS experienced improvement in ascites and liver chemistries, half of those with acute liver failure died soon after placement of the TIPS.[160] In another study of 14 patients who were treated with TIPS for BCS, all but 1 patient survived at a median follow-up time of 50 months, and none received subsequent liver transplantation.[161] A retrospective cohort study of 51 patients with BCS who underwent TIPS at a Chinese center revealed that survival rates at 1 year, 2 years, and 3 years were 83.8%, 81.2%, and 76.9%, respectively.[162] A similar analysis in an Indian cohort revealed survival rates of 93%, 89% and 84% at 1 year, 3 years, and 5 years, respectively.[163] A recent study reporting long-term outcomes in patients with BCS who underwent TIPS reveal transplant-free survival rates of 86%, 81%, and 76% at 1 year, 5 years and 10 years, respectively.[164]

TIPS is associated with several possible complications. In 1 study, 26% experienced periprocedural complications, including biliary puncture, intra-abdominal bleeding, acute TIPS thrombosis, and cardiopulmonary abnormalities.[155] Furthermore, 32% had early postprocedural complications within 1 week of TIPS placement, including subcapsular hematoma, intra-abdominal bleeding, acute TIPS thrombosis, or abnormal TIPS positioning.[155] Rates of hepatic encephalopathy after TIPS vary and in 1 analysis, 91%, 86%, and 86% of patients were unaffected by encephalopathy at 1 year, 3 years, and 5 years, respectively, after TIPS for BCS.[163]

Shunt dysfunction is common in patients who receive TIPS for BCS. In a study of 91 patients who underwent TIPS for acute or subacute BCS, improvement in liver chemistries and clinical symptoms, such as ascites, were noted,[165] although associated with shunt dysfunction in 11% of patients at 5 years postprocedure.[165] Another study of 54 patients who underwent TIPS for BCS revealed shunt dysfunction requiring TIPS revision in 42% of patients, within a mean follow-up time of 56 months.[155] Stents covered with polytetrafluoroethylene (PTFE) have been shown to have lower rates of dysfunction compared with bare stents.[166–168] A small study in which patients who received PTFE-covered stents compared with bare stents revealed that dysfunction occurred in 33% and 87% of cases, respectively, within a median follow-up period of 20.4 months.[169] A multicenter study of 124 consecutive patients with BCS who underwent TIPS between 1993 and 2006 revealed that transplant-free survival rates at 1 year and 5 years were 88% and 78%, respectively.[170] Although the stepwise approach to therapy in some centers has led to use of TIPSs only when medical therapy is ineffective in reversing liver dysfunction and portal hypertension, earlier consideration of TIPS may be given to reduce the risk of hepatic fibrosis that results from microvascular ischemia in ongoing HV obstruction.[171] On the other hand, endovascular approaches may yield similar outcomes with fewer complications compared with TIPSs.[172] Finally, TIPS also can be used as a bridge to liver transplantation.[173] Liver transplantation is considered in patients in whom symptoms of portal hypertension do not respond to TIPS placement.[170]

Surgery

Surgical options that involve the creation of a portosystemic shunt include side-to-side portacaval shunt and combined side-to-side portacaval and cavoatrial shunt.[174] The type of procedure that is performed depends on the pattern and location of venous occlusion. Such surgical procedures are less common with the more widespread use of TIPSs and endovascular therapies. Additional work-up, including angiography and portacaval venous pressure gradient measurements, are used to determine whether portacaval shunting is feasible.[31,174]

Early side-to-side portacaval shunt has been effective in patients with BCS, resulting from isolated HV thrombosis. In patients with concomitant obstruction of the vena cava, combined portacaval and cavoatrial shunt has been recommended.[175] Mesoatrial shunts were previously offered in this latter group, although associated with a higher rate of failure.[174,176,177] Portal decompression with these methods may prevent further hepatic decompensation and reduce the need for liver transplantation.[175] A series comparing outcomes in a series of patients who underwent surgical shunting revealed that patients had a 30-day survival rate of 97% to 100% and long-term survival rate of 95% to 100% at a mean follow-up time of 10 years to 15 years.[174] In another study, patients who underwent surgical shunting had an overall survival rates of 82%, 69%, and 62% at 1 year, 5 years, and 10 years, respectively.[178] Patients with the most favorable outcomes appeared to have intermediate prognosis at presentation based on symptoms and laboratory findings.[178] The types of shunts performed in this group were predominantly mesocaval shunts and less commonly portocaval shunts, mesoatrial shunts, mesoinnominate shunts, splenorenal shunts, cavoatrial shunts, and portoatrial shunts.[178] Shunt dysfunction increases the risk of refractory ascites, portal hypertensive bleeding, hepatic encephalopathy, progression of liver disease, and death.[179] Postprocedural anticoagulation is recommended to mitigate the risk of recurrent thrombosis.[180,181]

Surgical recanalization is performed more commonly in patients with occlusion involving the IVC and/or disruption of obstructing membranes or reconstruction of the IVC.[182] A study of thrombectomy and patch graft of the IVC revealed 5-year and 10 year survival rates of 89% and 70%, respectively.[129] A recent study describing open radical reconstruction of the HV and IVC using venovenous bypass in 83 patients revealed technical success in 96% of patients and survival rates of 91%, 90%, and 87% at 1 year, 3 years, and 5 years, respectively.[182]

Surgical approaches carry greater procedural risks than staged percutaneous therapy.[183] As experience with percutaneous and minimally invasive endovascular therapies has evolved, surgical shunting may become less common. A recent meta-analysis of pooled data of 2255 patients with BCS revealed that minimally invasive interventions using angioplasty, stenting, or TIPS were achieved successfully in 93.7% of patients, with mean survival rates of 92% and 76.4% at 1 year and 5 years.[184] Liver transplantation is considered when hepatic decompensation is fulminant and progressive or in cases of failure of percutaneous or surgical therapy.[180]

Liver Transplantation

Liver transplantation is considered as a last resort in cases of fulminant liver failure or decompensated cirrhosis with progressive hepatic decompensation resulting from BCS.[175,185] Although BCS is a rare indication for liver transplantation, outcomes have been favorable and have largely improved over time.[186] An analysis of data on

25 patients with underlying myeloproliferative disorder who received liver transplantation at a single center over a period of 20 years revealed 5-year patient and graft survival rates of 92% and 88%, respectively.[187] There was no significant difference in the incidence of vascular complications, such as splanchnic thrombosis, between those with and without BCS.[187] A more recent study has revealed no significant difference in long-term post-transplant survival in patients with BCS with or without underlying myeloproliferative disorder.[188] Compared with previous studies that reported 5-year patient survival rates of 65% to 71%,[189–191] recent analyses of post-transplant outcomes in patients with BCS revealed 10-year survival rates ranging between 68% and 84%.[192]

Risk factors for graft loss in patients who undergo liver transplantation for BCS include elevated bilirubin, elevated creatinine, age, hospitalization, life support, hospitalization, prior abdominal surgery or transplantation, donor age, donor death due to stroke, and prolonged cold ischemia time.[186] Life support, prior transplantation, and prolonged cold ischemia time also predict higher mortality.[186] Causes of early death after transplantation include infection, multiorgan dysfunction, graft failure, and hepatic artery thrombosis.[191]

In 1 series, 33% of patients who underwent liver transplantation for BCS developed recurrent thromboses affecting the liver.[193] The most common types of recurrent thromboses post-transplant include PV thrombosis (7%), HV thrombosis (2.4%), and thrombosis of the vena cava (2%).[191] In another small cohort of 11 patients, 3 suffered from recurrent BCS after transplantation, 3 developed other thromboembolic complications (eg, splenic vein thrombosis, PV thrombosis, and pulmonary embolism), and 4 experienced severe intra-abdominal bleeding.[189] The presence of the JAK2 V617F mutation is associated with a greater risk of thrombosis after liver transplantation.[193] Therefore, in patients with underlying myeloproliferative disorders, treatment with hydroxyurea and aspirin after transplantation is recommended to reduce the likelihood of recurrent thrombosis while avoiding the bleeding risk associated with anticoagulation.[187,194] Patients with other forms of hypercoagulability or unidentified precipitating factors for BCS, anticoagulation is recommended.[194] It has been reported that patients with BCS associated with PNH may be at greater risk of hematologic complications after liver transplantation, including bleeding and thrombosis.[195] A case of a patient with PNH treated with the monoclonal antibody eculizumab after liver transplantation and subsequent favorable post-transplant course provides some evidence that improved control of the underlying prothrombotic diathesis can modify post-transplant outcomes in this group.[196]

Living donor liver transplantation (LDLT) also has been successfully performed in patients with BCS.[197,198] In 1 series of patients, 39 patients treated with LDLT, only 2 developed recurrent BCS and 12 developed biliary anastomotic complications.[197]

PROGNOSIS AND LONG-TERM COMPLICATIONS

The overall in-hospital case fatality for patients with BCS is estimated at 4.9%.[14] Factors associated with mortality include male sex, increasing age, greater cardiopulmonary and metabolic comorbidities, and the presence of nonabdominal and hematologic malignancies.[14] A Swedish study reported a mortality of 44% at a median follow-up time of 2.7 years,[15] with liver failure representing the most common cause of death, followed by malignancy (eg, hepatocellular carcinoma [HCC]), gastrointestinal bleeding (eg, variceal hemorrhage), cardiac disease, pulmonary embolism, sepsis, and multiorgan failure.[15,17] Identification and treatment of the underlying cause or risk factor for BCS may be associated with improved outcomes.[199]

Patients with BCS associated with Behçet disease may experience poorer outcomes, with higher rates of acute liver failure and lower rates of survival compared with patients with BCS not associated with Behçet disease.[88,89] Furthermore, the prognosis of patients with BCS associated with myeloproliferative disorders often is driven by the underlying hematologic disorder.[200] In addition, patients with extensive splanchnic venous thromboses beyond HV thrombosis alone also may experience poorer outcomes. One report revealed a median survival of 1 month in patients with HV thrombosis combined with PV, splenic vein, superior mesenteric vein, or IVC thrombosis versus 6.3 years in patients with isolated HV thrombosis.[201]

Among patients who develop acute liver failure due to BCS, in-hospital mortality can be as high as 60%, although survival has improved over the past decade with the use of TIPSs and liver transplantation.[30] A review of 157 cases of BCS in Europe over a median follow-up period of 50 months revealed that 56% of patients required an invasive intervention, such as angioplasty, thrombolysis, TIPs, or liver transplantation.[202] A stepwise approach to treatment beginning with anticoagulation and medical therapy followed by progressive implementation of invasive techniques (percutaneous angioplasty, TIPSs, and surgical shunting) has improved the 5-year transplant-free survival and overall survival rates to 70% and 90%, respectively,[113,202,203] and 10-year survival rate of patients with BCS treated with a multimodal stepwise therapy at a Belgian center was 90%.[115]

In a large study of patients with BCS in China, recurrent disease occurred in 42% of patients at 5 years. Risk factors that increased the likelihood of recurrence included age less than 30 years, elevated lactate dehydrogenase, and advanced liver disease (CTP classes B and C).[204] In a retrospective study of 219 patients with BCS involving the IVC and requiring endovascular therapy and stenting, 28 developed recurrent disease,[205] largely due to stent thrombosis, obstruction above the stent, and HV obstruction exacerbated by stenting. Key risk factors for recurrence included younger age, advanced CTP score, higher Model for End-stage Liver Disease (MELD) score and higher total bilirubin.[205] Although rare, chronic BCS can lead to cirrhosis and is characterized by severe portal hypertension despite preserved liver synthetic function.[206]

Multiple prognostic models have been developed to predict outcomes in patients with BCS.[207,208] Although the MELD score provides valuable prognostic information in patients with cirrhosis, its performance in patients with primary BCS is comparatively poor due to its reliance on markers of hepatic synthetic function rather than manifestations of portal hypertension.[209] Nonetheless, a MELD score above 20 or CTP class C has been associated with increased 3-month mortality.[210] Other factors that affect prognosis include age, presence of ascites, creatinine, and features suggesting acute on chronic liver injury[211] as well as therapeutic response to diuretics.[208] The Rotterdam score, which takes into account the presence of ascites, encephalopathy, prothrombin time, and bilirubin, has been shown to reliably predict mortality at 3 months,[210] with Rotterdam score greater than 1.5 associated with 89% sensitivity and 63% specificity.[210] Whereas the Rotterdam score has been validated to predict intervention-free survival, the BCS-TIPS prognostic index score, which takes into account age, bilirubin, and INR, has been developed more recently to predict overall survival and performs similarly.[170,202] Furthermore, alanine aminotransferase (ALT) scores greater than 5 times the upper limit of normal are correlated with increased severity of liver disease and hepatocyte necrosis at presentation,[212] with greater likelihood of survival observed in those who experienced a decline in ALT by more than 50% within 3 days compared with those with slower ALT decline.[212]

HCC is a known complication of BCS-associated cirrhosis, with reported incidence rates similar to other etiologies of cirrhosis. A Japanese study revealed that HCC

Table 2
Society guidelines for the management of Budd-Chiari syndrome

AASLD guidelines[1]	Diagnostic work-up • Use ultrasound, CT, or MRI to rule out compressive lesions • Assess for prothrombotic risk factors, such as inherited and acquired thrombophilia, noting that multiple risk factors often are present and the discovery of a single risk factor should not preclude testing for others. • Assess for comorbidities that may increase risk of thrombosis. Therapy • Address underlying prothrombotic risk factors. • Begin anticoagulation immediately with LMWH titrated to anti-Xa activity of 0.5–0.8 IU/mL and transition to vitamin K antagonist with goal INR 2–3. • Indefinite anticoagulation unless contraindication exists. • Assess for and treat complications of portal hypertension. • Consider percutaneous angioplasty and stenting if feasible and appropriate based on nature of obstruction. • Consider TIPS in patients who do not improve with anticoagulation and/or angioplasty with stenting. • Collaborate with transplant center and consider liver transplantation in fulminant liver failure or progressive disease despite less-invasive therapies. • Monitor for development of HCC or progression of underlying disease if myeloproliferative disorder is identified.
EASL guidelines[2]	Diagnostic work-up • Consider BCS in all patients with acute or chronic liver disease. • Confirm diagnosis with Doppler ultrasound; confirm with CT or MRI, if indicated; and review radiology with expert radiologists. • Refer patients to expert tertiary care centers. • Rule out local precipitants of BCS, including intra-abdominal infection or thrombosis. • Assess for underlying prothrombotic risk factors, including inherited and acquired thrombophilias, such as myeloproliferative disorders, protein C or S deficiency, antithrombin deficiency, factor V Leiden mutation, prothrombin gene mutation, antiphospholipid syndrome, and PNH. • Testing for myeloproliferative disorders includes JAK2 V617F mutation testing initially, then CALR mutation testing if negative, and then bone marrow biopsy if both are negative in collaboration with hematology colleagues. Therapy • Treat underlying prothrombotic conditions. • Treat complications of portal hypertension. • Initiate indefinite anticoagulation with brief interruptions for invasive procedures. • Consider stepwise approach to treatment beginning with medical therapy and progressing sequentially to angioplasty with or without stenting and local thrombolysis, then TIPS using PTFE-covered stents, and then liver transplantation. • Closely monitor for clinical deterioration in order to escalate therapy as indicated. • Screen for HCC.

Adapted from DeLeve LD, Valla DC, Garcia-Tsao G, American Association for the Study Liver D. Vascular disorders of the liver. *Hepatology.* 2009;49(5):1729-1764; and European Association for the Study of the Liver. Electronic address eee. EASL Clinical Practice Guidelines: Vascular diseases of the liver. *J Hepatol.* 2016;64(1):179-202; with permission.

occurred in 6.4% of patients with BCS over a span of 15 years.[17] A South Korean study reported an annual HCC incidence of 2.8%.[213] In a series of 97 consecutive patients with BCS, liver nodules were discovered in 43 patients of whom HCC occurred in 11 cases,[214] with histologic cirrhosis identified on background liver biopsy in 9 of the 11 cases.[214] Risk factors associated with HCC include male sex, obstruction of the IVC and presence of factor V Leiden.[214] In another series, the cumulative incidence of HCC was 3.5% at 10 years, with cirrhosis and IVC thrombosis identified as risk factors.[215] A meta-analysis assessing the overall prevalence of HCC revealed a pooled prevalence of HCC of 15.4% among patients with BCS.[216]

Regenerative nodules are known to develop over time and may be difficult to differentiate from HCC.[217,218] The number of nodules may grow over time and some may develop a central scar.[219] Use of contrast-enhanced ultrasound or cross-sectional imaging with a liver protocol may differentiate types of nodules.[217,220] Hepatocellular adenomas also can occur and are associated with a risk for malignant transformation.[221] α-Fetoprotein levels above 15 ng/mL have been shown to differentiate HCC from benign nodules, with a positive predictive value of 100% and a negative predictive value of 91%.[214]

For women of child-bearing age with a history of BCS who are planning pregnancy, optimization of liver disease and portal hypertension is encouraged prior to gestation.[222,223] Patients should be screened for esophageal varices and prophylaxis should be initiated if otherwise indicated.[222] Anticoagulation with LWMH is especially important during and after pregnancy due to the higher risk of thrombosis, and involvement of a high-risk pregnancy team is advised.[222] In 1 series reporting the experience of 7 women with BCS who became pregnant and were treated with anticoagulation, 2 women were noted to have multiple fetal losses prior to 20 weeks' gestation.[224] There were 16 total pregnancies among the 7 women and, of these, 1 infant was delivered at 27 weeks whereas 9 infants were delivered at 32 weeks.[224] Fetuses carried beyond 20 weeks gestation are more likely to have a favorable outcome.[223,224]

SUMMARY

BCS is a rare entity characterized by obstruction of the HV outflow tract due to the presence of thrombosis, membranous change, or external compression and mass effect by tumor, infectious collections, or postsurgical changes.[3–5] Primary BCS resulting from venous thrombosis often occurs in the setting of multiple prothrombotic risk factors.[7] The presentation of BCS is heterogeneous, with variability in severity, onset, and chronicity of symptoms as well as laboratory parameters.[3] Management often requires a multidisciplinary, individualized, stepwise approach and includes anticoagulation, medical management, and optimization of complications of portal hypertension and treatment of underlying prothrombotic conditions as well as efforts to achieve venous recanalization or mechanical decompression using endovascular therapies, TIPSs, or surgical shunting[8] (**Table 2**). Liver transplantation is a salvage option for individuals with fulminant liver failure without response to medical therapy or persistent or progressive hepatic decompensation despite attempts at endovascular recanalization or surgical shunting.[185] Identification of BCS requires a high index of suspicion and should be considered when patients present with characteristic features, including ascites, hepatomegaly, or caudate lobe enlargement; prompt identification is key to appropriate management of this life-threatening condition.[6,7]

DISCLOSURE

The authors have no relevant disclosures.

REFERENCES

1. Budd G. On diseases of the liver. 1st edition. London: J. Churchill; 1845.
2. Chiari H. Ueber die selbstandige Phlebitis obliterans der Hauptstamme der Venae hepaticae als Todesursache. Beitr Pathol Anat 1899;26:1–18.
3. DeLeve LD, Valla DC, Garcia-Tsao G, American Association for the Study Liver Disease. Vascular disorders of the liver. Hepatology 2009;49(5):1729–64.
4. European Association for the Study of the Liver. Electronic address eee. EASL clinical Practice Guidelines: vascular diseases of the liver. J Hepatol 2016; 64(1):179–202.
5. de Franchis R, Baveno VIF. Expanding consensus in portal hypertension: report of the Baveno VI Consensus Workshop: stratifying risk and individualizing care for portal hypertension. J Hepatol 2015;63(3):743–52.
6. Hernandez-Gea V, De Gottardi A, Leebeek FWG, et al. Current knowledge in pathophysiology and management of Budd-Chiari syndrome and non-cirrhotic non-tumoral splanchnic vein thrombosis. J Hepatol 2019;71(1):175–99.
7. Valla DC. Budd-Chiari syndrome/hepatic venous outflow tract obstruction. Hepatol Int 2018;12(Suppl 1):168–80.
8. Khan F, Armstrong MJ, Mehrzad H, et al. Review article: a multidisciplinary approach to the diagnosis and management of Budd-Chiari syndrome. Aliment Pharmacol Ther 2019;49(7):840–63.
9. Valla D, Le MG, Poynard T, et al. Risk of hepatic vein thrombosis in relation to recent use of oral contraceptives. A case-control study. Gastroenterology 1986;90(4):807–11.
10. Zanetto A, Pellone M, Senzolo M. Milestones in the discovery of Budd-Chiari syndrome. Liver Int 2019;39(7):1180–5.
11. Mancuso A. Limits of evidence based medicine for rare diseases: the case of budd-chiari syndrome. Dig Liver Dis 2016;48(6):689.
12. Li Y, De Stefano V, Li H, et al. Epidemiology of Budd-Chiari syndrome: a systematic review and meta-analysis. Clin Res Hepatol Gastroenterol 2019;43(4): 468–74.
13. Ollivier-Hourmand I, Allaire M, Goutte N, et al. The epidemiology of Budd-Chiari syndrome in France. Dig Liver Dis 2018;50(9):931–7.
14. Ageno W, Dentali F, Pomero F, et al. Incidence rates and case fatality rates of portal vein thrombosis and Budd-Chiari Syndrome. Thromb Haemost 2017; 117(4):794–800.
15. Rajani R, Melin T, Bjornsson E, et al. Budd-Chiari syndrome in Sweden: epidemiology, clinical characteristics and survival - an 18-year experience. Liver Int 2009;29(2):253–9.
16. Shrestha SM, Okuda K, Uchida T, et al. Endemicity and clinical picture of liver disease due to obstruction of the hepatic portion of the inferior vena cava in Nepal. J Gastroenterol Hepatol 1996;11(2):170–9.
17. Okuda H, Yamagata H, Obata H, et al. Epidemiological and clinical features of Budd-Chiari syndrome in Japan. J Hepatol 1995;22(1):1–9.
18. Ki M, Choi HY, Kim KA, et al. Incidence, prevalence and complications of Budd-Chiari syndrome in South Korea: a nationwide, population-based study. Liver Int 2016;36(7):1067–73.
19. Mancuso A. Budd-Chiari syndrome in the West and the East: same syndrome, different diseases. Liver Int 2019;39(12):2417.

20. Zhang W, Qi X, Zhang X, et al. Budd-Chiari syndrome in China: a systematic analysis of epidemiological features based on the Chinese literature survey. Gastroenterol Res Pract 2015;2015:738548.
21. Heit JA. Epidemiology of venous thromboembolism. Nat Rev Cardiol 2015;12(8):464–74.
22. Nobre S, Khanna R, Bab N, et al. Primary budd-chiari syndrome in children: King's College hospital experience. J Pediatr Gastroenterol Nutr 2017;65(1):93–6.
23. Amarapurkar DN, Punamiya SJ, Patel ND. Changing spectrum of Budd-Chiari syndrome in India with special reference to non-surgical treatment. World J Gastroenterol 2008;14(2):278–85.
24. Eapen CE, Mammen T, Moses V, et al. Changing profile of budd chiari syndrome in India. Indian J Gastroenterol 2007;26(2):77–81.
25. Qi X, Guo X, Fan D. Difference in budd-chiari syndrome between the West and China. Hepatology 2015;62(2):656.
26. Okuda K. Inferior vena cava thrombosis at its hepatic portion (obliterative hepatocavopathy). Semin Liver Dis 2002;22(1):15–26.
27. Qi X, Han G, Guo X, et al. Review article: the aetiology of primary Budd-Chiari syndrome - differences between the West and China. Aliment Pharmacol Ther 2016;44(11–12):1152–67.
28. Cheng D, Xu H, Lu ZJ, et al. Clinical features and etiology of Budd-Chiari syndrome in Chinese patients: a single-center study. J Gastroenterol Hepatol 2013;28(6):1061–7.
29. Bhatt P, Gupta DK, Agrawal D, et al. Budd-Chiari syndrome with spontaneous intrahepatic portosystemic shunts: a case series. J Clin Exp Hepatol 2019;9(3):412–5.
30. Parekh J, Matei VM, Canas-Coto A, et al. Acute Liver Failure Study G. Budd-chiari syndrome causing acute liver failure: a multicenter case series. Liver Transpl 2017;23(2):135–42.
31. Menon KV, Shah V, Kamath PS. The Budd-Chiari syndrome. N Engl J Med 2004;350(6):578–85.
32. Dilawari JB, Bambery P, Chawla Y, et al. Hepatic outflow obstruction (Budd-Chiari syndrome). Experience with 177 patients and a review of the literature. Medicine (Baltimore) 1994;73(1):21–36.
33. Qi X, Han G. Images in clinical medicine. Abdominal-wall varices in the Budd-Chiari syndrome. N Engl J Med 2014;370(19):1829.
34. Qi X, Han G. Leg ulcer in budd-chiari syndrome. Am J Gastroenterol 2016;111(1):25.
35. Sakr M, Barakat E, Abdelhakam S, et al. Epidemiological aspects of Budd-Chiari in Egyptian patients: a single-center study. World J Gastroenterol 2011;17(42):4704–10.
36. Bansal V, Gupta P, Sinha S, et al. Budd-Chiari syndrome: imaging review. Br J Radiol 2018;91(1092):20180441.
37. Cheng D, Xu H, Hua R, et al. Comparative study of MRI manifestations of acute and chronic Budd-Chiari syndrome. Abdom Imaging 2015;40(1):76–84.
38. Erden A. Budd-Chiari syndrome: a review of imaging findings. Eur J Radiol 2007;61(1):44–56.
39. Bargallo X, Gilabert R, Nicolau C, et al. Sonography of the caudate vein: value in diagnosing Budd-Chiari syndrome. AJR Am J Roentgenol 2003;181(6):1641–5.
40. Brancatelli G, Vilgrain V, Federle MP, et al. Budd-Chiari syndrome: spectrum of imaging findings. AJR Am J Roentgenol 2007;188(2):W168–76.

41. Chaubal N, Dighe M, Hanchate V, et al. Sonography in budd-chiari syndrome. J Ultrasound Med 2006;25(3):373–9.
42. Lupescu IG, Dobromir C, Popa GA, et al. Spiral computed tomography and magnetic resonance angiography evaluation in Budd-Chiari syndrome. J Gastrointestin Liver Dis 2008;17(2):223–6.
43. Kamath PS. Budd-Chiari syndrome: radiologic findings. Liver Transpl 2006; 12(11 Suppl 2):S21–2.
44. Miller WJ, Federle MP, Straub WH, et al. Budd-Chiari syndrome: imaging with pathologic correlation. Abdom Imaging 1993;18(4):329–35.
45. Cazals-Hatem D, Vilgrain V, Genin P, et al. Arterial and portal circulation and parenchymal changes in Budd-Chiari syndrome: a study in 17 explanted livers. Hepatology 2003;37(3):510–9.
46. Riggio O, Marzano C, Papa A, et al. Small hepatic veins Budd-Chiari syndrome. J Thromb Thrombolysis 2014;37(4):536–9.
47. Tanaka M, Wanless IR. Pathology of the liver in Budd-Chiari syndrome: portal vein thrombosis and the histogenesis of veno-centric cirrhosis, veno-portal cirrhosis, and large regenerative nodules. Hepatology 1998;27(2):488–96.
48. Tang TJ, Batts KP, de Groen PC, et al. The prognostic value of histology in the assessment of patients with Budd-Chiari syndrome. J Hepatol 2001;35(3): 338–43.
49. Denninger MH, Chait Y, Casadevall N, et al. Cause of portal or hepatic venous thrombosis in adults: the role of multiple concurrent factors. Hepatology 2000; 31(3):587–91.
50. Primignani M, Mannucci PM. The role of thrombophilia in splanchnic vein thrombosis. Semin Liver Dis 2008;28(3):293–301.
51. Darwish Murad S, Plessier A, Hernandez-Guerra M, et al. Etiology, management, and outcome of the Budd-Chiari syndrome. Ann Intern Med 2009; 151(3):167–75.
52. Darwish Murad S, Valla DC, de Groen PC, et al. Pathogenesis and treatment of Budd-Chiari syndrome combined with portal vein thrombosis. Am J Gastroenterol 2006;101(1):83–90.
53. Hoekstra J, Guimaraes AH, Leebeek FW, et al. Impaired fibrinolysis as a risk factor for Budd-Chiari syndrome. Blood 2010;115(2):388–95.
54. Hernandez-Guerra M, Lopez E, Bellot P, et al. Systemic hemodynamics, vasoactive systems, and plasma volume in patients with severe Budd-Chiari syndrome. Hepatology 2006;43(1):27–33.
55. Campbell PJ, Green AR. The myeloproliferative disorders. N Engl J Med 2006; 355(23):2452–66.
56. De Stefano V, Fiorini A, Rossi E, et al. Incidence of the JAK2 V617F mutation among patients with splanchnic or cerebral venous thrombosis and without overt chronic myeloproliferative disorders. J Thromb Haemost 2007;5(4): 708–14.
57. McMahon C, Abu-Elmagd K, Bontempo FA, et al. JAK2 V617F mutation in patients with catastrophic intra-abdominal thromboses. Am J Clin Pathol 2007; 127(5):736–43.
58. Primignani M, Barosi G, Bergamaschi G, et al. Role of the JAK2 mutation in the diagnosis of chronic myeloproliferative disorders in splanchnic vein thrombosis. Hepatology 2006;44(6):1528–34.
59. Patel RK, Lea NC, Heneghan MA, et al. Prevalence of the activating JAK2 tyrosine kinase mutation V617F in the Budd-Chiari syndrome. Gastroenterology 2006;130(7):2031–8.

60. Marchetti M, Castoldi E, Spronk HM, et al. Thrombin generation and activated protein C resistance in patients with essential thrombocythemia and polycythemia vera. Blood 2008;112(10):4061–8.
61. How J, Zhou A, Oh ST. Splanchnic vein thrombosis in myeloproliferative neoplasms: pathophysiology and molecular mechanisms of disease. Ther Adv Hematol 2017;8(3):107–18.
62. Karakose S, Oruc N, Zengin M, et al. Diagnostic value of the JAK2 V617F mutation for latent chronic myeloproliferative disorders in patients with Budd-Chiari syndrome and/or portal vein thrombosis. Turk J Gastroenterol 2015;26(1):42–8.
63. Afredj N, Guessab N, Nani A, et al. Aetiological factors of Budd-Chiari syndrome in Algeria. World J Hepatol 2015;7(6):903–9.
64. Qi X, Zhang C, Han G, et al. Prevalence of the JAK2V617F mutation in Chinese patients with Budd-Chiari syndrome and portal vein thrombosis: a prospective study. J Gastroenterol Hepatol 2012;27(6):1036–43.
65. Smalberg JH, Koehler E, Darwish Murad S, et al. The JAK2 46/1 haplotype in Budd-Chiari syndrome and portal vein thrombosis. Blood 2011;117(15): 3968–73.
66. Klampfl T, Gisslinger H, Harutyunyan AS, et al. Somatic mutations of calreticulin in myeloproliferative neoplasms. N Engl J Med 2013;369(25):2379–90.
67. Jain A, Tibdewal P, Shukla A. Calreticulin mutations and their importance in Budd-Chiari syndrome. J Hepatol 2017;67(5):1111–2.
68. Nangalia J, Massie CE, Baxter EJ, et al. Somatic CALR mutations in myeloproliferative neoplasms with nonmutated JAK2. N Engl J Med 2013;369(25): 2391–405.
69. Poisson J, Plessier A, Kiladjian JJ, et al. Selective testing for calreticulin gene mutations in patients with splanchnic vein thrombosis: a prospective cohort study. J Hepatol 2017;67(3):501–7.
70. Plompen EP, Valk PJ, Chu I, et al. Somatic calreticulin mutations in patients with Budd-Chiari syndrome and portal vein thrombosis. Haematologica 2015;100(6): e226–8.
71. Turon F, Cervantes F, Colomer D, et al. Role of calreticulin mutations in the aetiological diagnosis of splanchnic vein thrombosis. J Hepatol 2015;62(1):72–4.
72. Li M, De Stefano V, Song T, et al. Prevalence of CALR mutations in splanchnic vein thrombosis: a systematic review and meta-analysis. Thromb Res 2018; 167:96–103.
73. Briere JB. Budd-Chiari syndrome and portal vein thrombosis associated with myeloproliferative disorders: diagnosis and management. Semin Thromb Hemost 2006;32(3):208–18.
74. Chait Y, Condat B, Cazals-Hatem D, et al. Relevance of the criteria commonly used to diagnose myeloproliferative disorder in patients with splanchnic vein thrombosis. Br J Haematol 2005;129(4):553–60.
75. Smalberg JH, Arends LR, Valla DC, et al. Myeloproliferative neoplasms in Budd-Chiari syndrome and portal vein thrombosis: a meta-analysis. Blood 2012; 120(25):4921–8.
76. De Stefano V, Vannucchi AM, Ruggeri M, et al. Splanchnic vein thrombosis in myeloproliferative neoplasms: risk factors for recurrences in a cohort of 181 patients. Blood Cancer J 2016;6(11):e493.
77. Janssen HL, Meinardi JR, Vleggaar FP, et al. Factor V Leiden mutation, prothrombin gene mutation, and deficiencies in coagulation inhibitors associated with Budd-Chiari syndrome and portal vein thrombosis: results of a case-control study. Blood 2000;96(7):2364–8.

78. Zhang P, Zhang J, Sun G, et al. Risk of Budd-Chiari syndrome associated with factor V Leiden and G20210A prothrombin mutation: a meta-analysis. PLoS One 2014;9(4):e95719.

79. Deltenre P, Denninger MH, Hillaire S, et al. Factor V Leiden related budd-chiari syndrome. Gut 2001;48(2):264–8.

80. Qi X, Ren W, De Stefano V, et al. Associations of coagulation factor V Leiden and prothrombin G20210A mutations with Budd-Chiari syndrome and portal vein thrombosis: a systematic review and meta-analysis. Clin Gastroenterol Hepatol 2014;12(11):1801–12.e7.

81. Mohanty D, Shetty S, Ghosh K, et al. Hereditary thrombophilia as a cause of Budd-Chiari syndrome: a study from Western India. Hepatology 2001;34(4 Pt 1):666–70.

82. Kumar SI, Kumar A, Srivastava S, et al. Low frequency of factor V Leiden and prothrombin G20210A mutations in patients with hepatic venous outflow tract obstruction in northern India: a case-control study. Indian J Gastroenterol 2005;24(5):211–5.

83. Qi X, De Stefano V, Wang J, et al. Prevalence of inherited antithrombin, protein C, and protein S deficiencies in portal vein system thrombosis and Budd-Chiari syndrome: a systematic review and meta-analysis of observational studies. J Gastroenterol Hepatol 2013;28(3):432–42.

84. Espinosa G, Font J, Garcia-Pagan JC, et al. Budd-Chiari syndrome secondary to antiphospholipid syndrome: clinical and immunologic characteristics of 43 patients. Medicine (Baltimore) 2001;80(6):345–54.

85. Giannakopoulos B, Krilis SA. The pathogenesis of the antiphospholipid syndrome. N Engl J Med 2013;368(11):1033–44.

86. Pelletier S, Landi B, Piette JC, et al. Antiphospholipid syndrome as the second cause of non-tumorous Budd-Chiari syndrome. J Hepatol 1994;21(1):76–80.

87. Carvalho D, Oikawa F, Matsuda NM, et al. Budd-Chiari syndrome in association with Behcet's disease: review of the literature. Sao Paulo Med J 2011;129(2):107–9.

88. Bismuth E, Hadengue A, Hammel P, et al. Hepatic vein thrombosis in Behcet's disease. Hepatology 1990;11(6):969–74.

89. Desbois AC, Rautou PE, Biard L, et al. Behcet's disease in Budd-Chiari syndrome. Orphanet J Rare Dis 2014;9:104.

90. Seyahi E, Caglar E, Ugurlu S, et al. An outcome survey of 43 patients with Budd-Chiari syndrome due to Behcet's syndrome followed up at a single, dedicated center. Semin Arthritis Rheum 2015;44(5):602–9.

91. Hoekstra J, Leebeek FW, Plessier A, et al. Paroxysmal nocturnal hemoglobinuria in Budd-Chiari syndrome: findings from a cohort study. J Hepatol 2009;51(4):696–706.

92. Leibowitz AI, Hartmann RC. The Budd-Chiari syndrome and paroxysmal nocturnal haemoglobinuria. Br J Haematol 1981;48(1):1–6.

93. Qi X, He C, Han G, et al. Prevalence of paroxysmal nocturnal hemoglobinuria in Chinese patients with Budd-Chiari syndrome or portal vein thrombosis. J Gastroenterol Hepatol 2013;28(1):148–52.

94. Qi X, Wu F, Ren W, et al. Thrombotic risk factors in Chinese Budd-Chiari syndrome patients. An observational study with a systematic review of the literature. Thromb Haemost 2013;109(5):878–84.

95. Qi X, Yang Z, De Stefano V, et al. Methylenetetrahydrofolate reductase C677T gene mutation and hyperhomocysteinemia in Budd-Chiari syndrome and portal

vein thrombosis: a systematic review and meta-analysis of observational studies. Hepatol Res 2014;44(14):E480–98.

96. Iba T, Levy JH. Inflammation and thrombosis: roles of neutrophils, platelets and endothelial cells and their interactions in thrombus formation during sepsis. J Thromb Haemost 2018;16(2):231–41.

97. Shrestha SM, Shrestha S. Hepatic vena cava disease: etiologic relation to bacterial infection. Hepatol Res 2007;37(3):196–204.

98. Bureau C, Laurent J, Robic MA, et al. Central obesity is associated with noncirrhotic portal vein thrombosis. J Hepatol 2016;64(2):427–32.

99. Fontana L, Eagon JC, Trujillo ME, et al. Visceral fat adipokine secretion is associated with systemic inflammation in obese humans. Diabetes 2007;56(4):1010–3.

100. Lentz SR. Thrombosis in the setting of obesity or inflammatory bowel disease. Hematology Am Soc Hematol Educ Program 2016;2016(1):180–7.

101. Vassiliadis T, Mpoumponaris A, Giouleme O, et al. Late onset ulcerative colitis complicating a patient with Budd-Chiari syndrome: a case report and review of the literature. Eur J Gastroenterol Hepatol 2009;21(1):109–13.

102. Kochhar R, Masoodi I, Dutta U, et al. Celiac disease and Budd Chiari syndrome: report of a case with review of literature. Eur J Gastroenterol Hepatol 2009;21(9):1092–4.

103. Deniz K, Ward SC, Rosen A, et al. Budd-Chiari syndrome in sarcoidosis involving liver. Liver Int 2008;28(4):580–1.

104. Falanga A, Russo L, Milesi V, et al. Mechanisms and risk factors of thrombosis in cancer. Crit Rev Oncol Hematol 2017;118:79–83.

105. Kracht M, Becquemin JP, Anglade MC, et al. Acute Budd-Chiari syndrome secondary to leiomyosarcoma of the inferior vena cava. Ann Vasc Surg 1989;3(3):268–72.

106. Kume H, Kameyama S, Kasuya Y, et al. Surgical treatment of renal cell carcinoma associated with Budd-Chiari syndrome: report of four cases and review of the literature. Eur J Surg Oncol 1999;25(1):71–5.

107. Ren W, Li X, Jia J, et al. Prevalence of Budd-Chiari syndrome during pregnancy or puerperium: a systematic review and meta-analysis. Gastroenterol Res Pract 2015;2015:839875.

108. Khuroo MS, Datta DV. Budd-Chiari syndrome following pregnancy. Report of 16 cases, with roentgenologic, hemodynamic and histologic studies of the hepatic outflow tract. Am J Med 1980;68(1):113–21.

109. Rautou PE, Plessier A, Bernuau J, et al. Pregnancy: a risk factor for Budd-Chiari syndrome? Gut 2009;58(4):606–8.

110. Maddrey WC. Hepatic vein thrombosis (Budd Chiari syndrome): possible association with the use of oral contraceptives. Semin Liver Dis 1987;7(1):32–9.

111. Chayanupatkul M, Rhee JH, Kumar AR, et al. Tamoxifen-associated Budd-Chiari syndrome complicated by heparin-induced thrombocytopenia and thrombosis: a case report and literature review. BMJ Case Rep 2012;2012.

112. Plessier A, Rautou PE, Valla DC. Management of hepatic vascular diseases. J Hepatol 2012;56(Suppl 1):S25–38.

113. Plessier A, Sibert A, Consigny Y, et al. Aiming at minimal invasiveness as a therapeutic strategy for Budd-Chiari syndrome. Hepatology 2006;44(5):1308–16.

114. Cura M, Haskal Z, Lopera J. Diagnostic and interventional radiology for Budd-Chiari syndrome. Radiographics 2009;29(3):669–81.

115. Martens P, Maleux GA, Devos T, et al. Budd-Chiari syndrome: reassessment of a step-wise treatment strategy. Acta Gastroenterol Belg 2015;78(3):299–305.

116. Kiladjian JJ, Cervantes F, Leebeek FW, et al. The impact of JAK2 and MPL mutations on diagnosis and prognosis of splanchnic vein thrombosis: a report on 241 cases. Blood 2008;111(10):4922–9.
117. Finazzi G, De Stefano V, Barbui T. Splanchnic vein thrombosis in myeloproliferative neoplasms: treatment algorithm 2018. Blood Cancer J 2018;8(7):64.
118. Shukla A, Bhatia SJ. Outcome of patients with primary hepatic venous obstruction treated with anticoagulants alone. Indian J Gastroenterol 2010;29(1):8–11.
119. De Gottardi A, Trebicka J, Klinger C, et al. Antithrombotic treatment with direct-acting oral anticoagulants in patients with splanchnic vein thrombosis and cirrhosis. Liver Int 2017;37(5):694–9.
120. Janczak DT, Mimier MK, McBane RD, et al. Rivaroxaban and apixaban for initial treatment of acute venous thromboembolism of atypical location. Mayo Clin Proc 2018;93(1):40–7.
121. Sharma S, Texeira A, Texeira P, et al. Pharmacological thrombolysis in Budd Chiari syndrome: a single centre experience and review of the literature. J Hepatol 2004;40(1):172–80.
122. Clark PJ, Slaughter RE, Radford DJ. Systemic thrombolysis for acute, severe Budd-Chiari syndrome. J Thromb Thrombolysis 2012;34(3):410–5.
123. Rautou PE, Douarin L, Denninger MH, et al. Bleeding in patients with Budd-Chiari syndrome. J Hepatol 2011;54(1):56–63.
124. De Stefano V, Qi X, Betti S, et al. Splanchnic vein thrombosis and myeloproliferative neoplasms: molecular-driven diagnosis and long-term treatment. Thromb Haemost 2016;115(2):240–9.
125. Sarin SK, Gupta N, Jha SK, et al. Equal efficacy of endoscopic variceal ligation and propranolol in preventing variceal bleeding in patients with noncirrhotic portal hypertension. Gastroenterology 2010;139(4):1238–45.
126. Wang ZG, Zhang FJ, Yi MQ, et al. Evolution of management for Budd-Chiari syndrome: a team's view from 2564 patients. ANZ J Surg 2005;75(1–2):55–63.
127. Xue H, Li YC, Shakya P, et al. The role of intravascular intervention in the management of Budd-Chiari syndrome. Dig Dis Sci 2010;55(9):2659–63.
128. Beckett D, Olliff S. Interventional radiology in the management of Budd Chiari syndrome. Cardiovasc Intervent Radiol 2008;31(5):839–47.
129. Hidaka M, Eguchi S. Budd-Chiari syndrome: focus on surgical treatment. Hepatol Res 2017;47(2):142–8.
130. Wu T, Wang L, Xiao Q, et al. Percutaneous balloon angioplasty of inferior vena cava in Budd-Chiari syndrome-R1. Int J Cardiol 2002;83(2):175–8.
131. Yang XL, Cheng TO, Chen CR. Successful treatment by percutaneous balloon angioplasty of Budd-Chiari syndrome caused by membranous obstruction of inferior vena cava: 8-year follow-up study. J Am Coll Cardiol 1996;28(7):1720–4.
132. Zhang B, Jiang ZB, Huang MS, et al. Effects of percutaneous transhepatic interventional treatment for symptomatic Budd-Chiari syndrome secondary to hepatic venous obstruction. J Vasc Surg Venous Lymphat Disord 2013;1(4):392–9.
133. Fan X, Liu K, Che Y, et al. Good clinical outcomes in budd-chiari syndrome with hepatic vein occlusion. Dig Dis Sci 2016;61(10):3054–60.
134. Cui YF, Fu YF, Li DC, et al. Percutaneous recanalization for hepatic vein-type Budd-Chiari syndrome: long-term patency and survival. Hepatol Int 2016;10(2):363–9.
135. Mukund A, Mittal K, Mondal A, et al. Anatomic recanalization of hepatic vein and inferior vena cava versus direct intrahepatic portosystemic shunt creation in budd-chiari syndrome: overall outcome and midterm transplant-free survival. J Vasc Interv Radiol 2018;29(6):790–9.

136. Cheng DL, Xu H, Li CL, et al. Interventional treatment strategy for primary budd-chiari syndrome with both inferior vena cava and hepatic vein involvement: patients from two centers in China. Cardiovasc Intervent Radiol 2019;42(9): 1311–21.

137. Fu YF, Xu H, Zhang K, et al. Accessory hepatic vein recanalization for treatment of Budd-Chiari syndrome due to long-segment obstruction of the hepatic vein: initial clinical experience. Diagn Interv Radiol 2015;21(2):148–53.

138. Fu YF, Li Y, Cui YF, et al. Percutaneous recanalization for combined-type Budd-Chiari syndrome: strategy and long-term outcome. Abdom Imaging 2015;40(8): 3240–7.

139. Bi Y, Chen H, Ding P, et al. Comparison of retrievable stents and permanent stents for Budd-Chiari syndrome due to obstructive inferior vena cava. J Gastroenterol Hepatol 2018;33(12):2015–21.

140. Qiao T, Liu CJ, Liu C, et al. Interventional endovascular treatment for Budd-Chiari syndrome with long-term follow-up. Swiss Med Wkly 2005;135(21–22): 318–26.

141. Ding PX, Han XW, Liu C, et al. Long-term outcomes of individualized treatment strategy in treatment of type I Budd-Chiari syndrome in 456 patients. Liver Int 2019;39(8):1577–86.

142. Ding PX, He X, Han XW, et al. An individualised strategy and long-term outcomes of endovascular treatment of budd-chiari syndrome complicated by inferior vena cava thrombosis. Eur J Vasc Endovasc Surg 2018;55(4):545–53.

143. Fu YF, Xu H, Wu Q, et al. Combined thrombus aspiration and recanalization in treating Budd-Chiari syndrome with inferior vena cava thrombosis. Radiol Med 2015;120(12):1094–9.

144. Han G, Qi X, Zhang W, et al. Percutaneous recanalization for Budd-Chiari syndrome: an 11-year retrospective study on patency and survival in 177 Chinese patients from a single center. Radiology 2013;266(2):657–67.

145. Zhang CQ, Fu LN, Xu L, et al. Long-term effect of stent placement in 115 patients with Budd-Chiari syndrome. World J Gastroenterol 2003;9(11):2587–91.

146. Yang F, Huang PC, Yan LL, et al. Catheter aspiration with recanalization for budd-chiari syndrome with inferior vena cava thrombosis. Surg Laparosc Endosc Percutan Tech 2019;29(4):304–7.

147. Wang Q, Li K, He C, et al. Angioplasty with versus without routine stent placement for Budd-Chiari syndrome: a randomised controlled trial. Lancet Gastroenterol Hepatol 2019;4(9):686–97.

148. Greenwood LH, Yrizarry JM, Hallett JW Jr, et al. Urokinase treatment of Budd-Chiari syndrome. AJR Am J Roentgenol 1983;141(5):1057–9.

149. Smalberg JH, Spaander MV, Jie KS, et al. Risks and benefits of transcatheter thrombolytic therapy in patients with splanchnic venous thrombosis. Thromb Haemost 2008;100(6):1084–8.

150. Li T, Zhang WW, Bai W, et al. Warfarin anticoagulation before angioplasty relieves thrombus burden in Budd-Chiari syndrome caused by inferior vena cava anatomic obstruction. J Vasc Surg 2010;52(5):1242–5.

151. Sun J, Zhang Q, Xu H, et al. Clinical outcomes of warfarin anticoagulation after balloon dilation alone for the treatment of Budd-Chiari syndrome complicated by old inferior vena cava thrombosis. Ann Vasc Surg 2014;28(8):1862–8.

152. Pelage JP, Denys A, Valla D, et al. Budd-Chiari syndrome due to prothrombotic disorder: mid-term patency and efficacy of endovascular stents. Eur Radiol 2003;13(2):286–93.

153. Sharma S, Kumar R, Rout G, et al. Dabigatran as an oral anticoagulant in patients with Budd-Chiari syndrome post-percutaneous endovascular intervention. J Gastroenterol Hepatol 2020;35(4):654–62.

154. Senzolo M, Cholongitas EC, Patch D, et al. Update on the classification, assessment of prognosis and therapy of Budd-Chiari syndrome. Nat Clin Pract Gastroenterol Hepatol 2005;2(4):182–90.

155. Hayek G, Ronot M, Plessier A, et al. Long-term outcome and analysis of dysfunction of transjugular intrahepatic portosystemic shunt placement in chronic primary Budd-Chiari syndrome. Radiology 2017;283(1):280–92.

156. Ochs A, Sellinger M, Haag K, et al. Transjugular intrahepatic portosystemic stent-shunt (TIPS) in the treatment of Budd-Chiari syndrome. J Hepatol 1993; 18(2):217–25.

157. Perello A, Garcia-Pagan JC, Gilabert R, et al. TIPS is a useful long-term derivative therapy for patients with Budd-Chiari syndrome uncontrolled by medical therapy. Hepatology 2002;35(1):132–9.

158. Rathod K, Deshmukh H, Shukla A, et al. Endovascular treatment of Budd-Chiari syndrome: single center experience. J Gastroenterol Hepatol 2017;32(1): 237–43.

159. Eapen CE, Velissaris D, Heydtmann M, et al. Favourable medium term outcome following hepatic vein recanalisation and/or transjugular intrahepatic portosystemic shunt for Budd Chiari syndrome. Gut 2006;55(6):878–84.

160. Mancuso A, Fung K, Mela M, et al. TIPS for acute and chronic Budd-Chiari syndrome: a single-centre experience. J Hepatol 2003;38(6):751–4.

161. Neumann AB, Andersen SD, Nielsen DT, et al. Treatment of Budd-Chiari syndrome with a focus on transjugular intrahepatic portosystemic shunt. World J Hepatol 2013;5(1):38–42.

162. Qi X, Guo W, He C, et al. Transjugular intrahepatic portosystemic shunt for Budd-Chiari syndrome: techniques, indications and results on 51 Chinese patients from a single centre. Liver Int 2014;34(8):1164–75.

163. Shalimar, Gamanagatti SR, Patel AH, et al. Long-term outcomes of transjugular intrahepatic portosystemic shunt in Indian patients with Budd-Chiari syndrome. Eur J Gastroenterol Hepatol 2017;29(10):1174–82.

164. Sonavane AD, Amarapurkar DN, Rathod KR, et al. Long term survival of patients undergoing TIPS in Budd-Chiari syndrome. J Clin Exp Hepatol 2019;9(1):56–61.

165. He F, Zhao H, Dai S, et al. Transjugular intrahepatic portosystemic shunt for Budd-Chiari syndrome with diffuse occlusion of hepatic veins. Sci Rep 2016; 6:36380.

166. Gandini R, Konda D, Simonetti G. Transjugular intrahepatic portosystemic shunt patency and clinical outcome in patients with Budd-Chiari syndrome: covered versus uncovered stents. Radiology 2006;241(1):298–305.

167. Olliff SP. Transjugular intrahepatic portosystemic shunt in the management of Budd Chiari syndrome. Eur J Gastroenterol Hepatol 2006;18(11):1151–4.

168. Tripathi D, Macnicholas R, Kothari C, et al. Good clinical outcomes following transjugular intrahepatic portosystemic stent-shunts in Budd-Chiari syndrome. Aliment Pharmacol Ther 2014;39(8):864–72.

169. Hernandez-Guerra M, Turnes J, Rubinstein P, et al. PTFE-covered stents improve TIPS patency in Budd-Chiari syndrome. Hepatology 2004;40(5): 1197–202.

170. Garcia-Pagan JC, Heydtmann M, Raffa S, et al. TIPS for Budd-Chiari syndrome: long-term results and prognostics factors in 124 patients. Gastroenterology 2008;135(3):808–15.

171. Mancuso A. Timing of transjugular intrahepatic portosystemic shunt for Budd-Chiari syndrome: an Italian hepatologist's perspective. J Transl Int Med 2017; 5(4):194–9.
172. Tripathi D, Sunderraj L, Vemala V, et al. Long-term outcomes following percutaneous hepatic vein recanalization for Budd-Chiari syndrome. Liver Int 2017; 37(1):111–20.
173. Ganger DR, Klapman JB, McDonald V, et al. Transjugular intrahepatic portosystemic shunt (TIPS) for Budd-Chiari syndrome or portal vein thrombosis: review of indications and problems. Am J Gastroenterol 1999;94(3):603–8.
174. Orloff MJ, Isenberg JI, Wheeler HO, et al. Budd-Chiari syndrome revisited: 38 years' experience with surgical portal decompression. J Gastrointest Surg 2012;16(2):286–300 [discussion: 300].
175. Orloff MJ, Daily PO, Orloff SL, et al. Surgical treatment of Budd-Chiari syndrome–when is liver transplant indicated? Transplant Proc 2001;33(1–2):1435.
176. Cameron JL, Herlong HF, Sanfey H, et al. The Budd-Chiari syndrome. Treatment by mesenteric-systemic venous shunts. Ann Surg 1983;198(3):335–46.
177. Chen H, Zhang F, Ye Y, et al. Long-term follow-up study and comparison of meso-atrial shunts and meso-cavo-atrial shunts for treatment of combined Budd-Chiari syndrome. J Surg Res 2011;168(1):162–6.
178. Darwish Murad S, Valla DC, de Groen PC, et al. Determinants of survival and the effect of portosystemic shunting in patients with Budd-Chiari syndrome. Hepatology 2004;39(2):500–8.
179. Bachet JB, Condat B, Hagege H, et al. Long-term portosystemic shunt patency as a determinant of outcome in Budd-Chiari syndrome. J Hepatol 2007; 46(1):60–8.
180. Hemming AW, Langer B, Greig P, et al. Treatment of Budd-Chiari syndrome with portosystemic shunt or liver transplantation. Am J Surg 1996;171(1):176–80 [discussion: 180–1].
181. Klein AS, Molmenti EP. Surgical treatment of Budd-Chiari syndrome. Liver Transpl 2003;9(9):891–6.
182. Li Q, Zhang T, Wang D, et al. Radical surgical treatment of Budd-Chiari syndrome through entire exposure of hepatic inferior vena cava. J Vasc Surg Venous Lymphat Disord 2019;7(1):74–81.
183. Yu C, Gao Y, Nie Z, et al. Effectiveness and postoperative prognosis of using preopening and staged percutaneous transluminal angioplasty of the inferior vena cava in treating Budd-Chiari syndrome accompanied with inferior vena cava thrombosis. Ann Vasc Surg 2019;60:52–60.
184. Zhang F, Wang C, Li Y. The outcomes of interventional treatment for Budd-Chiari syndrome: systematic review and meta-analysis. Abdom Imaging 2015;40(3): 601–8.
185. Mancuso A. Time to resize the role of liver transplant for Budd-Chiari syndrome. Liver Int 2015;35(10):2339.
186. Segev DL, Nguyen GC, Locke JE, et al. Twenty years of liver transplantation for Budd-Chiari syndrome: a national registry analysis. Liver Transpl 2007;13(9): 1285–94.
187. Chinnakotla S, Klintmalm GB, Kim P, et al. Long-term follow-up of liver transplantation for Budd-Chiari syndrome with antithrombotic therapy based on the etiology. Transplantation 2011;92(3):341–5.
188. Potthoff A, Attia D, Pischke S, et al. Long-term outcome of liver transplant patients with Budd-Chiari syndrome secondary to myeloproliferative neoplasms. Liver Int 2015;35(8):2042–9.

189. Cruz E, Ascher NL, Roberts JP, et al. High incidence of recurrence and hematologic events following liver transplantation for Budd-Chiari syndrome. Clin Transpl 2005;19(4):501–6.

190. Dogrul AB, Yankol Y, Mecit N, et al. Orthotopic liver transplant for Budd-Chiari syndrome: an analysis of 14 cases. Exp Clin Transplant 2016;14(6):641–5.

191. Mentha G, Giostra E, Majno PE, et al. Liver transplantation for Budd-Chiari syndrome: a European study on 248 patients from 51 centres. J Hepatol 2006; 44(3):520–8.

192. Ulrich F, Pratschke J, Neumann U, et al. Eighteen years of liver transplantation experience in patients with advanced Budd-Chiari syndrome. Liver Transpl 2008;14(2):144–50.

193. Westbrook RH, Lea NC, Mohamedali AM, et al. Prevalence and clinical outcomes of the 46/1 haplotype, Janus kinase 2 mutations, and ten-eleven translocation 2 mutations in Budd-Chiari syndrome and their impact on thrombotic complications post liver transplantation. Liver Transpl 2012;18(7):819–27.

194. Melear JM, Goldstein RM, Levy MF, et al. Hematologic aspects of liver transplantation for Budd-Chiari syndrome with special reference to myeloproliferative disorders. Transplantation 2002;74(8):1090–5.

195. Bahr MJ, Schubert J, Bleck JS, et al. Recurrence of Budd-Chiari syndrome after liver transplantation in paroxysmal nocturnal hemoglobinuria. Transpl Int 2003; 16(12):890–4.

196. Singer AL, Locke JE, Stewart ZA, et al. Successful liver transplantation for Budd-Chiari syndrome in a patient with paroxysmal nocturnal hemoglobinuria treated with the anti-complement antibody eculizumab. Liver Transpl 2009;15(5):540–3.

197. Ara C, Akbulut S, Ince V, et al. Living donor liver transplantation for Budd-Chiari syndrome: overcoming a troublesome situation. Medicine (Baltimore) 2016; 95(43):e5136.

198. Karaca C, Yilmaz C, Ferecov R, et al. Living-donor liver transplantation for Budd-Chiari syndrome: case series. Transplant Proc 2017;49(8):1841–7.

199. Min AD, Atillasoy EO, Schwartz ME, et al. Reassessing the role of medical therapy in the management of hepatic vein thrombosis. Liver Transpl Surg 1997; 3(4):423–9.

200. Lavu S, Szuber N, Mudireddy M, et al. Splanchnic vein thrombosis in patients with myeloproliferative neoplasms: the Mayo clinic experience with 84 consecutive cases. Am J Hematol 2018;93(3):E61–4.

201. Mahmoud AE, Helmy AS, Billingham L, et al. Poor prognosis and limited therapeutic options in patients with Budd-Chiari syndrome and portal venous system thrombosis. Eur J Gastroenterol Hepatol 1997;9(5):485–9.

202. Seijo S, Plessier A, Hoekstra J, et al. Good long-term outcome of Budd-Chiari syndrome with a step-wise management. Hepatology 2013;57(5):1962–8.

203. Akamatsu N, Sugawara Y, Kokudo N. Budd-Chiari syndrome and liver transplantation. Intractable Rare Dis Res 2015;4(1):24–32.

204. Gao X, Gui E, Lu Z, et al. Risk factors of recurrence among 471 Chinese patients with Budd-Chiari syndrome. Clin Res Hepatol Gastroenterol 2015;39(5):620–6.

205. Li WD, Yu HY, Qian AM, et al. Risk factors for and causes and treatment of recurrence of inferior vena cava type of Budd-Chiari syndrome after stenting in China: a retrospective analysis of a large cohort. Eur Radiol 2017;27(3):1227–37.

206. Lin M, Zhang F, Wang Y, et al. Liver cirrhosis caused by chronic Budd-Chiari syndrome. Medicine (Baltimore) 2017;96(34):e7425.

207. Rautou PE, Moucari R, Escolano S, et al. Prognostic indices for Budd-Chiari syndrome: valid for clinical studies but insufficient for individual management. Am J Gastroenterol 2009;104(5):1140–6.
208. Zeitoun G, Escolano S, Hadengue A, et al. Outcome of Budd-Chiari syndrome: a multivariate analysis of factors related to survival including surgical portosystemic shunting. Hepatology 1999;30(1):84–9.
209. Darwish Murad S, Kim WR, de Groen PC, et al. Can the model for end-stage liver disease be used to predict the prognosis in patients with Budd-Chiari syndrome? Liver Transpl 2007;13(6):867–74.
210. Montano-Loza AJ, Tandon P, Kneteman N, et al. Rotterdam score predicts early mortality in Budd-Chiari syndrome, and surgical shunting prolongs transplant-free survival. Aliment Pharmacol Ther 2009;30(10):1060–9.
211. Langlet P, Escolano S, Valla D, et al. Clinicopathological forms and prognostic index in Budd-Chiari syndrome. J Hepatol 2003;39(4):496–501.
212. Rautou PE, Moucari R, Cazals-Hatem D, et al. Levels and initial course of serum alanine aminotransferase can predict outcome of patients with Budd-Chiari syndrome. Clin Gastroenterol Hepatol 2009;7(11):1230–5.
213. Park H, Yoon JY, Park KH, et al. Hepatocellular carcinoma in Budd-Chiari syndrome: a single center experience with long-term follow-up in South Korea. World J Gastroenterol 2012;18(16):1946–52.
214. Moucari R, Rautou PE, Cazals-Hatem D, et al. Hepatocellular carcinoma in Budd-Chiari syndrome: characteristics and risk factors. Gut 2008;57(6):828–35.
215. Paul SB, Shalimar, Sreenivas V, et al. Incidence and risk factors of hepatocellular carcinoma in patients with hepatic venous outflow tract obstruction. Aliment Pharmacol Ther 2015;41(10):961–71.
216. Ren W, Qi X, Yang Z, et al. Prevalence and risk factors of hepatocellular carcinoma in Budd-Chiari syndrome: a systematic review. Eur J Gastroenterol Hepatol 2013;25(7):830–41.
217. Brancatelli G, Federle MP, Grazioli L, et al. Large regenerative nodules in Budd-Chiari syndrome and other vascular disorders of the liver: CT and MR imaging findings with clinicopathologic correlation. AJR Am J Roentgenol 2002;178(4):877–83.
218. de Sousa JM, Portmann B, Williams R. Nodular regenerative hyperplasia of the liver and the Budd-Chiari syndrome. Case report, review of the literature and reappraisal of pathogenesis. J Hepatol 1991;12(1):28–35.
219. Flor N, Zuin M, Brovelli F, et al. Regenerative nodules in patients with chronic Budd-Chiari syndrome: a longitudinal study using multiphase contrast-enhanced multidetector CT. Eur J Radiol 2010;73(3):588–93.
220. Zhang R, Qin S, Zhou Y, et al. Comparison of imaging characteristics between hepatic benign regenerative nodules and hepatocellular carcinomas associated with Budd-Chiari syndrome by contrast enhanced ultrasound. Eur J Radiol 2012;81(11):2984–9.
221. Sempoux C, Paradis V, Komuta M, et al. Hepatocellular nodules expressing markers of hepatocellular adenomas in Budd-Chiari syndrome and other rare hepatic vascular disorders. J Hepatol 2015;63(5):1173–80.
222. Bissonnette J, Durand F, de Raucourt E, et al. Pregnancy and vascular liver disease. J Clin Exp Hepatol 2015;5(1):41–50.
223. Rautou PE, Angermayr B, Garcia-Pagan JC, et al. Pregnancy in women with known and treated Budd-Chiari syndrome: maternal and fetal outcomes. J Hepatol 2009;51(1):47–54.
224. Khan F, Rowe I, Martin B, et al. Outcomes of pregnancy in patients with known Budd-Chiari syndrome. World J Hepatol 2017;9(21):945–52.

Alpha1-Antitrypsin Deficiency

A Cause of Chronic Liver Disease

Vignan Manne, MD[a], Kris V. Kowdley, MD, AGAF[b],*

KEYWORDS

- Alpha1-antitrypsin • Cirrhosis • *SERPINA1*

KEY POINTS

- Alpha1-antitrypsin deficiency (A1ATD) is a genetic disorder that can cause liver and lung disease that can present at any age but follows a bimodal age distribution.
- A1ATD seems to be more common than other liver diseases, such as autoimmune hepatitis or Wilson disease, but is still under-recognized.
- A1ATD has multiple alleles but the most important disease-causing genotypes are PI*ZZ and PI*SZ.
- Diagnosis of A1ATD requires measuring serum levels and the phenotype or genotype, although serum levels may be influenced by many factors and are therefore insufficient for diagnosis.
- Although no medical therapy for A1ATD-related liver disease is currently available, monitoring for complications of liver disease can be useful so diagnosis is critical.

INTRODUCTION

Alpha1-antitrypsin (A1AT) is a serum glycoprotein, encoded by the gene *SERPINA1*, that belongs to a family of proteins known as serine protease inhibitors, or serpins.[1] The major function of A1AT is to inhibit serine proteases secreted by neutrophils, such as neutrophil elastase, usually in response to inflammation.[1] The protein is produced in many cell types but principally in hepatocytes and then released into circulation where it performs its inhibitory function primarily in the blood and lungs.[1,2] A1AT deficiency (A1ATD) can lead to a constellation of disease states, with lung and liver disease being the most common.[1,2]

A1ATD is a genetic disorder caused by mutations in *SERPINA1* that lead to deficiency in the circulating levels of A1AT.[3] The decreased level of A1AT leads to unopposed proteolytic degradation of lung tissue and can cause emphysema and chronic

[a] Sunrise Health Consortium GME, 2880 North Tenaya Way, Las Vegas, NV 89128, USA; [b] 3216 Northeast 45th Place Suite 212, Seattle, WA 98105, USA
* Corresponding author.
E-mail address: kris.kowdley@swedish.org

Clin Liver Dis 24 (2020) 483–492
https://doi.org/10.1016/j.cld.2020.04.010
1089-3261/20/© 2020 Elsevier Inc. All rights reserved.

bronchitis.[1] In contrast, the accumulation of abnormal A1AT polymers in hepatocytes is the key feature associated with the development of liver disease.[2] The development of liver disease seems to be independent of lung disease.[2] A1ATD-linked chronic liver disease is a frequently unrecognized and underdiagnosed cause of chronic liver disease.[1–4] The focus of this article is to aid gastroenterologists in the diagnosis and management of A1ATD-linked chronic liver disease.

GENETICS OF ALPHA1-ANTITRYPSIN DEFICIENCY
Genotypes and Phenotypes of Alpha1-Antitrypsin Deficiency

The gene SERPINA1 is located on the long arm of chromosome 14 and is highly polymorphic with more than 100 germ-line mutations identified.[2,3,5] Despite the diversified nature of SERPINA1, the phenotypic expression of A1AT is generally in 4 different groups: normal, decreased, dysfunctional, or null variants based on circulating levels of A1AT.[2,6] The null phenotypic variant is associated with severe lung disease but not liver disease, because this variant is linked to an absence of A1AT, not just a deficiency,[2] because abnormal polymerization and accumulation of mutant A1AT is necessary to develop A1ATD-linked liver disease, which is absent in null phenotypic variants.[2,3,5,7] The dysfunctional variant has also not been associated with liver disease because, again, this variant does not seem to cause intrahepatic accumulation.[6] Therefore, A1ATD-linked liver disease has been mostly described in the decreased phenotypic variant.[2,3]

SERPINA1 is inherited in an autosomal codominant pattern, meaning that each allele plays a role in determining the final circulating levels of the protein.[3] The standard nomenclature used to describe the genotype and phenotype is denoted with the abbreviation PI (protease inhibitor), followed by the 2 alleles (ie, PI*MM). The normal wild-type allele is denominated with the letter M and the most common alleles associated with A1ATD are designated Z and S.[2] Most A1ATD-linked liver disease is seen in patients who are homozygous for the Z allele, or PI*ZZ.[1–3,5] The compound heterozygote phenotype, PI*SZ, is also implicated in A1ATD liver disease, although it is far less common.[7,8] There have been several other phenotypes associated with liver disease (**Table 1**), but these are notably rare.[7]

Compound Heterozygotes Without Alpha1-Antitrypsin Deficiency

Another phenomenon that has been well described is the association of the Z allele as a risk factor for progression of liver disease in patients with preexisting cirrhosis.[9–11] The phenotypes PI*MZ and PI*SZ are known to have decreased levels of A1AT, roughly 55% of normal and 40% of normal respectively, but may not be below the threshold used to diagnose A1ATD and therefore are not always associated with liver or lung disease.[12] Prior research seemed to show a link between heterozygosity of the Z allele increasing the risk for development of chronic liver disease,[9] but this was not borne out in follow-up studies.[10,11] Even so, data indicate that, in patients with

Table 1 Alleles associated with alpha-1 antitrypsin deficiency	
Most common disease alleles[2,7]	Z[a], S[b]
Rare disease alleles[c]	M$_{malton}$,[53] Siiyama,[54] King[55]

[a] The genotype/phenotype PI*ZZ accounts for roughly 95% of A1ATD.
[b] The genotype/phenotype PI*SZ accounts for roughly 4% of A1ATD.
[c] Rare phenotypes account for less than 1% of A1ATD.

cirrhosis from other causes, the Z allele seemed to increase the risk of liver disease progression.[10,11] A recent study conducted by Schaefer and colleagues[11] showed that patients with cirrhosis of any cause and with the PI*MZ phenotype had higher model for end-stage of liver disease (MELD) scores, were more likely to have decompensating events, and had higher rates of liver transplant or death. The implication of the Z allele in causing progression of liver disease is not entirely understood.[11] Furthermore, whether these data should lead to screening for the A1AT phenotype in patients with cirrhosis is unclear and not addressed by major guidelines.[1,12]

EPIDEMIOLOGY OF ALPHA1-ANTITRYPSIN DEFICIENCY
Prevalence of Select Alleles and Phenotypes

Data on the frequency of the myriad rare alleles are not readily available; however, several epidemiologic studies have examined the most common disease-causing alleles, Z and S, and the phenotypes PI*ZZ and PI*SZ.[13,14] Blanco and colleagues[13] compiled data from 93 countries to show that the frequency of the Z allele seems highest in countries with large white populations. More importantly, the prevalence of the PI*ZZ phenotype was noted to be from 1:2000 to 1:5000 in areas with the highest frequency of Z alleles.[13] For context, the PI*ZZ phenotype is significantly more common than other causes of liver disease, such as Wilson disease, which is noted to be close to 1:30,000 to 1:100,000,[15] or autoimmune hepatitis, with a prevalence of 1:5900 to 1:9100.[16] Furthermore, the PI*SZ phenotype seems to be even more common and not only includes white populations but also seems to include a Hispanic population, with prevalence data suggesting from 1:700 to 1:3000 have this phenotype in areas of highest allelic frequency.[14] Despite having phenotypes associated with disease, only a small proportion of patients develop chronic liver disease that can occur at any age.[2,3]

Neonatal and Pediatric Alpha1-Antitrypsin Deficiency

A1ATD-linked liver disease can present at any age and is the most common presentation in neonatal and pediatric populations because lung disease takes decades to develop.[17] Even so, not all children who have a disease-associated phenotype develop liver disease.[17] For example, a study in Sweden that identified children at birth with a phenotype that could result in A1ATD were followed up to 6 months, and liver abnormalities occurred in up to 50% of these children.[18] The liver abnormalities were variable, and ranged from mild increases in transaminase levels to neonatal jaundice up to and including significant portal hypertension and cirrhosis requiring pediatric liver transplant.[18] This same cohort was followed until age 12 years and most of the liver abnormalities among patients without cirrhosis resolved, and the overall risk of fibrosis and cirrhosis was noted to be only 2% to 3%.[19] A recent systematic review also suggested that cirrhosis develops in fewer than 10% of pediatric patients (0–18 years old) despite having an abnormal phenotype associated with A1ATD.[20] The most notable risk factors for progression of liver disease in the pediatric population were increased aspartate transaminase level, persistent or recurrent jaundice, and increased gamma-glutamyltransferase level.[20]

Adult Alpha1-Antitrypsin Deficiency

The prevalence of chronic liver disease in adults seems to mirror the prevalence in the pediatric population.[20,21] The systematic review done in children was also performed in adults and similarly noted that roughly 10% of adults with a phenotype associated with A1ATD developed complications of liver disease.[20] A newly released retrospective, longitudinal study conducted in Sweden by Tanash and Piitulainen[21] also supported this conclusion.[21] The study included more than 1500 adult patients with the PI*ZZ phenotype and found that 7% had developed cirrhosis and an additional 2% had developed hepatocellular carcinoma (HCC) over a mean follow-up of 12 years.

Risk factors for progression of liver disease in adults varied from the pediatric population.[20] The most consistent risk factors found in the review were male gender and increased body mass index.[20,22] The study by Tanash and Piitulainen[21] concurred that male gender was a risk factor for progression but also noted that age greater than 50 years and diabetes also increased the risk. This finding suggests that A1ATD-linked chronic liver disease has an aggressive and an indolent form that can appear very early in age or much later in life and is consistent with a large body of evidence that shows A1ATD has a bimodal age distribution.[20]

PATHOPHYSIOLOGY
Polymerization and Accumulation of Alpha1-Antitrypsin Deficiency

As noted earlier, the polymerization of the mutant A1AT protein is necessary for development of liver disease, whereas the absence of the protein leads to lung disease.[1–3] To form polymers, the abnormal genes first make a normal nascent protein that then is translocated to the endoplasmic reticulum (ER).[2,3] In the ER, the mutant protein, especially in the case of the Z alleles, takes longer to fold properly compared with the normal M allele[2,3] (**Fig. 1**). The inefficiently folded protein is detected by the

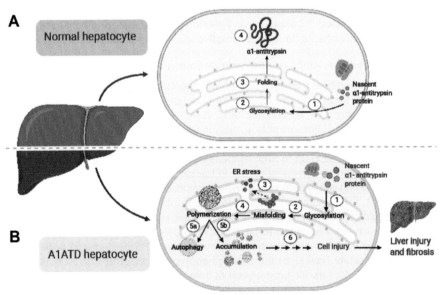

Fig. 1. Mechanism of liver injury in A1ATD. (*A*) The normal folding of the A1AT protein in the ER from (1) transport of nascent polypeptide to the ER, (2) glycosylation of the protein and entry into the ER, (3) normal folding, (4) transport of the protein out of the cell. (*B*) The abnormal nascent protein is (1) transported to the ER and (2) glycosylated. The protein undergoes abnormal folding leading to (3) ER stress and proteolytic degradation or (4) polymerization of multiple misfolded proteins. These proteins can either be further degraded by (5a) autophagy and other cellular mechanisms or (5b) continue to accumulate. The accumulation eventually leads to (6) cell injury and, thus, liver injury, fibrosis, and ultimately cirrhosis.

hepatocyte and is usually targeted for degradation, but some of the proteins escape this degradation by forming thermodynamically stable polymers with other mutant proteins.[23–25] These stable polymers can continue to accumulate and form characteristic globules that can be stained and seen under light microscopy[3] (**Fig. 2**). Other cell types can also produce the mutant A1AT and undergo the same pathophysiology as in hepatocytes, but the level of production is too low for these intracellular polymers to be seen.[26]

Rough Endoplasmic Reticulum Stress, Proteolytic Degradation, and Autophagy

The accumulation of inefficiently folded proteins and protein polymers within the ER causes ER stress.[2] The presence of ER stress activates a series of proteolytic degradation pathways[27–31] (**Fig. 1**). These pathways break down nonpolymerized mutant proteins and attempt to degrade the polymerized proteins, but not as adeptly, and variation in the efficiency of these multiple pathways is thought to be one reason for hepatocellular injury.[27,32] Another proteolytic pathway is a process known as autophagy.[33] This process involves specialized vacuoles that degrade abnormal proteins and larger structures, including large polymers of abnormal A1AT.[33–35] Experimental murine models have found that inducing autophagy may be one approach to degrade large polymers and reduce the likelihood of hepatocellular injury.[33–35]

DIAGNOSIS OF ALPHA1-ANTITRYPSIN DEFICIENCY–LINKED LIVER DISEASE
Under-Recognized Cause of Liver Disease

A1ATD is widely known to be under-recognized and underdiagnosed.[1–3,12,36] For example, the burden of A1ATD in the United States is estimated to be more than 70,000, and more than 250,000 people have the PI*ZZ and PI*SZ phenotypes, respectively.[13,14,37] Research indicates that fewer than 10% of the affected population have been diagnosed with A1ATD,[36] with the average delay in diagnosis being roughly 6 years.[38] These data are not specific to the United States and have mirrored research from other countries as well.[39]

Although it is not entirely clear why there is such a large gap in diagnosis, there are a few known problems. Awareness about A1ATD is increasing among providers but there are still several gaps in knowledge that can lead to under-recognition.[4] In addition, adherence to current guidelines may not be optimal.[39–41]

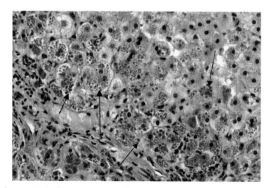

Fig. 2. Polymers of A1ATD in hepatocytes. Photomicrograph of a liver biopsy from a patient with A1ATD. The stain (*black arrows*) shows the diastase-resistant pink globules that are characteristic of this disease (periodic acid–Schiff with diastase, original magnification ×100). (*Courtesy of* Jerad M Gardner, MD.)

Screening

Current guidelines do not support screening for A1ATD in the pediatric population without overt signs of liver disease[1] because of a paucity of unbiased evidence.[1] Neonatal screening decreased long-term smoking rates in patients who tested positive for A1ATD.[42,43] Nevertheless, the cost-effectiveness of screening all newborns is unclear; therefore, it may be prudent to consider screening children who have persistent neonatal jaundice, other liver abnormalities, or parents who have been previously diagnosed with A1ATD.[17]

In adults, screening for A1ATD is supported by guidelines in all patients with unexplained increased aminotransferase levels or who have evidence of chronic liver disease.[1,12] The young adult population, between the ages of 18 and 40 years, generally do not manifest evidence of liver disease with A1ATD, but it may be useful to screen for A1ATD given that having a heterozygous phenotype with a Z allele seems to increase the risk of progression of preexisting liver disease.[10,11]

Diagnostic Studies

Diagnostic testing for A1ATD has evolved over the last few decades. Simply measuring A1AT levels is not sufficient to diagnose A1ATD.[1,12,44] A1AT is an acute phase reactant and circulating levels can vary dramatically based on genotype in acute illness.[1,44] Due to this variability, guidelines recommend adjunct testing for genotype or phenotype in addition to circulating levels.[1,44]

A routinely used test to identify the phenotype is isoelectric focusing.[12,44] This test uses speed of migration of the A1AT protein in gel electrophoresis to identify the different phenotypes.[44] Isoelectric focusing can identify the most common phenotypes, such as PI*MM or PI*ZZ, as well as some rarer phenotypes.[44] One limitation of this method is that certain rare deficient and null phenotypes have normal MM protein migration, giving discordant results, so clinical context is important when using this test.[44]

Genotyping of specific alleles can also be done using polymerase chain reaction. Because most A1ATD is seen in patients with the Z and S alleles, specific primers for these alleles have been developed for genotyping.[1] The main drawback of genotyping is the lack of primers for more rare phenotypes, although this will likely improve over time.[44] Whole-gene sequencing or expanded genotyping to test for known abnormal alleles is becoming more widely available, less expensive, and may become the standard of care for diagnosis in the future.[1,44]

Liver biopsy may also be a useful adjunct test for A1ATD, although this is not commonly recommended by guidelines.[1,12] The classic periodic acid–Schiff–positive and diastase-resistant granules of accumulated protein polymers (see **Fig. 2**) are not always seen on biopsy because of some of the granules being 1 μm or less.[12] Liver biopsy may be best used to rule out other causes of liver disease if there is uncertainty about the diagnosis.[45]

MANAGEMENT
Monitoring

Monitoring patients with A1ATD has proven benefits in patients with lung disease.[1,12,44] Its utility in patients without advanced liver disease is not well understood.[2] A study conducted by Tanash and colleagues[46] found that liver-related mortality in a Swedish population who were never-smokers was as high as 28% in adults. Most patients had passed away from complications of decompensated liver disease, with 38% having complications of HCC.[46] Of note, the rate of HCC in A1ATD is not increased compared with other causes of cirrhosis.[17,20,46] However, current guidelines recommend monitoring laboratory tests and doing an ultrasonography scan annually given the high mortality associated with development of liver disease.[1,12] An additional benefit to monitoring patients with A1ATD is to prevent the development of another cause of liver disease. Vaccinating against hepatitis A and B, moderating alcohol consumption, and minimizing the risk of metabolic diseases are reasonable recommendations as well.[2]

Medical Therapies

At present, there are no approved medical therapies for the management of A1ATD-linked liver disease.[2,3] Several therapies are currently under investigation.[2,3] One pathway that shows promise is enhancement of cellular autophagy to degrade intracellular A1AT protein polymers.[33] In murine models, the antiepileptic medication carbamazepine has been shown to be effective in augmenting this process,[34,35] and a phase 2 clinical trial is currently underway to evaluate the effect of this medication in patients with severe A1ATD-linked liver disease.[47] Another therapy that has also shown promise uses small-interfering RNAs (siRNAs) to disrupt the transcription of messenger RNA generated from the SERPINA1 gene leading to decreased levels of mutant proteins.[48] The caveat to this approach is that although it may help liver disease, it will continue to cause a deficiency of A1AT so it must be used in conjunction with other therapies to augment intravascular A1AT levels.[2]

Other potential targets include attempting to improve efficiency in folding of mutant proteins to prevent polymerization and trying to inhibit the polymerization process itself.[2] These targets are not as well studied and there is still more work needed to address the clinical application of these methods.[2]

Liver Transplant

In patients with cirrhosis and cirrhosis-related complications from A1ATD-linked liver disease, liver transplant is another potential option. Liver transplant in pediatrics for A1ATD is a common indication with excellent outcomes.[49] A 15-year follow-up study in 42 pediatric patients transplanted for A1ATD found survival to be more than 75%, which was notably better than liver transplant for biliary atresia in the same center.[49] Most deaths occurred within the first 6 months with infection, hemorrhage and graft failure being the most likely causes of death.[49]

Even in adults, liver transplant seems to have good outcomes for A1ATD-linked disease.[50] Transplant for A1ATD-linked cirrhosis accounts for only a small proportion of transplants, roughly 1%.[51] A retrospective study including 73 patients with A1ATD-linked cirrhosis from 1987 to 2012 conducted by Carey and colleagues[50] showed that the posttransplant outcomes at 1, 3, 5, and 10 years were 90%, 88%, 85%, and 78%, respectively. These results are on par with the most recent transplant outcomes for other causes of liver disease.[52] Some patients continued to have worsening lung function despite having a new liver that could produce normal A1AT.[50] The reasons for this are not yet fully understood but, overall, the use of liver transplant is a viable option for A1ATD-linked cirrhosis.

SUMMARY

A1ATD-linked liver disease is an under-recognized cause of chronic liver disease. It is hoped that improvements in education and awareness will improve diagnosis of this common disease. More work is necessary to recognize patients who are at risk earlier, especially because new and exciting therapies may be available in the near future for management of this disease.

DISCLOSURE

Nothing to disclose for V. Manne or K.V. Kowdley.

REFERENCES

1. Sandhaus RA, Turino G, Brantly ML, et al. The diagnosis and management of alpha-1 antitrypsin deficiency in the adult. Chronic Obstr Pulm Dis 2016;3(3): 668–82.
2. Greene CM, Marciniak SJ, Teckman JH, et al. α1-antitrypsin deficiency. Nat Rev Dis Primers 2016;2:16051.
3. Teckman JH, Jain A. Advances in alpha-1 antitrypsin deficiency liver disease. Curr Gastroenterol Rep 2014;16(1):367.
4. Stoller JK, Brantly M. The challenge of detecting alpha-1 antitrypsin deficiency. COPD 2013;10(Suppl 1):26–34.
5. Blanco I, de Serres FJ, Carcaba V, et al. Alpha-1 antitrypsin deficiency PI*Z and PI*S gene frequency distribution using on maps of the world by an inverse distance weighting (IDW) multivariate interpolation method. Hepat Mon 2012; 12(10 HCC):e7434.
6. Stoller JK, Aboussouan LS. A review of α1-antitrypsin deficiency. Am J Respir Crit Care Med 2012;185(3):246–59.
7. Gooptu B, Dickens JA, Lomas DA. The molecular and cellular pathology of α1-antitrypsin deficiency. Trends Mol Med 2014;20(2):116–27.
8. Mahadeva R, Chang WS, Dafforn TR, et al. Heteropolymerization of S, I, and Z alpha1-antitrypsin and liver cirrhosis. J Clin Invest 1999;103(7):999–1006.
9. Graziadei IW, Joseph JJ, Weisner RH, et al. Increased risk of chronic liver failure in adults with heterozygous alpha1-antitrypsin deficiency. Hepatology 1998;28: 1058–63.
10. Regev A, Guaqueta C, Molina EG, et al. Does the heterozygous state of alpha-1 antitrypsin deficiency have a role in chronic liver disease? Interim results of a large case-control study. J Pediatr Gastroenterol Nutr 2006;43(Suppl 1):S30–5.
11. Schaefer B, Mandorfer M, Viveiros A, et al. Heterozygosity for the alpha1-antitrypsin Z allele in cirrhosis is associated with more advanced disease. Liver Transpl 2018;24(6):744–51.
12. American Thoracic Society, European Respiratory Society. American Thoracic Society/European Respiratory Society statement: standards for the diagnosis and management of individuals with alpha-1 antitrypsin deficiency. Am J Respir Crit Care Med 2003;168(7):818–900.
13. Blanco I, Bueno P, Diego I, et al. Alpha-1 antitrypsin PI*Z gene frequency and PI*ZZ genotype numbers worldwide: an update. Int J Chron Obstruct Pulmon Dis 2017;12:561–9.
14. Blanco I, Bueno P, Diego I, et al. Alpha-1 antitrypsin Pi*SZ genotype: estimated prevalence and number of SZ subjects worldwide. Int J Chron Obstruct Pulmon Dis 2017;12:1683–94.
15. Ala A, Walker AP, Ashkan K, et al. Wilson's disease. Lancet 2007;369(9559): 397–408.
16. Heneghan MA, Yeoman AD, Verma S, et al. Autoimmune hepatitis. Lancet 2013; 382(9902):1433–44.
17. Torres-Duran M, Lopez-Campos JL, Barrecheguren M, et al. Alpha-1 antitrypsin deficiency: outstanding questions and future directions. Orphanet J Rare Dis 2018;13(1):114.

18. Sveger T. Liver disease in alpha1-antitrypsin deficiency detected by screening of 200,000 infants. N Engl J Med 1976;294(24):1316–21.
19. Sveger T. The natural history of liver disease in alpha1-antitrypsin deficient children. Acta Paediatr Scand 1988;77(6):847–51.
20. Townsend SA, Edgar RG, Ellis PR, et al. Systematic review: the natural history of alpha-1 antitrypsin deficiency, and associated liver disease. Aliment Pharmacol Ther 2018;47(7):877–85.
21. Tanash HA, Piitulainen E. Liver disease in adults with severe alpha1-antitrypsin deficiency. J Gastroenterol 2019;54(6):541–8.
22. Bowlus CL, Willner I, Zern MA, et al. Factors associated with advanced liver disease in adults with alpha1-antitrypsin deficiency. Clin Gastroenterol Hepatol 2005;3(4):390–6.
23. Lomas DA, Evans DL, Finch JT, et al. The mechanism of Z alpha 1-antitrypsin accumulation in the liver. Nature 1992;357(6379):605–7.
24. Dafforn TR, Mahadeva R, Elliot PR, et al. A kinetic mechanism for the polymerization of alpha1-antitrypsin. J Biol Chem 1999;274(14):9548–55.
25. Lomas DA, Mahadeva R. Alpha1-antitrypsin polymerization and serpinopathies: pathobiology and prospects for therapy. J Clin Invest 2002;110(11):1585–90.
26. Van't Wout EF, Dickens JA, van Schadewijk A, et al. Increased ERK signaling molecules promotes inflammatory signaling in primary airway epithelial cell expressing Z α1-antitrypsin. Hum Mol Genet 2014;23(4):929–41.
27. Cabral CM, Choudhury P, Liu Y, et al. Processing by endoplasmic reticulum mannosidases partitions a secretion-impaired glycoprotein into distinct disposal pathways. J Biol Chem 2000;275(32):25015–22.
28. Teckman JH, Burrows J, Hidvegi T, et al. The proteasome participates in degradation of mutant alpha 1- antitrypsin Z in the endoplasmic reticulum of hepatoma-derived hepatocytes. J Biol Chem 2001;276(48):44865–72.
29. Teckman JH, Perlmutter DH. Retention of mutant alpha(1)- antitrypsin Z in endoplasmic reticulum is associated with an autophagic response. Am J Physiol Gastrointest Liver Physiol 2000;279(5):G961–74.
30. Sifers RN. Cell biology. Protein degradation unlocked. Science 2003;299(5611):1330–1.
31. Qu D, Teckman JH, Omura S, et al. Degradation of a mutant secretory protein, alpha1-antitrypsin Z, in the endoplasmic reticulum requires proteasome activity. J Biol Chem 1996;271(37):22791–5.
32. Cabral CM, Liu Y, Moremen KW, et al. Organizational diversity among distinct glycoprotein endoplasmic reticulum-associated degradation programs. Mol Biol Cell 2002;13(8):2639–50.
33. Marciniak SJ, Lomas DA. Alpha1-antitrypsin deficiency and autophagy. N Engl J Med 2010;363(19):1863–4.
34. Hidvegi T, Ewing M, Hale P, et al. An autophagy-enhancing drug promotes degradation of mutant alpha1-antitrypsin Z and reduces hepatic fibrosis. Science 2010;329(5988):229–32.
35. Kaushal S, Annamali M, Blomenkamp K, et al. Rapamycin reduces intrahepatic alpha-1- antitrypsin mutant Z protein polymers and liver injury in a mouse model. Exp Biol Med (Maywood) 2010;235(6):700–9.
36. Silverman EK, Sandhaus RA. Clinical practice. Alpha1-antitrypsin deficiency. N Engl J Med 2009;360(26):2749–57.
37. Howden L, Meyer J. Age and sex composition: 2010. 2010 census briefs [Internet]. C2010BR-03. c2011. Available at: http://www.census.gov/prod/cen2010/briefs/c2010br-09.pdf. Accessed November 29, 2019.

38. Stoller JK, Sandhaus RA, Turino G, et al. Delay in diagnosis of alpha1-antitrypsin deficiency: a continuing problem. Chest 2005;128(4):1989–94.
39. Greulich T, Ottaviani S, Bals R, et al. Alpha1-antitrypsin deficiency-diagnostic testing and disease awareness in Germany and Italy. Respir Med 2013;107(9): 1400–8.
40. Rubenfeld GD, Cooper C, Carter G, et al. Barriers to providing lung-protective ventilation to patients with acute lung injury. Crit Care Med 2004;32(6):1289–93.
41. Cabana MD, Rand CS, Powe NR, et al. Why don't physicians follow clinical practice guidelines? A framework for improvement. JAMA 1999;282:1458–65.
42. Thelin T, Sveger T, Mcneil TF. Primary prevention in a high-risk group: smoking habits in adolescents with homozygous alpha-1-antitrypsin deficiency (ATD). Acta Paediatr 1996;85(10):1207–12.
43. Wall M, Moe E, Eisenberg J, et al. Long-term follow-up of a cohort of children with alpha-1-antitrypsin deficiency. J Pediatr 1990;116(2):248–51.
44. Miravitlles M, Dirksen A, Ferrarotti I, et al. European Respiratory Society statement: diagnosis and treatment of pulmonary α1-antitrypsin deficiency. Eur Respir J 2017;50(5) [pii.1700610].
45. Nelson D, Teckman J, Di Bisceglie A, et al. Diagnosis and management of patients with a1-antitrypsin (A1AT) deficiency. Clin Gastroenterol Hepatol 2012; 10(6):575–80.
46. Tanash HA, Nilsson PM, Nilsson JA, et al. Clinical course and prognosis of never-smokers with severe alpha-1-antitrypsin deficiency (PiZZ). Thorax 2008;63(12): 1091–5.
47. Carbamazepine in severe liver disease due to alpha-1 antitrypsin deficiency (CBZ). Available at: https://clinicaltrials.gov/ct2/show/NCT01379469. Accessed November 29, 2019.
48. Guo S, Booten SL, Aghajan M, et al. Antisense oligonucleotide treatment ameliorates alpha-1 antitrypsin-related liver disease in mice. J Clin Invest 2014;124(1): 251–61.
49. Hughes MG Jr, Khan KM, Gruessner AC, et al. Long-term outcome in 42 pediatric liver transplant patients with alpha 1-antitrypsin deficiency: a single-center experience. Clin Transplant 2011;25(5):731–6.
50. Carey EJ, Iyer EN, Nelson DR, et al. Outcomes for recipients of liver transplantation for alpha-1-antitrypsin deficiency-related cirrhosis. Liver Transpl 2013;19(12): 1370–6.
51. Kemmer N, Kaiser T, Zacharias V, et al. Alpha-1 Antitrypsin deficiency: outcomes after liver transplantation. Transplant Proc 2008;40:1492–4.
52. Kim WR, Lake JR, Smith JM, et al. OPTN/SRTR 2017 annual data report: liver. Am J Transplant 2019;19(Suppl 2):184–283.
53. Miranda E, Perez J, Ekeowa UI, et al. A novel monoclonal antibody to characterize polymers in liver disease associated with alpha1-antitrypsin deficiency. Hepatology 2010;52(3):1078–88.
54. Lomas DA, Finch JT, Seyama K, et al. α1-Antitrypsin Siiyama (Ser53→Phe); further evidence for intracellular loop-sheet polymerization. J Biol Chem 1993; 268(21):15333–5.
55. Lomas DA, Elliot PR, Sidhar SK, et al. α1-Antitrypsin Mmalton (Phe52- deleted) forms loop-sheet polymers in vivo: evidence for the C sheet mechanism of polymerization. J Biol Chem 1995;270(28):16864–70.

Microbiome

Emerging Concepts in Patients with Chronic Liver Disease

Bradley Reuter, MD, Jasmohan S. Bajaj, MD, MS*

KEYWORDS

- Outcomes • Fecal transplant • Cirrhosis • Hepatic encephalopathy

KEY POINTS

- The gut microbiome is a major research focus in chronic liver disease owing to alterations in gut–liver and gut–brain axes.
- Changes in microbiota structure and function across disease stages can be analyzed in differing samples using techniques that vary in depth of sequencing and cost.
- There are consistent microbiota functional changes (bile acids, endotoxin, short chain fatty acids) and composition changes as liver disease progresses and patients develop cirrhosis and complications.
- Alteration in the microbiota with therapies for hepatic encephalopathy, diet, periodontal therapy, and fecal transplant can help in selected patients with chronic liver disease.

INTRODUCTION

Cirrhosis and liver cancer account for 3.5% of all deaths worldwide, and an estimated 50 million adults are affected with chronic liver disease.[1,2] In addition to mortality, chronic liver diseases carry a significant economic impact and low quality of life.[3]

GUT MICROBIOME

It is first important to distinguish between the human microbiota and the microbiome. The microbiota is the overall collection of microbes within the body including bacteria, archaea, fungi, microbial eukaryotes, and viruses and phages.[4] In total the microbiota consists of up to 100 trillion cells.[5] The microbiome is a term for a specific collection of microbes and their genes that exist within a specific system in the body (like the gut).[6] Although the gut microbiome has been studied and linked to many diseases, this review specifically focuses on its link to chronic liver

Division of Gastroenterology, Hepatology and Nutrition, Virginia Commonwealth University, McGuire VA Medical Center, 1201 Broad Rock Boulevard, Richmond, VA 23249, USA
* Corresponding author.
E-mail address: jasmohan.bajaj@vcuhealth.org
Twitter: @jasmohanbajaj (J.S.B.)

Clin Liver Dis 24 (2020) 493–520
https://doi.org/10.1016/j.cld.2020.04.006
1089-3261/20/© 2020 Elsevier Inc. All rights reserved.

liver.theclinics.com

disease. Specifically, the gut microbiome has been shown to influence nonalcoholic steatohepatitis, nonalcoholic fatty liver disease, alcoholic hepatitis, primary sclerosing cholangitis, cirrhosis, and hepatocellular carcinoma (HCC).[6] The healthy human gut microbiome contains an abundance of bacteria with only a small minority of nonbacterial microbes.[4] Although there is considerable variation of gut microbiome composition between even healthy individuals, the majority of bacteria are members of the phyla Bacteroidetes and Firmicutes with the combined percentage of approximately 95%.[7] Other phyla present at lower levels are Actinobacteria, Fusobacteria, Verrucomicrobia, and Proteobacteria, and facultative anaerobes 6. When functioning properly, the autochthonous taxa and nonautochthonous taxa are responsible for a wide variety of functions, including production of short chain fatty acids for gut barrier integrity and colonocyte nutrients,[8] secondary bile acid synthesis,[9] and protection against pathogens.[10] Dysbiosis is the term used to describe the alteration of a patient's normal microbiome that can result in disadvantageous changes to physiologic functions. In dysbiosis, the balance in gut microdiversity changes as beneficial microbes (symbionts) decrease and harmful (pathobionts) increase.[6] When dysbiosis occurs in cirrhosis, there is a propagation of the disease and an increase in complications.[8]

Microbiome Sample Collection for Analysis

There is no perfect answer to this question owing to differences in studies that vary in depth and collection practices. Considerations include feasibility, cost, and how the subsequent analysis of the sample will be performed. Stool is the most commonly collected and accessible material. The disadvantage with stool is that it does not capture all gut microbes, especially ones that adhere well to the mucosa and small intestine microbes.[11,12] The typical protocol for stool sampling is to collect the whole stool, homogenize it as soon as possible, then flash freeze it, with an aliquot preserved in 20% glycerol in Lysogeny broth for culturing.[4] If RNA analysis is planned the sample should be placed in an RNA later solution for nucleic acid protection. Once collected the samples can be analyzed for bacterial RNA or DNA. There are a variety of microbiome analysis techniques depending on the goal of the study (**Table 1**).

Data Analysis

The choice for data comparison depends on the question that needs to be answered. Initially the raw DNA sequence data needs to be to organized into a table/chart showing how many of each species, gene, or strain is seen per sample. Analysis is then performed at the whole microbiome level and the individual taxa and genes level.[4] Whole microbiome analysis uses alpha and beta diversity. Alpha diversity shows a number of different types of microbial taxa within a group.[18] Beta diversity shows differences in diversity between groups. Individual taxa differences discriminant analysis effect size or by nonparametric tests. Tests of function are separated into direct and indirect testing. Indirect analysis shows gene expressions based on metagenomic data, whereas direct tests are functional correlates of microbial function (endotoxemia, secondary bile acid production, etc).[18] It is important to remember that different methods provide different results, even with using the sample or raw DNA.[4] Owing to this factor, there is not a large clinical role for these techniques at this time. Pathogen diagnosis should still rely on traditional cultures and assay (polymerase chain reaction vs antibody).[4] Finally, these data are linked to relevant clinical variables in order for an analysis to occur.

Table 1
Microbiome analysis techniques

Type	Overview	Strengths	Weaknesses	Microbes Studied	Throughput, Time, and Cost
Culture	Classical system of isolating and growing specific microbes on specific medias under aerobic conditions	The most sensitive detection method for organisms with well-characterized selective culture conditions Can use multiple sample types (stool, blood, skin) Helpful to detect the absolute abundance of viable organisms, antibiotic sensitivities/resistances, and phenotypic classification[13]	Limited scope of which microbes can be successfully cultured Not helpful for majority of anaerobic gut microbiome	Bacteria Fungi Archaea Viruses	Low throughput One sample per media used 24–48 h $
Assay/ PCR panels Examples: qPCR and RT-PCR[14]	Target a set of known bacteria, viruses, parasites, or functional genes Samples (stool) go through nucleic acid extraction followed by complementary DNA synthesis and amplification The end result (genomic DNA vs PCR product) is then qualified and	Provides absolute abundance of each taxon per gram or milliliter of input material Has a high dynamic range	Panels are only targeted so they will miss undiscovered gut taxa	Viruses Some other selective organisms pending the panel used	Low throughput 1–24 samples[15] 1–5 h[15] $$

(continued on next page)

Table 1
(continued)

quantified using the panel

Type	Overview	Strengths	Weaknesses	Microbes Studied	Throughput, Time, and Cost
Metataxonomics/ amplicon sequencing (16S rRNA gene sequencing)	Samples undergo extraction of nuclear material then PCR amplification is done using gene matched primers (usually the 16S rRNA for bacteria and archaea) This allows for amplifications of all variants bookended by the primers, hypervariable gene sequences are targeted Samples are then compared with large databases of microbial profiles and additional bioinformatic analysis is done based on clinical question	Assessment of microbiome diversity and composition at the genus level Can be used to assess functional changes Relatively cheaper than alterative techniques	Difficult to apply to viruses owing to there being no common viral gene[5] Each genus has a wide range of strains that are genomically distinct, which cannot be adequately appreciated using this method Can typically only go as far as the genus level[4] Bacteria have different numbers copies of 16S rRNA gene, influences relative abundance[4]	16S (bacteria, some archaea) 18S (eukaryotes) ITS (fungi)	High throughput 384 samples per run 48 h $$

Method	Description	Informs	Challenges	Organisms	Throughput
Shotgun metagenomics	Untargeted DNA sequencing of the whole genome. All DNA from a sample is broken down into fragments. These fragments are then sequenced, then software attempts to combine the fragments into a view of the whole microbiome[16]	Informs composition including species and strain. Gives functional insight. Gives a complete list of microbial strains present in the microbiome and how abundant each strain is[5]	Considerable technical challenges. All DNA will be sequenced, including human DNA (not a good option for biopsy specimens and required human DNA analysis consent)	All Organisms including host	High throughput. 384 samples per run. 48 h. $$$
Metaproteomics (protein), metatranscriptomics (RNA)	Metaproteomics: uses mass spectrometry to sort out the wide range of proteins in a sample[5]. Metatranscriptomics: sequencing of microbial RNA	Very broad: this includes all protein or RNA made by all the organisms present. Can be used to assess functional changes and can read gene expression	Lacks a link to specific organisms. Most bacterial transcripts only last a few minutes[17]. Poor correlation between gene expression and actual proteins in the gut	RNA viruses and all organisms including host	High throughput. 96–384 samples per run. 48 h. $$$$
Metabolomics (targeted vs nontargeted)	Study of the nonprotein small molecules including products of metabolism[5]. Metabolic responses of an individual or population	Relates directly to the function of the community	Limited list of discovered targeted molecules. Difficult to annotate untargeted metabolomics	All organisms including host	High throughput. 96 samples per run. 48 h. $$$

Abbreviations: PCR, polymerase chain reaction; qPCR, quantitative polymerase chain reaction; RT-PCR, reverse transcriptase polymerase chain reaction.

LIVER DISEASES AND THE MICROBIOME

The gut, the intestinal microbiota, and the liver are uniquely matched to have a bidirectional relationship. The liver receives 75% of its blood supply via the portal vein from the intestines, and the liver releases bile acids into the biliary tract to the intestine.[19] Major mechanisms in which the intestinal microbiota effects the liver include bile acid metabolism, intestinal permeability, chronic inflammation, immune system activation, short chain fatty acids, choline, and ethanol.[20] The etiology of the dysbiosis associated with chronic liver disease remains unknown, but there are some working theories proposed. The first is that in chronic liver disease there is a decreased production of bile acids and thus less reaches the duodenum. This is important owing to the antimicrobial properties of bile acids. Bile acids have a detergent action, making them toxic to bacteria.[21] Bile acids also have an effect on the intestinal mucosa, influencing the production of peptides critical for bacterial control.[22,23] These changes allow for an environment suspectable to the development of small bacterial intestinal overgrowth. This factor leads to an increased quantity of bacteria, functional bacteria changes, and an increased intestinal permeability.[24] Cirrhosis microbiome composition has shown a wide amount of study to study variability. In a typical dysbiosis pattern, potentially pathogenic bacteria (Enterobacteriaceae Veillonellaceae, and Streptococcaceae) increase and beneficial bacteria (Proteobacteria and Fusobacteria) decrease.[25] The cirrhosis dysbiosis ratio tool was designed to estimate dysbiosis in cirrhotics.[8] This study showed a worsening in cirrhosis dysbiosis ratio in the setting of disease progression. There has been significant work done to increase the understanding of the gut microbiome in relation to specific etiologies of liver disease (**Table 2**).

CIRRHOSIS COMPLICATIONS AND HOW MICROBES MAY BE RELATED
Hepatic Encephalopathy

The gut microbiota most likely has a strong link to the pathophysiology of hepatic encephalopathy (HE), specifically endotoxemia.[53] Intestinal microbiota studies have shown a decrease in *Lachnospiraceae* and *Ruminococcacae* and an increase in *Enterobacteriaceae*, *Streptococcaceae*, and *Porphyromonadaceae* associated with HE. Specifically, *Lachnospiraceae* and *Ruminococcaceae* negatively correlated, whereas *Enterobactericeae* positively correlated with ammonia-associated astrocyte swelling.[54] White matter changes on brain MRI were positively associated with *Porphyromonadaceae*.[54] Another study showed a positive correlation with cognitive impairment with *Alcaligenaceae* and *Porphyromonadaceae*, versus *Prevotella*, which was linked to improvement in cognition and decreased inflammation.[53] Studies have shown that evaluation of the intestinal microbiota can help to predict overt HE development in cirrhotic inpatients.[55] Specifically, this patient population has higher endoxemia, lower cirrhosis dysbiosis ratios, and increased levels of *Enterobacteriaceae*.[55] This study initially looked at changes on admission for cirrhotic patients, whereas another study also showed that patients with overt HE have distinct changes in their microbiota during hospital stays, and these changes have the ability to predict HE recurrence.[56] There is an increased percentage of urease active bacteria in patients with cirrhosis, specifically *Streptococcaceae*.[57] These changes are thought to lead to increased ammonia production and contribute to the development of HE.[58,59]

Hepatocellular Carcinoma

There has been growing evidence that dysbiosis and intestinal microbiota changes impact the development of HCC by increasing steatosis, oxidative stress, and inflammation.[60] Multiple studies have shown that there are intestinal microbiota changes

Table 2
Specific liver diseases and the gut microbiome

	Findings	Take Away Points
Alcohol-related liver disease	Studies have looked at the entire spectrum of disease up to alcoholic hepatitis[26]	Possible pathway exists in which alcohol itself leads to an initial dysbiosis through increased gut permeability
	Chronic use of alcohol results in increased intestinal permeability, thus initial gut microbial changes are provoked by the use of alcohol itself[27]	Once this dysbiosis is established, it affects gut permeability further, allowing for this altered microbiome to enter the portal circulation along with endotoxins
	Progression through the spectrum correlates in proportion with bacterial and fungal composition	Once in the portal circulation, this could trigger hepatic inflammation contributing to progression of liver fibrosis
	Alcohol consumption itself provokes microbiome changes leading eventually to dysbiosis[28] (stool)[29]	If patients stop drinking, many of these microbiome changes are reversible
	There is a proportional increase in secondary bacterial products like secondary bile acids,[30] biopsy	
	As liver disease worsens, the correlating dysbiosis shows an unfavorable increase in Enterobacteriaceae and Enterococcaceae, both of which increase the risk of gut translocation[31] (biopsy),[32] (stool)	
	Bifidobacterium, *Enterobacterium*, and *Lactobacillus* are all decreased in ALD[33] (stool),[34] (stool),[35] while cirrhotic patients with ALD show the typical trend of lower levels of Bacteroidetes and Firmicutes phyla[30] (biopsy),[36] (biopsy)[37]	
	Alcoholism predisposes people to small intestinal bacterial overgrowth which leads in increased risk for spontaneous bacterial peritonitis and worse severity of alcoholic cirrhosis[38] (breath test),[39] (breath test)	
	Fortunately, studies have shown these negative changes can be reversed with alcohol cessation[40] (stool)	

(continued on next page)

Table 2
(continued)

	Findings	Take Away Points
NAFLD and nonalcoholic steatohepatitis	Difficult area to study owing to overlap with other components of metabolic syndromes (DM, obesity)[41] As disease progresses studies have shown a proportional increase in Enterobacteraceae[42] (stool) Studies have shown endogenous bacteria have the ability to produce alcohol[43] (stool), this may contribute to fatty liver disease initiation and progression There appears to be differences in intestinal microbiota between nonalcoholic steatohepatitis and NAFLD patients NAFLD patients have decreased Bacteroidetes and Firmicutes, along with increased Lactobacillus[44] (stool) Bacteroidetes levels were found to be lower in nonalcoholic steatohepatitis patients in one study[45] (stool) and decreased Ruminococcus, Faecalibacterium prausnitzii, and Coprococcus in another[44] (stool) When comparing nonalcoholic steatohepatitis to NAFLD populations, there has been a link showing Bacteroides associated functionality by promote nonalcoholic steatohepatitis[46]	Very difficult area to study and interpret owing to the difficult nature of studying it independently of other components of obesity and metabolic syndromes May be a link between dysbiosis leading to bacterial byproducts production (ethanol and 3- phenylpropanoate) and disease progression Significant additional work needs to be done within this area

PBC	Decreased levels of Bacteroidetes species[47] (stool) Increased levels of Fusobacteria, *Haemophilus*, *Veillonella*, *Clostridium*, *Lactobacillus*, *Streptococcus*, *Pseudomonas*, *Klebsiella*, Enterobacteriaceae, and Proteobacteria species[47] (stool) Changes in the intestinal microbiota in PBC have been associated with increased liver injury indicators and proinflammatory cytokines This may indicate a role for altered intestinal microbiota in the development or progression of PBC itself[48] (stool) Have shown differences in patients being treated or not treated with UDCA After UDCA treatment, there was found to be decreased levels of *Haemophilus* spp, *Streptococcus* spp, and *Pseudomonas* spp and increased levels of *Bacteroidetes* spp, *Sutterella* spp, and *Oscillospira* spp[49]	Clear microbiome changes have been seen between PBC patients and controls Some early data suggest that intestinal microbiota changes may be linked to disease formation/progression Treatment with UDCA has been showed to alter the intestinal microbiota and reverse dysbiosis
Primary sclerosing cholangitis	Studies thus have shown a lot of inconsistency in changes to the intestinal microbiota with dysbiosis with different genus and species populations and relative changes[50] Multiple studies have shown that there is an abundance of *Veillonella*[51] (stool) Dysbiosis leads to bacterobilia, which leads to increased cholangiocyte inflammation and progression to fibrosis[52]	Conflicting data about the exact changes in dysbiosis in this population Overall thought is that dysbiosis leads to bacterobilia, which in turns leads to cholangiocyte inflammation and fibrosis

Abbreviations: ALD, alcoholic liver disease; DM, diabetes mellitus; NAFLD, nonalcoholic fatty liver disease; PBC, primary biliary sclerosis; UDCA, ursodeoxycholic acid.

between cirrhotic patients and patients who develop HCC.[61–63] A recent study looked to microbial diversity as a possible noninvasive biomarker for HCC.[62] This study showed an increase in *Actinobacteria* and a decrease in *Verrucomicrobia*. In looking specifically at cirrhotic patients with nonalcoholic steatohepatitis with HCC, increased levels of *Bacteroides* and *Ruminococcaceae* and decreased levels of *Akkermansia* and *Bifidobacterium* were seen in comparison with cirrhotics who did not develop HCC.[61] Correlations with calprotectin concentrations and systemic inflammation were also seen in tandem with these microbiome changes.[61] When looking specifically at hepatitis B virus–related HCC, these patients have increased levels of proinflammatory bacteria, which was thought to result in reduced levels of anti-inflammatory short-chain fatty acids.[64] There remains a lot of questions in this area especially concerning gut translocation of specific bacteria and the role of toll-like receptors (especially toll-like receptor 4) in HCC pathogenesis.[65]

Spontaneous Bacterial Peritonitis

It is logical to assume that dysbiosis would be linked to spontaneous bacterial peritonitis in the context of all the known data concerning increased gut permeability and translocation. In patients with ascites, their serum microbiome showed higher levels of lipopolysaccharide binding protein (a biomarker for translocation). This finding was associated with a higher abundance of Clostridiales and an unknown genus belonging to the Cyanobacteria phylum.[66] These patients may have a more significant deterioration of their intestinal barrier integrity and increase rates of translocation, placing them more at risk for development of spontaneous bacterial peritonitis. In cirrhotics, there is an increase in the gram-negative taxa, specifically components of Enterobacteriaceae (the major causative organisms in the pathogenesis of spontaneous bacterial peritonitis).[67]

TREATMENTS BASED ON THE MICROBIOTA

Numerous strategies have been developed to modulate the gut microbiome. They can be delineated by lifestyle modifications versus clinical interventions. Lifestyle modifications include nutritional intervention and modification, caloric restriction, and exercise. Clinical interventions include fecal microbiota transfer, antibiotics, prebiotics, probiotics, pharmabiotics, laxatives, and bile acid/fibroblast growth factor analogues.[68]

Antibiotics

Any antibiotic that is oral or undergoes biliary excretion and enterohepatic circulation has the capability to impact the gut microbiota.[68] The obvious concern is for elimination of beneficial phyla and the expansion of harmful phyla, contributing to dysbiosis. This process can lead to antibiotic resistance, *Clostridium difficile* infection, small bowel bacterial overgrowth, and fungal overgrowth. Antibiotics have also been shown to both positively and negatively impact microbiota factors including inflammation, metabolism, and tumorigenesis.[69–71]

Owing to the harmful microbiome effects of broad-spectrum antibiotics there has been a push for more narrow-spectrum treatments which treat the target pathogen but allow the commensals unharmed.[72] Quorum sensing inhibition[73] and antitoxin drugs[74] offer promise, but there have been no significant studies looking at the use of these drugs in chronic liver disease. For this limited review, we only focus on trials in which agents that influence gut microbiota with analyses of gut microbiota composition before and after therapy (**Table 3**). Several trials that only studied microbial interventions without testing for microbiota composition were not included.

Table 3
Microbiota altering therapeutic trial in chronic liver disease

Patient Population	Study	Intervention	Microbiota Analysis After the Intervention	Conclusions
Probiotics				
Mild alcohol-induced liver injury and subgroup of mild alcoholic hepatitis	Kirpich et al,[75] 2008	5 d of *Bifidobacterium bifidum* and *Lactobacillus plantarum* 8PA3 vs standard therapy alone (abstinence plus vitamins)	Alcoholic patients had significantly increased numbers of both bifidobacteria and lactobacilli	In the mild alcoholic hepatitis subgroup therapy associated with reduction in ALT, AST, GGT, LDH and total bilirubin Therapy showed restoration of the bowel flora and greater improvement in alcohol-induced liver injury
Cirrhosis and MHE	Bajaj et al,[76] 2014	*Lactobacillus* GG vs placebo in 30 patients with cirrhosis and MHE, followed for 8 wk	Improvement in dysbiosis (reduced Enterobacteriaceae and increased *Clostridiales incertae* Sedis XIV and *Lachnospiraceae*) and bacterial composition and function No improvement in cognition Safely tolerated	*Lactobacillus* GG is safe and can improve dysbiosis and microbial functionality on metabolomics

(continued on next page)

Table 3
(continued)

Patient Population	Study	Intervention	Microbiota Analysis After the Intervention	Conclusions
HBV-induced cirrhosis with MHE	Xia et al,[77] 2018	*Clostridium butyricum* and *Bifidobacterium infantis* in MHE (n = 30) vs no treatment (n = 37) for 3 mo	*Clostridium* and *Bifidobacterium* increased while Enterococcus and Enterobacteriaceae decreased Cognition improved Decrease in venous ammonia Improvement in intestinal mucosal barrier	MHE in patients with HBV-induced cirrhosis improved after probiotics
Outpatients with cirrhosis and cognitive dysfunction	Roman et al,[78] 2019	One-half of patients had fecal microbiome analysis (n = 9 probiotic group, n = 8 placebo group)	No significant changes seen at a phylum, genus, or species level	Improved cognitive function, risk of falls, and inflammatory response

Synbiotics

NAFLD	Scorletti et al,[81] 2020	Synbiotic agents (fructo-oligosaccharides, 4 g twice per day, plus Bifidobacterium animalis subspecies lactis BB-12; n = 55) or placebo (n = 49) for 10–14 mo	Synbiotic patients had higher proportions of Bifidobacterium and Faecalibacterium species, and reductions in *Oscillibacter* and *Alistipes* species Changes in the composition of fecal microbiota were not associated with liver fat or markers of fibrosis	Treatment altered the microbiome but did not decrease liver fat content or markers of liver fibrosis
Adult outpatients with nonalcoholic steatohepatitis	Manzhalii et al,[82] 2017	Experiment group (n = 38) vs control (n = 37) Low-fat diet plus LBSF synbiotic for 12 wk (*L casei, L rhamnosus, L bulgaris, B longum,* and *S thermophilus* with fructooligo-saccharides)	A shift toward a more normal microbiome in the treatment group with increases in Bifidobacteria, lactobacillus, *E coli*, etc	Treatment showed improvement in liver inflammation without adverse events

(continued on next page)

Table 3
(continued)

Patient Population	Study	Intervention	Microbiota Analysis After the Intervention	Conclusions
Diet				
Outpatients with cirrhosis (compensated and decompensated)	Bajaj et al,[83] 2018	United States patients (n = 157), Turkish patients (n = 139) Compared differing dietary habits on gut microbiota and clinical outcomes	The Turkish cohort had a significantly higher microbial diversity No change between controls and cirrhotics in the Turkish group In contrast, microbial diversity changed in the US-based cohort and was the lowest in decompensated patients	A diet rich in fermented milk, vegetables, cereals, coffee, and tea is associated with a higher microbial diversity Microbial diversity was associated with an independently lower risk of 90-d hospitalizations
Outpatient cirrhosis (compensated and decompensated)	Bajaj et al,[84] 2020	Compared American and Mexican diet cohorts to assess hospitalization and MHE (n = 275)	On regression, Prevotellaceae, Ruminococcaceae, and Lachnospiraceae lowered hospitalization Risk independent of MELD and ascites MHE rate was similar MELD, decompensation increased, whereas the cirrhosis dysbiosis ratio and Prevotellaceae decreased the risk of MHE	Changes in diet and microbiota, especially related to animal fat and protein intake and Prevotellaceae, are associated with MHE and hospitalizations in Mexican patients with cirrhosis compared with an American cohort

Periodontal therapy

Cirrhotics with chronic gingivitis and/or mild or moderate period-ontitis	Bajaj et al,[86] 2018	N = 30 cirrhosis and N = 20 noncirrhotic controls, 30 d of periodontal therapy	Treatment resulted in favorable changes with higher relative abundance of autochthonous taxa (Ruminococcaceae and Lachnospiraceae) and reduction in potentially pathogenic (Enterobacteriaceae) and oral-origin taxa (Porphyromonadaceae and Streptococcaceae)	Systematic periodontal therapy in cirrhotic outpatients improved endotoxemia, as well as systemic and local inflammation, and modulated salivary and stool microbial dysbiosis

Fecal/intestinal microbiota transplantation

PSC patients concurrent IBD	Allegretti et al,[88] 2019	Ten patients underwent a single FMT by colonoscopy Primary outcome was safety Secondary outcome was decreased ALP levels and metabonomic dynamics assessed	Diversity and similarity to donor increased in all patients after FMT, with changes seen as early as week 1 and maintained an upward trend throughout week 24	FMT in PSC is safe In addition, increases in bacterial diversity and engraftment may correlate with an improvement in ALP among patients with PSC

(continued on next page)

Table 3
(continued)

Patient Population	Study	Intervention	Microbiota Analysis After the Intervention	Conclusions
ALD	Phillips et al,[89] 2018	16 patients with ALD received FMT, were compared with other treatment modalities (corticosteroids, nutrition support only, and pentoxifylline)	After FMT, Actinobacteria and Proteobacteria decreased substantially with a increase in Firmicutes Persisted at day 30 and 90 after transplantation	Healthy donor FMT for SAH improves survival compared with current therapies
Severe alcoholic hepatitis	Phillips et al,[90] 2017	Eight male patients ineligible for corticosteroids given 1 wk of daily FMT	Microbiota analysis showed no difference in phyla composition of donors and recipients at baseline Firmicutes dominated in donors and recipients at 1 y, Proteobacteria reduced, and Actinobacteria increased after FMT in recipients Certain pathogenic species were also reduced after FMT at 1 year	FMT was safe and improved liver disease severity and survival at 1 y

Chronic hepatitis B	Ren et al,[91] 2017	Patients who remained persistently positive for HBeAg after >3 y of ongoing ETV- or TDF-based antiviral therapy (FMT = 5, control = 13) End point was effect of FMT on HBV antigen titers	Monthly FMT treatment decrease HBeAg titers and 2/5 patients achieved HBeAg clearance No change in HBV surface antigen	There is a potential role for modulating gut microbiota in chronic hepatitis B treatment
Patients with cirrhosis with recurrent HE	Bajaj et al,[92] 2017	SOC (n = 10) vs FMT (n = 10) Primary outcome was safety Secondary were serious adverse events, cognition, microbiota and metabolomic changes	Eight SOC patients had 11 SAEs vs 2 FMT patients had SAEs Five SOC and no FMT patients developed further HE FMT increased diversity and beneficial taxa	FMT in HE patients is safe and reduced hospitalizations, improved cognition and dysbiosis in cirrhosis with recurrent HE

(continued on next page)

Table 3
(continued)

Patient Population	Study	Intervention	Microbiota Analysis After the Intervention	Conclusions
Antibiotics				
Cirrhotic patient with refractory ascites	Lv et al,[93] 2020	Rifaximin and IV antibiotics	Rifaximin alone reduced the levels of *Roseburia*, *Haemophilus*, and *Prevotella* The combination of rifaximin and IV antibiotics resulted in a decrease in *Lachnospiraceae_noname*, *Subdoligranulum*, and *Dorea* and increase in *Coprobacillus* Gene expression of virulence factors was significantly reduced after treatment in both groups	Through microbiota alterations rifaximin may mitigate ascites and improve survival in cirrhotic patients with refractory ascites
HE and MHE therapies				
Cirrhosis	Bajaj et al,[94] 2013	Rifaximin	Small decrease in eillonellaceae and increase in Eubacteriaceae Reduction in network connectivity, specifically Enterobacteriaceae, Porphyromonadaceae, and Bacteroidaceae Increase in serum fatty acids	Rifaximin was associated with improvements in cognitive function and endotoxemia in MHE
Cirrhosis	Bajaj et al,[95] 2012	Lactulose N = 7 Men who were controlled on lactulose compared with their baseline after lactulose withdrawn over 30 d	Small decrease in Fecalibacterium and Veillonellaceae but no change in diversity There were metabolomics changes seen	Lactulose may a have important noncompositional effect on the gut microbiome

Cirrhosis	Bajaj et al,[8] 2014, Lactulose initiation	Lactulose N = 7 Compared before and after lactulose given for OHE Re-analyzed after 30 d of treatment	Enterobacteriacea increased and cirrhosis dysbiosis ration decreased after HE developed	Starting lactulose was not able to change the microbiome changes typically seen with cirrhosis progression
Cirrhosis	Sarangi et al,[96] 2017 Lactulose initiation in outpatients	Lactulose N = 21 Compared before and after lactulose was started on outpatient cirrhotics Looked at metagenomic changes and differences between patients who responded to lactulose	No change in any microbial output	Consistent with other studies with respect to resistance of change to the microbial and bacterial composition

(continued on next page)

Table 3
(continued)

Patient Population	Study	Intervention	Microbiota Analysis After the Intervention	Conclusions
		and those who did not		
Cirrhosis	Wang et al,[97] 2019, multicenter study in MHE	Lactulose N = 67 Multicenter study Compared metagenomic changes and lactose responsiveness before and after lactulose adjusted to MHE reversal	Increased levels of Firmicutes in lactulose responders No significant changes before and after lactulose therapy	There may be a link between lactulose response and microbiome differences but this needs additional studies
Cirrhosis	Bajaj et al,[94] 2013, rifaximin before vs after in MHE	Rifaximin N = 20 Compared before and after 8 wk of rifaximin (550 mg BID) Assessed microbiota, cognition, metabolomics, and endotoxemia, changes in brain function, and MRI	As cognition improved there was seen a transition toward more beneficial metabolite links compared with pathogenic (Enterobacteriaceae, Porphyromonadaceae and Bacteroidaceae) Although a link was seen between decreased endotoxemia and improved cognition, no significant composition changes were noted, just metabolomics	Bacteria function was improved with rifaximin

| Cirrhosis (decompensated) | Kaji et al,[98] 2017 | Rifaximin N = 20 Compared microbiota, endotoxema, ammonia, and cognition before and after treatment (440 mg TID) | No changes in microbiome diversity but improved cognition, endotoxin, and ammonia levels Minor reductions seen in levels of Veillonella and Streptococcus | No significant change in microbiome composition, but improved cognition and decreased endotoxin activity with treatment |
| Cirrhosis | Schulz et al,[99] 2019 | Rifaximin (550 mg BID) with or without lactulose N = 5 MHE patients treated for 3 months Assessed cognition, duodenal, and fecal microbiota changes | MHE improved but there were no changes seen in the samples (duodenal and fecal) | There was no change in microbiome composition but there was a improvement in cognition |

Abbreviations: ALD, alcoholic liver disease; ALP, alkaline phosphatase; ALT, alanine aminotransferase; AST, aspartate aminotransferase; BID, 2 times per day; ETV, entecavir; FMT, fecal microbiota transplantation; GGT, gamma glutamyl transferase; HBeAg, hepatitis B virus e antigen; HBV, hepatitis B virus; HE, hepatic encephalopathy; IBD, inflammatory bowel disease; IV, intravenous; LDH, lactate dehydrogenase; MELD, Model for End Stage Liver Disease; MHE, minimal hepatic encephalopathy; OHE, overt hepatic encephalopathy; PSC, primary sclerosing cholangitis; SAH, subarachnoid hemorrhage; SOC, standard of care; TDF, tenofovir; TID, 3 times per day.

Probiotics

Probiotics are defined as live microorganisms that, when given in the correct dosing, confer a health benefit on the host.[75] Probiotics have been studied in a wide variety of human diseases as a way to modulate the gut microbiota. There has been a growing body of evidence for the use of probiotics in the treatment of chronic liver disease (see **Table 3**).

Prebiotics

Prebiotics consistent of nondigestive food ingredients that are fermented in the gut, the largest subgroup being prebiotic fibers, which are usually nondigestible carbohydrates. They then can modulate the microbiome in beneficial ways to the host. It has been shown that prebiotics can modify gut barrier integrity and endotoxin translocation.[79] Prebiotics have been showed to be able to stimulate bacterial production of short chain fatty acids, stimulate growth of *Bifidobacteria* and *Lactobacilli*, and provide additional pathogen protection by lowering the luminal pH.[80] Although there have been numerous studies looking at the use of prebiotics in chronic liver disease, there have been no definitive studies that meet our criteria (human, adult, pretreatment and post-treatment microbiome analysis). There are some ongoing clinical trials and promising rodent studies, however, that show encouraging treatment with prebiotics, including pectin.

Synbiotics

Synbiotics are combinations of prebiotics and probiotics, used to gain the benefit of both. A wave of new studies has decided to use this strategy in the hopes of maximizing the benefit of both interventions (see **Table 3**).

Diet

The studies looking at diet for possible microbiota therapy in chronic liver disease are relatively new and have looked at how different cultural diets impact microbial diversity.[83] There has been interest to see how animal fat and protein intake impacts the microbiota and impactions compensated and compensated cirrhotic patient[84] (see **Table 3**). As more information is gathered in this area, hopefully new dietary guidelines can be generated for cirrhotic patients.

Periodontal therapy

Periodontitis leads to destruction of tooth-supporting structures through inflammation and a dysregulation of the immune response to a dysbiotic biofilm.[85] There is concern that a prolonged inflammatory response may lead to systemic complications. This possible therapeutic target has been investigated in cirrhotic patients (see **Table 3**).

Fecal/Intestinal Microbiota Transplantation

Although there is robust literature for the use of fecal microbiota transplantation for treatment of refractory *C difficile* infection, its use in chronic liver disease is relatively new. One major difference between these 2 illness groups is that because the microbiome has been destroyed by antibiotics in refractory *C difficile* infection, normalization can often be obtained after a single inoculation and with a small dose of donor material.[90] The etiology of liver disease-associated intestinal microbiota is much more complex. It thus makes attempts at normalization more difficult and there remains a significant amount of questions surrounding what the target microbiota composition and functionality should be in chronic liver disease overall and for individual disease etiologies. It is unclear what the optimal treatment regiments are, including the length of treatment, amount of material, and identification of treatment end-points.[87] fecal microbiota transplantation has been studied in a wide variety of chronic liver disease patients (see **Table 3**).

Hepatic Encephalopathy and Minimal Hepatic Encephalopathy

Although lactulose and rifaximin are mainstays in the treatment of HE and minimal HE, there remains poor understanding of their underlying mechanisms in the disease process. Numerous studies have looked at better understanding HE pathophysiology and how these treatments impact the microbiome (see **Table 3**).

SUMMARY

Gut microbiota analysis and interpretation is now a major part of clinical and translational research in chronic diseases, including liver disease and cirrhosis. There are specific areas in liver disease where gut microbiota composition and functional changes can be cost effective,[100] but further work needs to be done to translate these changes into clinical practice.

DISCLOSURE

None for B. Reuter, JSB's institution received research grants from Salix Pharmaceuticals and he has served on advisory boards for Norgine and Merz Pharmaceuticals.

REFERENCES

1. Asrani SK, Devarbhavi H, Eaton J, et al. Burden of liver diseases in the world. J Hepatol 2019;70(1):151–71.
2. Global burden of liver disease: a true burden on health sciences and economies!! World Gastroenterology Organisation. Available at: https://www.worldgastroenterology.org/publications/e-wgn/e-wgn-expert-point-of-view-articles-collection/global-burden-of-liver-disease-a-true-burden-on-health-sciences-and-economies. Accessed April 1, 2020.
3. Stepanova M, De Avila L, Afendy M, et al. Direct and indirect economic burden of chronic liver disease in the United States. Clin Gastroenterol Hepatol 2017; 15(5):759–66.e5.
4. Allaband C, McDonald D, Vázquez-Baeza Y, et al. Microbiome 101: studying, analyzing, and interpreting gut microbiome data for clinicians. Clin Gastroenterol Hepatol 2019;17(2):218–30.
5. Marchesi JR, Ravel J. The vocabulary of microbiome research: a proposal. Microbiome 2015;3(1):31.
6. Mullish BH, Quraishi MN, Segal JP, et al. The gut microbiome: what every gastroenterologist needs to know. Frontline Gastroenterol 2020. https://doi.org/10.1136/flgastro-2019-101376.
7. Huttenhower C, Gevers D, Knight R, et al. Structure, function and diversity of the healthy human microbiome. Nature 2012;486(7402):207–14.
8. Bajaj JS, Heuman DM, Hylemon PB, et al. Altered profile of human gut microbiome is associated with cirrhosis and its complications. J Hepatol 2014; 60(5):940–7.
9. Ridlon JM, Kang DJ, Hylemon PB. Bile salt biotransformations by human intestinal bacteria. J Lipid Res 2006;47(2):241–59.
10. Libertucci J, Young VB. The role of the microbiota in infectious diseases. Nat Microbiol 2019;4(1):35–45.

11. Eckburg PB, Bik EM, Bernstein CN, et al. Microbiology: diversity of the human intestinal microbial flora. Science 2005;308(5728):1635–8.

12. De Cárcer DA, Cuív PÓ, Wang T, et al. Numerical ecology validates a biogeographical distribution and gender-based effect on mucosa-associated bacteria along the human colon. ISME J 2011;5(5):801–9.

13. Váradi L, Luo JL, Hibbs DE, et al. Methods for the detection and identification of pathogenic bacteria: past, present, and future. Chem Soc Rev 2017;46(16): 4818–32.

14. Zautner AE, Groß U, Emele MF, et al. More pathogenicity or just more pathogens? -On the interpretation problem of multiple pathogen detections with diagnostic multiplex assays. Front Microbiol 2017;8(JUN):1210.

15. Huang RSP, Johnson CL, Pritchard L, et al. Performance of the Verigene® enteric pathogens test, Biofire FilmArray™ gastrointestinal panel and Luminex xTAG® gastrointestinal pathogen panel for detection of common enteric pathogens. Diagn Microbiol Infect Dis 2016;86(4):336–9.

16. Riesenfeld CS, Schloss PD, Handelsman J. Metagenomics: genomic analysis of microbial communities. Annu Rev Genet 2004;38(1):525–52.

17. Har-El R, Silberstein A, Kuhn J, et al. Synthesis and degradation of lac mRNA in E. coli depleted of 30S ribosomal subunits. Mol Gen Genet 1979;173(2):135–44.

18. Acharya C, Bajaj JS. Altered microbiome in patients with cirrhosis and complications. Clin Gastroenterol Hepatol 2019;17(2):307–21.

19. Henao-Mejia J, Elinav E, Thaiss CA, et al. Role of the intestinal microbiome in liver disease. J Autoimmun 2013;46:66–73.

20. Schwenger KJ, Clermont-Dejean N, Allard JP. The role of the gut microbiome in chronic liver disease: the clinical evidence revised. JHEP Rep 2019;1(3): 214–26.

21. Begley M, Gahan CGM, Hill C. The interaction between bacteria and bile. FEMS Microbiol Rev 2005;29(4):625–51.

22. Vlahcevic ZR, Buhac I, Bell CC, et al. Abnormal metabolism of secondary bile acids in patients with cirrhosis. Gut 1970;11(5):420–2.

23. Swann JR, Want EJ, Geier FM, et al. Systemic gut microbial modulation of bile acid metabolism in host tissue compartments. Proc Natl Acad Sci U S A 2011;108(SUPPL. 1):4523–30.

24. Wigg AJ, Roberts-Thomson IC, Grose RH, et al. The role of small intestinal bacterial overgrowth, intestinal permeability, endotoxaemia, and tumour necrosis factor α in the pathogenesis of non-alcoholic steatohepatitis. Gut 2001;48(2): 206–11.

25. Chen Y, Yang F, Lu H, et al. Characterization of fecal microbial communities in patients with liver cirrhosis. Hepatology 2011;54(2):562–72.

26. Bajaj JS. Alcohol, liver disease and the gut microbiota. Nat Rev Gastroenterol Hepatol 2019;16(4):235–46.

27. Leclercq S, Cani PD, Neyrinck AM, et al. Role of intestinal permeability and inflammation in the biological and behavioral control of alcohol-dependent subjects. Brain Behav Immun 2012;26(6):911–8.

28. Yang AM, Inamine T, Hochrath K, et al. Intestinal fungi contribute to development of alcoholic liver disease. J Clin Invest 2017;127(7):2829–41.

29. Li F, Duan K, Wang C, et al. Probiotics and alcoholic liver disease: treatment and potential mechanisms. Gastroenterol Res Pract 2016;2016:5491465.

30. Mutlu EA, Gillevet PM, Rangwala H, et al. Colonic microbiome is altered in alcoholism. Am J Physiol Gastrointest Liver Physiol 2012;302(9):G966–78.

31. Llopis M, Cassard AM, Wrzosek L, et al. Intestinal microbiota contributes to individual susceptibility to alcoholic liver disease. Gut 2016;65(5):830–9.

32. Llorente C, Jepsen P, Inamine T, et al. Gastric acid suppression promotes alcoholic liver disease by inducing overgrowth of intestinal Enterococcus. Nat Commun 2017;8(1):837.

33. Bull-Otterson L, Feng W, Kirpich I, et al. Metagenomic analyses of alcohol induced pathogenic alterations in the intestinal microbiome and the effect of lactobacillus rhamnosus GG treatment. PLoS One 2013;8(1):e53028.

34. Tuomisto S, Pessi T, Collin P, et al. Changes in gut bacterial populations and their translocation into liver and ascites in alcoholic liver cirrhotics. BMC Gastroenterol 2014;14(1). https://doi.org/10.1186/1471-230X-14-40.

35. Bluemel S, Williams B, Knight R, et al. Precision medicine in alcoholic and nonalcoholic fatty liver disease via modulating the gut microbiota. Am J Physiol Gastrointest Liver Physiol 2016;311(6):G1018–36.

36. Kakiyama G, Hylemon PB, Zhou H, et al. Colonic inflammation and secondary bile acids in alcoholic cirrhosis. Am J Physiol Gastrointest Liver Physiol 2014; 306(11). https://doi.org/10.1152/ajpgi.00315.2013.

37. Hartmann P, Seebauer CT, Schnabl B. Alcoholic liver disease: the gut microbiome and liver cross talk. Alcohol Clin Exp Res 2015;39(5):763–75.

38. Bode C, Kolepke R, Schafer K, et al. Breath hydrogen excretion in patients with alcoholic liver disease - evidence of small intestinal bacterial overgrowth. Z Gastroenterol 1993;31(1):3–7.

39. Casafont Morencos F, de las Heras Castaño G, Martín Ramos L, et al. Small bowel bacterial overgrowth in patients with alcoholic cirrhosis. Dig Dis Sci 1996;41(3):552–6.

40. Leclercq S, Matamoros S, Cani PD, et al. Intestinal permeability, gut-bacterial dysbiosis, and behavioral markers of alcohol-dependence severity. Proc Natl Acad Sci U S A 2014;111(42):E4485–93.

41. Young VB. The role of the microbiome in human health and disease: an introduction for clinicians. BMJ 2017;356:j831.

42. Boursier J, Mueller O, Barret M, et al. The severity of nonalcoholic fatty liver disease is associated with gut dysbiosis and shift in the metabolic function of the gut microbiota. Hepatology 2016;63(3):764–75.

43. Zhu L, Baker SS, Gill C, et al. Characterization of gut microbiomes in nonalcoholic steatohepatitis (NASH) patients: a connection between endogenous alcohol and NASH. Hepatology 2013;57(2):601–9.

44. Da Silva HE, Teterina A, Comelli EM, et al. Nonalcoholic fatty liver disease is associated with dysbiosis independent of body mass index and insulin resistance. Sci Rep 2018;8(1):1466.

45. Mouzaki M, Comelli EM, Arendt BM, et al. Intestinal microbiota in patients with nonalcoholic fatty liver disease. Hepatology 2013;58(1):120–7.

46. Shawcross DL, Wright GAK, Stadlbauer V, et al. Ammonia impairs neutrophil phagocytic function in liver disease. Hepatology 2008;48(4):1202–12.

47. Tang R, Wei Y, Li Y, et al. Gut microbial profile is altered in primary biliary cholangitis and partially restored after UDCA therapy. Gut 2018;67(3):534–71.

48. Lv LX, Fang DQ, Shi D, et al. Alterations and correlations of the gut microbiome, metabolism and immunity in patients with primary biliary cirrhosis. Environ Microbiol 2016;18(7):2272–86.

49. Seidler S, Zimmermann HW, Weiskirchen R, et al. Elevated circulating soluble interleukin-2 receptor in patients with chronic liver diseases is associated with non-classical monocytes. BMC Gastroenterol 2012;12:38.

50. Karlsen TH. Primary sclerosing cholangitis: 50?years of a gut-liver relationship and still no love? Gut 2016;65(10):1579–81.

51. Kummen M, Holm K, Anmarkrud JA, et al. The gut microbial profile in patients with primary sclerosing cholangitis is distinct from patients with ulcerative colitis without biliary disease and healthy controls. Gut 2017;66(4):611–9.

52. Role of the microbiota and antibiotics in primary sclerosing cholangitis. Available at: https://www.ncbi.nlm.nih.gov/pubmed/24232746. Accessed April 2, 2020.

53. Bajaj JS, Ridlon JM, Hylemon PB, et al. Linkage of gut microbiome with cognition in hepatic encephalopathy. Am J Physiol Gastrointest Liver Physiol 2012; 302(1):G168–75.

54. Ahluwalia V, Betrapally NS, Hylemon PB, et al. Impaired gut-liver-brain Axis in patients with cirrhosis. Sci Rep 2016;6. https://doi.org/10.1038/srep26800.

55. Bajaj JS, Vargas HE, Reddy KR, et al. Association between intestinal microbiota collected at hospital admission and outcomes of patients with cirrhosis. Clin Gastroenterol Hepatol 2019;17(4):756–65.e3.

56. Sung CM, Chen KF, Lin Y, et al. Predicting clinical Outcomes of cirrhosis patients with hepatic encephalopathy from the fecal microbiome. Cell Mol Gastroenterol Hepatol 2019;8(2):301–18.e2.

57. Zhang Z, Zhai H, Geng J, et al. Large-scale survey of gut microbiota associated with MHE via 16S rRNA-based pyrosequencing. Am J Gastroenterol 2013; 108(10):1601–11.

58. Rai R, Saraswat VA, Dhiman RK. Gut microbiota: its role in hepatic encephalopathy. J Clin Exp Hepatol 2015;5(S1):S29–36.

59. Hansen BA, Vilstrup H. Increased intestinal hydrolysis of urea in patients with alcoholic cirrhosis. Scand J Gastroenterol 1985;20(3):346–50.

60. Tripathi A, Debelius J, Brenner DA, et al. The gut-liver axis and the intersection with the microbiome. Nat Rev Gastroenterol Hepatol 2018;15(7):397–411.

61. Ponziani FR, Bhoori S, Castelli C, et al. Hepatocellular carcinoma is associated with gut microbiota profile and inflammation in nonalcoholic fatty liver disease. Hepatology 2019;69(1):107–20.

62. Ren Z, Li A, Jiang J, et al. Gut microbiome analysis as a tool towards targeted non-invasive biomarkers for early hepatocellular carcinoma. Gut 2019;68(6): 1014–23.

63. Grąt M, Wronka KM, Krasnodębski M, et al. Profile of gut microbiota associated with the presence of hepatocellular cancer in patients with liver cirrhosis. Transplant Proc 2016;48(5):1687–91.

64. Liu Q, Li F, Zhuang Y, et al. Alteration in gut microbiota associated with hepatitis B and non-hepatitis virus related hepatocellular carcinoma. Gut Pathog 2019; 11(1):1.

65. Tao X, Wang N, Qin W. Gut microbiota and hepatocellular carcinoma. Gastrointest Tumors 2015;2(1):33–40.

66. Santiago A, Pozuelo M, Poca M, et al. Alteration of the serum microbiome composition in cirrhotic patients with ascites. Sci Rep 2016;6:25001.

67. Tandon P, Garcia-Tsao G. Bacterial infections, sepsis, and multiorgan failure in cirrhosis. Semin Liver Dis 2008;28(1):26–42.

68. Quigley EMM, Gajula P. Recent advances in modulating the microbiome. F1000Res 2020;9. https://doi.org/10.12688/f1000research.20204.1.

69. Pérez-Cobas AE, Gosalbes MJ, Friedrichs A, et al. Gut microbiota disturbance during antibiotic therapy: a multi-omic approach. Gut 2013;62(11):1591–601.

70. Fujisaka S, Ussar S, Clish C, et al. Antibiotic effects on gut microbiota and metabolism are host dependent. J Clin Invest 2016;126(12):4430–43.

71. Zackular JP, Baxter NT, Iverson KD, et al. The gut microbiome modulates colon tumorigenesis. MBio 2013;4(6).

72. Langdon A, Crook N, Dantas G. The effects of antibiotics on the microbiome throughout development and alternative approaches for therapeutic modulation. Genome Med 2016;8(1). https://doi.org/10.1186/s13073-016-0294-z.

73. Miller MB, Bassler BL. Quorum sensing in bacteria. Annu Rev Microbiol 2001; 55(1):165–99.

74. Bender KO, Garland M, Ferreyra JA, et al. A small-molecule antivirulence agent for treating Clostridium difficile infection. Sci Transl Med 2015;7(306):306ra148.

75. Kirpich IA, Solovieva NV, Leikhter SN, et al. Probiotics restore bowel flora and improve liver enzymes in human alcohol-induced liver injury: a pilot study. Alcohol 2008;42(8):675–82.

76. Bajaj JS, Heuman DM, Hylemon PB, et al. Randomised clinical trial: lactobacillus GG modulates gut microbiome, metabolome and endotoxemia in patients with cirrhosis. Aliment Pharmacol Ther 2014;39(10):1113–25.

77. Xia X, Chen J, Xia J, et al. Role of probiotics in the treatment of minimal hepatic encephalopathy in patients with HBV-induced liver cirrhosis. J Int Med Res 2018;46(9):3596–604.

78. Román E, Nieto JC, Gely C, et al. Effect of a multistrain probiotic on cognitive function and risk of Falls in patients with cirrhosis: a randomized trial. Hepatol Commun 2019;3(5):632–45.

79. Dewulf EM, Cani PD, Claus SP, et al. Insight into the prebiotic concept: lessons from an exploratory, double blind intervention study with inulin-type fructans in obese women. Gut 2013;62(8):1112–21.

80. Macfarlane S, Macfarlane GT, Cummings JH. Review article: prebiotics in the gastrointestinal tract. Aliment Pharmacol Ther 2006;24(5):701–14.

81. Scorletti E, Afolabi PR, Miles EA, et al. Synbiotic alters fecal microbiomes, but not liver fat or fibrosis, in a randomized trial of patients with non-alcoholic fatty liver disease. Gastroenterology 2020. https://doi.org/10.1053/j.gastro.2020. 01.031.

82. Manzhalii E, Virchenko O, Falalyeyeva T, et al. Treatment efficacy of a probiotic preparation for non-alcoholic steatohepatitis: a pilot trial. J Dig Dis 2017;18(12): 698–703.

83. Bajaj JS, Idilman R, Mabudian L, et al. Diet affects gut microbiota and modulates hospitalization risk differentially in an international cirrhosis cohort. Hepatology 2018;68(1):234–47.

84. Bajaj JS, Torre A, Lara Rojas M, et al. Cognition and hospitalizations are linked with salivary and fecal microbiota in cirrhosis cohorts from USA and Mexico. Liver Int 2020;liv:14437.

85. Hajishengallis G. Immunomicrobial pathogenesis of periodontitis: keystones, pathobionts, and host response. Trends Immunol 2014;35(1):3–11.

86. Bajaj JS, Matin P, White MB, et al. Periodontal therapy favorably modulates the oral-gut-hepatic axis in cirrhosis. Am J Physiol Gastrointest Liver Physiol 2018; 315(5):G824–37.

87. Bajaj JS, Khoruts A. Microbiota changes and intestinal microbiota transplantation in liver diseases and cirrhosis. J Hepatol 2020. https://doi.org/10.1016/j. jhep.2020.01.017.

88. Allegretti JR, Kassam Z, Carrellas M, et al. Fecal microbiota transplantation in patients with primary sclerosing cholangitis: a pilot clinical trial. Am J Gastroenterol 2019;114(7):1071–9.

89. Philips CA, Phadke N, Ganesan K, et al. Corticosteroids, nutrition, pentoxifylline, or fecal microbiota transplantation for severe alcoholic hepatitis. Indian J Gastroenterol 2018;37(3):215–25.

90. Philips CA, Pande A, Shasthry SM, et al. Healthy donor fecal microbiota transplantation in steroid-ineligible severe alcoholic hepatitis: a pilot study. Clin Gastroenterol Hepatol 2017;15(4):600–2.

91. Ren YD, Ye ZS, Yang LZ, et al. Fecal microbiota transplantation induces hepatitis B virus e-antigen (HBeAg) clearance in patients with positive HBeAg after long-term antiviral therapy. Hepatology 2017;65(5):1765–8.

92. Bajaj JS, Kassam Z, Fagan A, et al. Fecal microbiota transplant from a rational stool donor improves hepatic encephalopathy: a randomized clinical trial. Hepatology 2017;66(6):1727–38.

93. Lv X-Y, Ding H-G, Zheng J-F, et al. Rifaximin improves survival in cirrhotic patients with refractory ascites: a real-world study. World J Gastroenterol 2020; 26(2):199–218.

94. Bajaj JS, Heuman DM, Sanyal AJ, et al. Modulation of the metabiome by rifaximin in patients with cirrhosis and minimal hepatic encephalopathy. PLoS One 2013;8(4):e60042.

95. Bajaj JS, Gillevet PM, Patel NR, et al. A longitudinal systems biology analysis of lactulose withdrawal in hepatic encephalopathy. Metab Brain Dis 2012;27(2): 205–15.

96. Sarangi AN, Goel A, Singh A, et al. Faecal bacterial microbiota in patients with cirrhosis and the effect of lactulose administration. BMC Gastroenterol 2017; 17(1):125.

97. Wang JY, Bajaj JS, Wang J Bin, et al. Lactulose improves cognition, quality of life, and gut microbiota in minimal hepatic encephalopathy: a multicenter, randomized controlled trial. J Dig Dis 2019;20(10):547–56.

98. Kaji K, Takaya H, Saikawa S, et al. Rifaximin ameliorates hepatic encephalopathy and endotoxemia without affecting the gut microbiome diversity. World J Gastroenterol 2017;23(47):8355–66.

99. Schulz C, Schütte K, Vilchez-Vargas R, et al. Long-term effect of rifaximin with and without lactulose on the active bacterial assemblages in the Proximal small bowel and Faeces in patients with minimal hepatic encephalopathy. Dig Dis 2019;37(2):161–9.

100. Bajaj JS, Acharya C, Sikaroodi M, et al. Cost-effectiveness of integrating gut microbiota analysis into hospitalisation prediction in cirrhosis. GastroHep 2020; 2(2):79–86.

Acute on Chronic Liver Failure: Definition and Implications

Ariel Aday, MD[a], Jacqueline G. O'Leary, MD, MPH[a,b,*]

KEYWORDS

- Acute on chronic liver failure • Cirrhosis • Dysbiosis • Organ failure • Liver transplant

KEY POINTS

- ACLF is a distinct entity unique from acute decompensation that requires underlying liver disease, occurs secondary to inflammation, and is defined by organ failures.
- Mortality is high in ACLF and increases with severity and number of organ failures.
- Given the increased risk for infection, proton pump inhibitors should be discontinued when clear indication is lacking.
- Identify and treat infections early, as each hour delay of antibiotic administration worsens outcome.
- Refer appropriate patients for liver transplant evaluation early to improve mortality.

INTRODUCTION

As the prevalence of chronic liver disease increases worldwide, more patients with chronic liver disease are hospitalized with complications of cirrhosis. Many complications of liver disease result in decompensation, defined as the development of hepatic encephalopathy, ascites, hepatorenal syndrome, or variceal hemorrhage. However, acute on chronic liver failure (ACLF) has arisen as a separate complication of liver disease, often occurring after a precipitating event, and heralding a high risk of short-term mortality. Although 3 main definitions exist, they all require organ failures with worsening mortality as the number of organ failures increases.

DEFINITIONS

ACLF is a unique condition distinct from acute liver failure (ALF) and acute decompensation (AD). ALF is an infrequent syndrome defined as acute liver injury within 8 weeks (fulminant) or 26 weeks (subfulminant) manifested by hepatic encephalopathy, coagulopathy (international normalized ratio [INR] $\geq$1.5), and jaundice (serum total bilirubin

[a] University of Texas Southwestern, 5323 Harry Hines Blvd, Dallas, TX 75390, USA; [b] Dallas Veterans Affairs Medical Center, 4500 South Lancaster Road, Dallas, TX 75216, USA
* Corresponding author. Dallas VA Medical Center, 4500 South Lancaster Road, Dallas, TX 75216.
E-mail address: dr_jackieo@yahoo.com

Clin Liver Dis 24 (2020) 521–534
https://doi.org/10.1016/j.cld.2020.04.004
1089-3261/20/Published by Elsevier Inc.

liver.theclinics.com

≥2 mg/dL) in a patient without preexisting liver disease, with the notable exception of Wilson disease.[1] AD refers to the new development of ascites, hepatic encephalopathy, hepatorenal syndrome, or variceal hemorrhage in a patient with underlying cirrhosis.[2] Although these symptoms are often present in patients with ACLF, AD only requires 1 of the aforementioned events, does not require any organ failure, and may or may not require hospital admission.

Consensus has been reached that ACLF is defined by the number and type of hepatic and extrahepatic organ failures and only occurs in patients with underlying liver disease. Although numerous nuanced definitions with even more prognostic scoring systems have been published worldwide,[3] 3 definitions predominate (**Table 1**).

The Asian Pacific Association for the Study of the Liver (APASL) was the first consensus group to define ACLF using the following criteria[4]:

1. Underlying liver disease, although cirrhosis is not required
2. Hepatic insult resulting in jaundice (defined as a serum bilirubin ≥5 mg/dL) and coagulopathy (INR ≥1.5)
3. Complicated within 4 weeks by ascites and/or hepatic encephalopathy

The APASL definition reflects the patient population most commonly seen in Asia, specifically, acute insults (eg, HBV reactivation), and hepatitis A virus (HAV), hepatitis D virus (HDV), or hepatitis E virus (HEV) superinfection occurring in patients with chronic HBV. Using these criteria, there is an estimated 25% to 37% 30-day mortality.[5]

Second, the European Association for the Study of the Liver (EASL) formed the Chronic Liver Failure (CLIF) consortium, which created the EASL-CLIF definition of ACLF.[6] Cirrhosis is a prerequisite, and the prognosis depends on the number of organ failures that develop (up to 6). Organ failures are defined as:

1. Liver failure if the serum total bilirubin is ≥ 12.0 mg/dL.
2. Kidney failure if the serum creatinine is ≥ 2.0 mg/dL or the patient requires dialysis.
3. Cerebral failure if the West-Haven grade of hepatic encephalopathy is 3 or 4.
4. Coagulation failure if the INR is ≥ 2.5 or platelets are ≤ 20×10^9/L.
5. Circulatory failure if a vasopressor (dopamine, dobutamine, epinephrine, or norepinephrine) or terlipressin is used.
6. Respiratory failure if the PaO/Fio_2 ratio is ≤ 200 or the SpO_2/Fio_2 ratio is ≤ 214.

The CLIF Consortium-Organ Failure scoring system (CLIF-C OF score) incorporates a grading system contingent on the number of organ failures present (**Fig. 1**):

- ACLF-1 occurs in patients with a single organ kidney failure, a single nonrenal organ failure with kidney dysfunction (serum creatine 1.5-1.9 mg/dL) and/or West Haven grade I-II hepatic encephalopathy, or a single cerebral failure with kidney dysfunction (serum creatine 1.5-1.9 mg/dL).
- ACLF-2 occurs in patients with 2 organ failures.
- ACLF-3 occurs in patients with 3 or more organ failures.

Using a prospective European cohort, hospitalized cirrhotic patients with acute decompensation were further characterized to assist in creation of diagnostic criteria, stages, and natural history. In addition to the characteristics used in their organ failure scoring system, other factors were found to play a significant role in patient prognosis with ACLF development[6]; prognosis declined as white blood cell count (WBC) at presentation increased. This finding was impactful even within the laboratory normal range, since patients with cirrhosis tend to have low WBCs count at baseline.[6] The probability of death was also higher in patients without a prior history of AD compared to those with a history of AD. Although this finding seems counterintuitive, the major

Table 1
Comparison of available definitions for acute on chronic liver failure

	APASL	EASL/CLIF	NACSELD
Definition and severity scoring	Hepatic insult resulting in jaundice (bilirubin ≥5 mg/dL) and coagulopathy (INR ≥1.5) complicated within 4 weeks by ascites and/or hepatic encephalopathy	Prognosis dependent on the number of organ failures that develop (up to 6 organs – liver, kidney, lung, cerebral, coagulation, circulation) Graded by number of organ failures present: • ACLF-1: kidney failure alone; another organ failure with kidney dysfunction* and/or hepatic encephalopathy;** or cerebral failure with kidney dysfunction.* • ACLF-2: 2 organ failures • ACLF-3: 3 or more organ failures	Prognosis dependent on the number of organ failures present; ACLF requires at least 2 organ failures
Cohort			
Inclusion criteria	• Chronic liver disease or Compensated cirrhosis	• Compensated and decompensated cirrhosis	• Cirrhosis with a complication necessitating hospital admission
Exclusion criteria	• Bacterial infections • History of hepatic decompensation	• Human immunodeficiency virus (HIV) infection • HCC outside Milan criteria • Severe, chronic diseases of extrahepatic origin • Elective/scheduled admissions	• HIV infection • Prior organ transplant • Untreated or widespread malignancies • Elective/scheduled admissions
Study design	Consensus group, observational	Prospective, observational study	Prospective, observational study
Comment	Common precipitants including reactivation HBV as well as superinfections with HAV, HDV, HEV	Unknown trigger in approximately 40% Alcoholic hepatitis and infections common	Infections included

* Kidney dysfunction defined as a serum creatinine 1.5-1.9 mg/dL.
** Hepatic encephalopathy defined here as West Haven grade I and II.

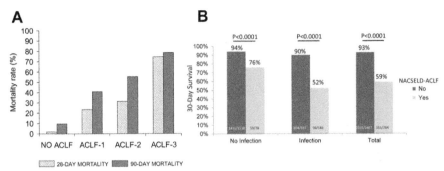

Fig. 1. (*A*) Mortality rate at 28 days and 90 days based on grade of the ACLF. (*B*) 30-day survival for infected and noninfected patients by NACSELD-ACLF. (*From* [*A*] Moreau R, et al. Acute-on-chronic liver failure is a distinct syndrome that develops in patients with acute decompensation of cirrhosis. Gastroenterology 2013;144(7):1426-37; with permission; and [*B*] O'Leary, J.G., et al., *NACSELD acute-on-chronic liver failure (NACSELD-ACLF) score predicts 30-day survival in hospitalized patients with cirrhosis.* Hepatology, 2018. **67**(6): p. 2367-2374; with permission.)

driver of ACLF is inflammation. As cirrhosis progresses, patients become functionally more immunocompromised. Therefore, the authors hypothesize that patients without a history of AD may have a more vigorous immunologic response to any given insult than patients with a history of prior AD.

To make the diagnosis more user friendly, the North American Consortium for the Study of End-stage Liver Disease (NACSELD) proposed and validated simplified criteria for ACLF based on organ failures (see **Fig. 1**)[7,8]:

1. Kidney failure was defined as requiring dialysis.
2. Brain failure was defined as West Haven grade 3 or 4 hepatic encephalopathy.
3. Respiratory failure was defined as requiring mechanical ventilation or bilevel positive airway pressure.
4. Circulatory failure was defined as the need for pressor support, mean arterial pressure less than 60 mm Hg, or a reduction in systolic blood pressure by 40 mm Hg from baseline despite adequate fluid resuscitation.

ACLF was defined as the development of 2 or more organ failures. This classification was developed using a prospective multicenter Canadian and American cohort of nonelectively admitted patients with cirrhosis who presented with or developed an infection during their index hospitalization.[7] These criteria were validated using a separate prospectively enrolled cohort of 2675 patients with and without infections.[8] As a result of this later analysis, this definition of ACLF was deemed valid in infected and uninfected cirrhotic patients. A separate group independently validated this definition on the nationwide inpatient sample of approximately 1.9 million admitted cirrhotic patients.[9] Although the study was performed using ICD (International Classification of Diseases)-9 codes, 31% of the patients were infected; 5.4% had ACLF, and the c-statistic remained high at 0.75. Of note, nonalcoholic steatohepatitis (NASH) appears to be the most rapidly growing etiology of ACLF in this region of the world.[10]

These 3 groups use definitions largely reflective of the types of underlying liver disease and precipitating events seen in their respective regions.[2] Given the ambiguity and heterogeneity in diagnostic criteria for ACLF between the 3 groups, a consensus conference proposed classifying ACLF into 3 subtypes based on the severity of underlying liver disease (type A noncirrhotic, type B compensated cirrhosis, and type C decompensated cirrhosis).[3] Consensus was reached on the common precipitants of all subtypes, which are viral infection, superinfection or reactivation, alcohol consumption, drug-induced liver injury, ischemia, surgery, and sepsis. In addition, consensus was also reached on the final common pathway toward ACLF of these subtypes being mediated by inflammation and resulting in organ failure(s), and that the number and type of organ failures determine outcome.

Regardless of how ACLF is defined, the number of hospitalizations for patients that have or develop ACLF is growing nationwide.[11] This rise is occurring on the backbone of an increasing rate of admissions and readmissions for patients with cirrhosis. Of note, half of patients with cirrhosis admitted to the hospital experience readmission within 90 days.[12] Patients at highest risk for readmission in multivariable modeling had higher model for end-stage liver disease (MELD) scores at index admission, diabetes, and hepatic encephalopathy; those taking prophylactic antibiotics and those who had nosocomial infections during index hospitalization also had a high risk of readmission.

Precipitating factors for ACLF are only identified in 50% of cases and often do not predict prognosis even when recognized.[13] Infections are frequent precipitants of hospital admission and readmissions; notably, one-third of hospitalized patients with cirrhosis either present with or develop infections during their admission and on readmission.[14,15] There can be an exaggerated immunologic response to infection, which can lead to organ failure. After successful resolution of infection, the compensatory anti-inflammatory response syndrome (CARS) can create an immune paralysis.[16] This immune dysregulation leaves patients vulnerable to subsequent infections.[17] In fact, 45% of patients discharged from the hospital after successful treatment of an infection develop another infection over the next 3 months. Because three-quarters of these infections occur in a different location from the first infection, it is believed that subsequent infection is caused by an increased susceptibility to infection and not inadequate treatment from the first infection.[18] Risk factors for recurrent infections include older age, proton-pump inhibitor (PPI) use, development of the first infection while on spontaneous bacterial peritonitis (SBP) prophylaxis, and a higher MELD score at admission.

Given the detrimental effects infections have on prognosis, early initiation of primary SBP prophylaxis is tempting. However, as patients with cirrhosis live longer, there has been an increase in multidrug resistant infections in this population.[19] When outcomes of admitted patients on primary versus secondary SBP prophylaxis were compared after propensity score matching for admission MELD and serum albumin, patients on primary prophylaxis had a worse outcome than those on secondary prophylaxis.[20] Specifically, they had a higher risk for acute kidney injury (AKI), death, and liver transplant. Therefore it is essential to strictly adhere to the guidelines for initiation of primary SBP prophylaxis[21]: ascites total protein of no more than 1.5 g/dL and Child-Turcotte-Pugh score of at least 9 and serum total bilirubin of at least 3 mg/dL or serum creatinine of at least 1.2 mg/dL, serum Na no more than 130 meq/L or serum urea nitrogen (BUN) of at least 25 mg/dL. In addition, there is an urgent need to identify agents for use in patients who fail primary or secondary SBP prophylaxis. In the future, it will be essential to develop new ways of preventing infections without the use of antibiotics. Established methods to reduce healthcare-associated infections in these patients should be employed aggressively on admission, including avoidance of urinary catheter placement unless clearly indicated and prompt removal when clinically appropriate, avoidance of long-term indwelling central line catheters, and avoidance of initiation of PPI therapy unless strongly indicated.[22]

RISK FACTORS FOR ACUTE ON CHRONIC LIVER FAILURE

Cirrhotic patients are at risk for ACLF for many reasons. First, cirrhotic patients have gut microbiome dysbiosis, which progressively worsens as liver disease progresses.[23] The cirrhotic dysbiosis ratio (CBR) or the ratio of good bacteria to bad bacteria was developed to evaluate the severity of dysbiosis in this population, and it was demonstrated that this ratio progressively declines from normal outpatients, to compensated outpatients, to decompensated outpatients, and is worst in cirrhotic inpatients.[24] Of note, this ratio is also worse in patients with NASH compared with other types of liver disease. However, although highly correlated with the severity of liver disease, it has never been shown to cause progression of liver disease, nor have alterations been associated with altered outcomes.

Second, not only do patients with cirrhosis have dysbiosis, but they are at risk for small intestinal bacterial overgrowth (SIBO). Risk factors for SIBO include[25] advancing age, antisecretory drugs, altered intestinal motility, and fatty liver. Cirrhotic patients have significant delays in gastric emptying and small bowel transit time at baseline, and this dysmotility worsens with decompensation.[26] Bacterial translocation is seen more commonly in patients with cirrhosis, especially when there is evidence of portal hypertension, which allows the dysbiotic gut microbiota to capitalize on the intestinal permeability as a gateway into the systemic circulation where further damage can be deployed on the poorly armed immune system.[27]

Third, patients with cirrhosis are functionally immunocompromised. The majority of the reticuloendothelial system is located within the liver, where the normal function is to clear endotoxins, bacteria, and cytokines. With portosystemic shunting, blood is directed away from the liver, resulting in disruption of this essential housekeeping function. Furthermore, there are also impairments in intrinsic factors crucial to normal immune function including phagocytosis and chemotaxis.[28]

GUT-HEPATIC ACCESS

The role of intestinal bacteria and their biproducts has garnered increasing attention in the cirrhotic patient population largely because of investigations to better understand the gut-liver access and implications. The intestinal microbiome composition has been shown to be associated with adverse outcomes in patients with cirrhosis. Specifically, increased abundance of the taxa Proteobacteria (Enterobacteriaceae, Campylobacteriaceae, and Pasteurellaceae) on admission has been associated with an increased risk of extra-hepatic organ failure, ACLF and death.[29] Intestinal products also influence hepatic lipid metabolism, glucose regulation, and bile acid synthesis, which play contributory roles in influencing microbial composition in the gut.[30] Normal hepatic function serves as the first stop in filtration and detoxification of circulating bacterial biproducts, but this defense mechanism is impaired in cirrhotic patients, allowing for entry into the systemic circulation and resulting in an inflammatory response.[31] With increases in intestinal permeability, this inflammatory cascade can cause or exacerbate decompensation and/or ACLF.

PREVENTION OF ACUTE ON CHRONIC LIVER FAILURE

Because the outcome of ACLF is poor, it is essential to identify mechanisms for prevention. This section highlights suggested ways to mitigate the risk of ACLF development in patients with cirrhosis.

Discontinue Proton Pump Inhibitors

Most patients with cirrhosis are on a PPI for an unknown reason or poor indication. PPIs block the oxidative burst of the neutrophil, thereby causing further immuno-suppression in an already immunocompromised host.[32] Many patients are started on a PPI while hospitalized either as prophylaxis or during a gastrointestinal (GI) bleed. As a result, they can and should be discontinued whenever possible. Of note, H2 blockers do not cause immunosuppression, and therefore when acid suppression is required, H2 blockers are a good alternative.[33] PPIs are associated with higher rates of readmission independent of comorbidities, other medications, age, and admission MELD.[34] PPIs also alter the gut microbiome; initiation increases the oral-origin microbiota, which are more pathogenic, and discontinuation de-creases these bacteria in overall composition.[34] Discontinuing PPIs in patients without clear indications for them will lower patients' risk for infection and readmissions.[18,33,34]

Use Nonselective Beta-Blockers as Primary Prophylaxis for Variceal Bleeding

Options include: propranolol, nadolol, and carvedilol. Although banding to obliteration and nonselective beta-blocker (NSBB) use are both considered equally efficacious as primary prophylaxis for variceal bleeding, NSBB use is more cost-effective and may improve outcome in patients with ACLF.[35,36] Endoscopic screening for varices is indi-cated in patients with cirrhosis with platelets less than 150×10^9/L or with a liver stiff-ness measurement (LSM) of greater than 20 kPa on ultrasound elastography.[36] Primary prophylaxis should be started in all patients with CTP class A and B cirrhosis with large varices and all patients with CTP class C cirrhosis with small or large vari-ces.[36] However, emerging data have shown patients with compensated cirrhosis and clinically significant portal hypertension (defined by hepatic venous pressure gradient [HVPG]) had a lower risk for decompensation when randomized to an NSBB.[37] This is supported by meta-analysis data showing a lower risk for clinical events (ascites, var-iceal hemorrhage, or encephalopathy) in patients who have an HVPG response to NSBBs.[38] Although NSBBs have proven efficacy, some patients are not candidates for treatment with them. Patients with ascites with either a systolic blood pressure less than 90 mm Hg or type 2 hepatorenal syndrome are at increased risk for death from NSBB use, and therefore cannot be treated with NSBBs.[39] Especially during admission, NSBB should be discontinued in patients with a low MAP, but reinitiated once the MAP increases.[40]

When selecting an NSBB consider:

a. Propranolol is the least effective and combined with its inconvenient dosing often leads to noncompliance.
b. Nadolol is conveniently dosed once per day, and its lower central nervous system penetration decreases the risk for depression.
c. Carvedilol is the most potent NSBB because of its alpha component; however, this feature can also exacerbate volume overload in CTP B and C patients. Therefore, carvedilol is usually reserved for CTP A patients.[41]

NSBBs have even been found beneficial in patients with ACLF; patients admitted on NSBB had improved 28-mortality.[35] In addition, a trial of 136 patients with ACLF and no or small varices but HVPG of at least 12 showed patients randomized to carvedilol had a lower risk for AKI, SBP, and 28-day mortality but not 90-day mortality.[42]

Although the precise mechanism for improved outcomes in patients with ACLF on NSBBs is unknown, NSBBs have been shown to decrease intestinal permeability and therefore may decrease the translocation of dysbiotic bacteria into the systemic circulation that may initiate or exacerbate SIRS.[43]

Diagnose and Treat Renal Dysfunction Early

Cirrhotic patients live and die by their kidneys. The new definition of AKI in patients with cirrhosis is an increase in serum creatinine of at least 0.3 mg/dL in 48 hours or an increase in serum creatinine of at least 1.5 fold over baseline.[44,45] Even with complete resolution, a small short-term increase can have a lasting negative impact on prognosis. Similarly, even a peak serum creatinine of less than 1.5 mg/dL can be harmful and worsen prognosis.[46] Although all increases in serum creatinine negatively impact prognosis, some are worse than others.[47] AKI-hepatorenal syndrome (AKI-HRS) and infection-related AKI have the worst prognosis and similar prognostic implications, and parenchymal nephropathy has the least impact on patient survival.[48] However, both have the same impact on the MELD score, which is likely why the MELD score currently has lower predictive power than in the past.[49]

When AKI occurs, it is essential to eliminate all nephrotoxins including nonsteroidal anti-inflammatory drugs (NSAIDS) and aspirin, stop diuretics, and ensure the patient is not intravascularly depleted.[44] A low threshold to initiate intravenous albumin therapy should be utilized even in patients with extravascular hypervolemia, as it is the first-line therapy for AKI, even in patients whose peak creatinine is less than 1.0 mg/dL.[44]

In patients with more advanced AKI with AKI-HRS, vasopressors (terlipressin is first-line treatment in countries where it is available, and norepinephrine is first-line treatment in countries where it is not) in combination with intravenous albumin are indicated.[44,50] This is because vasopressors have been proven superior to midodrine, octreotide and intravenous albumin therapy.[51]

Patients who require dialysis should be considered for liver transplantation. However, in inpatients with decompensated cirrhosis who are not liver transplant candidates, dialysis is most often considered futile, because[52] these patients cannot be adequately dialyzed as an outpatient secondary to low blood pressure limiting fluid removal, and the mortality is approximately 90% at 3 months.

Identify and Treat Infections Early

Most infected cirrhotic patients do not mount a fever, and up to one-third of patients with SBP are asymptomatic. As a result, it is imperative to have a high level of suspicion for an infection when any new symptom of decompensation or organ failure develops. Every hour antibiotics are delayed increases mortality,[53] and therefore, prompt work-up followed by swift antibiotic administration is essential.

Nosocomial infections are frequent (approximately 15%) and increase the risk for death in admitted patients with cirrhosis. Nosocomial infections occur more frequently in patients admitted with an infection, those with an admission MELD greater than 20, those with SIRS, and those taking PPIs, rifaximin, and/or lactulose.[54] Recurrent infections after discharge occur in almost half of admitted cirrhotic patients, but because three-fourths of these infections occur in a different location than the first infection, it simply reflects the host's inability to fight infection rather than a failure of therapy.[18]

Use Intravenous Albumin When Indicated

Intravenous albumin was first used to treat ascites and edema in patients with cirrhosis in 1946 with some success.[55] Patients with cirrhosis not only have inadequate levels but poor quality albumin.[56] Of late, a resurgence of interest in expanding the indication for use of intravenous albumin has occurred. The recent ANSWER trial documented improved mortality in 440 cirrhotic outpatients with uncomplicated ascites over 18 months with chronic outpatient administration of 40 g of intravenous albumin weekly (hazard ratio [HR] = 0.62; 95% confidence interval [CI] 0.40–0.95).[57] This concept is under further study in the PRECIOSA trial of weight-based (up to 100 g) intravenous albumin treatment every 10 days to patients with uncomplicated ascites and recent hospital admission.[58] Of note, in the published pilot-PRECIOSA study, high-dose intravenous albumin improved circulatory function and left ventricular function and reduced plasma levels of multiple cytokines without increasing portal pressures.

Currently, intravenous albumin is an approved therapy for several indications:

- To prevent paracentesis-induced circulatory dysfunction (PICD) when more than 5 L are removed during a paracentesis
- To prevent AKI in patients with SBP
- To treat AKI

Other unapproved indications include:

- Treatment of hospitalized patients with non-SBP infections to improve survival[59]
- Use in combination with diuretics to improve volume status and prevent renal dysfunction
- Treatment of hyponatremia[60]
- To prevent PICD when less than 5 L are removed during a paracentesis in patients with ACLF[61]

Relative Adrenal Insufficiency

A single prospective clinical trial of admitted cirrhotic patients found almost half had relative adrenal insufficiency. Unfortunately, relative adrenal insufficiency increased the risk for death and doubled the risk for ACLF.[62] Therefore, one should be hypervigilant to ensure this diagnosis is made early in a patient's course.

ACUTE ON CHRONIC LIVER FAILURE AND LIVER TRANSPLANTATION

Given the high mortality and decrease in transplant-free survival once ACLF develops, liver transplantation remains an important rescue therapy for many individuals.[6,8] Some ACLF patients who meet criteria for transplant have higher mortality after transplant compared to those transplanted without ACLF.[63] The severity of ACLF appears to have a negative impact on outcomes after liver transplant, with ACLF grade 3 having the most profound negative impact. In a retrospective study of 72,316 admissions for decompensated cirrhosis in the Veterans Affairs (VA) system spanning over a decade, 26% of admissions met EASL-CLIF criteria for ACLF. Higher mortality was associated with older age, white race, HCC, MELD-Na, and admission to a nontransplant facility. Furthermore, over the 10-year period, ACLF prevalence decreased, while mortality for ACLF-3 increased.[64] Selection of candidates for transplant and post-transplant outcomes are also negatively impacted by the number of organ failures present during an episode of ACLF. Although consistent data show that increasing numbers of organ failures result in increased costs after transplant, most (but not all) data show an increased risk for death after transplant with ACLF grade 3.[63,65–67] In a prospective multinational study performed by NACSELD, 2793 cirrhotic patients were hospitalized, 27.5% were listed for transplant, and 35% of those listed underwent a liver transplant. The patients who were listed were more likely to be younger, have ACLF, AKI, and a higher MELD than the nonlisted patients. ACLF was most prevalent in the dead or delisted patients. In this study, despite the ACLF group having higher preliver transplant creatinine and perioperative dialysis, the postliver transplant creatinine at 3- and 6-month follow-up was no different than those transplanted patients without ACLF exhibiting excellent renal recovery in both groups.[68] Of note, stabilization with ACLF resolution[67] or sepsis resolution[66] or improvement in MELD may mitigate the increased mortality.[8,69]

SUMMARY

There are significant challenges in appropriately identifying and managing patients with ACLF given rising rates of hospitalizations and high mortality rates. Prevention of ACLF is only possible if clinicians are aware of this clinical entity and its implications. As the outcome can be poor, preventive strategies in patients with cirrhosis are crucial and include:

- Early identification of infections
- Discontinuation of PPI therapy when clear ongoing need is not found and removal of indwelling catheters unless strongly indicated
- Use of intravenous albumin for volume expansion per guidelines
- Early diagnosis and treatment of AKI
- NSBB use for primary prophylaxis of variceal hemorrhage whenever possible

Current available definitions of ACLF allow clinicians to stratify these patients in order to target therapeutic approaches and make more accurate assessments of prognosis. Reassessments throughout the disease course should be implemented in order to select for patients who may benefit from tertiary interventions such as transplant, and those who have reached medical futility. Multiple organ failures can develop rapidly and portend poor outcomes, thus necessitating close monitoring and potentially early transfer to a tertiary care center as transplant has been shown to be a viable option in highly selected patients. Further investigations are needed to elucidate if there is a beneficial response to steroid supplementation in patients with relative adrenal insufficiency, which remains common. Future therapeutic targets may need to address the detrimental effects of intestinal dysbiosis and the impaired systemic inflammatory response in these patients.

REFERENCES

1. Stravitz RT, Lee WM. Acute liver failure. Lancet 2019;394(10201):869–81.
2. Gustot T, Moreau R. Acute-on-chronic liver failure vs. traditional acute decompensation of cirrhosis. J Hepatol 2018;69(6):1384–93.
3. Jalan R, et al. Toward an improved definition of acute-on-chronic liver failure. Gastroenterology 2014;147(1):4–10.
4. Sarin SK, et al. Acute-on-chronic liver failure: consensus recommendations of the Asian Pacific Association for the study of the liver (APASL). Hepatol Int 2009;3(1):269–82.
5. Dhiman RK, et al. Chronic liver failure-Sequential organ failure assessment is better than the Asia-Pacific association for the study of liver criteria for defining acute-on-chronic liver failure and predicting outcome. World J Gastroenterol 2014;20(40):14934–41.
6. Moreau R, et al. Acute-on-chronic liver failure is a distinct syndrome that develops in patients with acute decompensation of cirrhosis. Gastroenterology 2013;144(7):1426–37.
7. Bajaj JS, et al. Survival in infection-related acute-on-chronic liver failure is defined by extrahepatic organ failures. Hepatology 2014;60(1):250–6.

8. O'Leary JG, et al. NACSELD acute-on-chronic liver failure (NACSELD-ACLF) score predicts 30-day survival in hospitalized patients with cirrhosis. Hepatology 2018;67(6):2367–74.

9. Rosenblatt R, S.Z., Tafesh Z, et al. Oral abstracts (Abstract 284): validating the results of the NACSELD-ACLF score using a nationally-representative inpatient database. Hepatology 2018;68(S1):1–74A.

10. Axley P, et al. NASH is the most rapidly growing etiology for acute-on-chronic liver failure-related hospitalization and disease burden in the United States: a population-based study. Liver Transpl 2019;25(5):695–705.

11. Allen AM, et al. Time trends in the health care burden and mortality of acute on chronic liver failure in the United States. Hepatology 2016;64(6):2165–72.

12. Bajaj JS, et al. The 3-month readmission rate remains unacceptably high in a large North American cohort of patients with cirrhosis. Hepatology 2016;64(1):200–8.

13. Hernaez R, et al. Acute-on-chronic liver failure: an update. Gut 2017;66(3):541–53.

14. Bajaj JS, et al. Second infections independently increase mortality in hospitalized patients with cirrhosis: the North American consortium for the study of end-stage liver disease (NACSELD) experience. Hepatology 2012;56(6):2328–35.

15. Tapper EB, Halbert B, Mellinger J. Rates of and reasons for hospital readmissions in patients with cirrhosis: a multistate population-based cohort study. Clin Gastroenterol Hepatol 2016;14(8):1181–8.

16. Jalan R, et al. Acute-on chronic liver failure. J Hepatol 2012;57(6):1336–48.

17. Fernandez J, Gustot T. Management of bacterial infections in cirrhosis. J Hepatol 2012;56(Suppl 1):S1–12.

18. O'Leary JG, et al. Long-term use of antibiotics and proton pump inhibitors predict development of infections in patients with cirrhosis. Clin Gastroenterol Hepatol 2015;13(4):753–9.

19. Fernandez J, et al. Multidrug-resistant bacterial infections in patients with decompensated cirrhosis and with acute-on-chronic liver failure in Europe. J Hepatol 2019;70(3):398–411.

20. Bajaj JS, et al. Outcomes in patients with cirrhosis on primary compared to secondary prophylaxis for spontaneous bacterial peritonitis. Am J Gastroenterol 2019;114(4):599–606.

21. Runyon BA, A.P.G. Committee. Management of adult patients with ascites due to cirrhosis: an update. Hepatology 2009;49(6):2087–107.

22. Sargenti K, et al. Healthcare-associated and nosocomial bacterial infections in cirrhosis: predictors and impact on outcome. Liver Int 2015;35(2):391–400.

23. Bajaj JS, et al. Altered profile of human gut microbiome is associated with cirrhosis and its complications. J Hepatol 2014;60(5):940–7.

24. Rai R, Saraswat VA, Dhiman RK. Gut microbiota: its role in hepatic encephalopathy. J Clin Exp Hepatol 2015;5(Suppl 1):S29–36.

25. Shanab AA, et al. Small intestinal bacterial overgrowth in nonalcoholic steatohepatitis: association with toll-like receptor 4 expression and plasma levels of interleukin 8. Dig Dis Sci 2011;56(5):1524–34.

26. Chander Roland B, et al. Decompensated cirrhotics have slower intestinal transit times as compared with compensated cirrhotics and healthy controls. J Clin Gastroenterol 2013;47(10):888–93.

27. Acharya C,, Bajaj JS. Altered microbiome in patients with cirrhosis and complications. Clin Gastroenterol Hepatol 2019;17(2):307–21.

28. Bonnel AR, Bunchorntavakul C, Reddy KR. Immune dysfunction and infections in patients with cirrhosis. Clin Gastroenterol Hepatol 2011;9(9):727–38.
29. Bajaj JS, et al. Association between intestinal microbiota collected at hospital admission and outcomes of patients with cirrhosis. Clin Gastroenterol Hepatol 2019;17(4):756–65.
30. Tripathi A, et al. The gut-liver axis and the intersection with the microbiome. Nat Rev Gastroenterol Hepatol 2018;15(7):397–411.
31. Fukui H. Gut-liver axis in liver cirrhosis: how to manage leaky gut and endotoxemia. World J Hepatol 2015;7(3):425–42.
32. Garcia-Martinez I, et al. Use of proton pump inhibitors decrease cellular oxidative burst in patients with decompensated cirrhosis. J Gastroenterol Hepatol 2015; 30(1):147–54.
33. Bajaj JS, et al. Proton pump inhibitors are associated with a high rate of serious infections in veterans with decompensated cirrhosis. Aliment Pharmacol Ther 2012;36(9):866–74.
34. Bajaj JS, et al. Proton pump inhibitor initiation and withdrawal affects gut microbiota and readmission risk in cirrhosis. Am J Gastroenterol 2018;113(8):1177–86.
35. Mookerjee RP, et al. Treatment with non-selective beta blockers is associated with reduced severity of systemic inflammation and improved survival of patients with acute-on-chronic liver failure. J Hepatol 2016;64(3):574–82.
36. Garcia-Tsao G, et al. Portal hypertensive bleeding in cirrhosis: risk stratification, diagnosis, and management: 2016 practice guidance by the American Association for the study of liver diseases. Hepatology 2017;65(1):310–35.
37. Villanueva C, et al. Beta blockers to prevent decompensation of cirrhosis in patients with clinically significant portal hypertension (PREDESCI): a randomised, double-blind, placebo-controlled, multicentre trial. Lancet 2019;393(10181): 1597–608.
38. Turco L, et al. Lowering portal pressure improves outcomes of patients with cirrhosis, with or without ascites: a meta-analysis. Clin Gastroenterol Hepatol 2020;18(2):313–27.
39. Serste T, et al. Deleterious effects of beta-blockers on survival in patients with cirrhosis and refractory ascites. Hepatology 2010;52(3):1017–22.
40. Bhutta AQ, et al. Beta-blockers in hospitalised patients with cirrhosis and ascites: mortality and factors determining discontinuation and reinitiation. Aliment Pharmacol Ther 2018;47(1):78–85.
41. Giannelli V, et al. Beta-blockers in liver cirrhosis. Ann Gastroenterol 2014; 27(1):20–6.
42. Kumar M, et al. Treatment with carvedilol improves survival of patients with acute-on-chronic liver failure: a randomized controlled trial. Hepatol Int 2019;13(6): 800–13.
43. Reiberger T, et al. Non-selective betablocker therapy decreases intestinal permeability and serum levels of LBP and IL-6 in patients with cirrhosis. J Hepatol 2013; 58(5):911–21.
44. Angeli P, et al. Diagnosis and management of acute kidney injury in patients with cirrhosis: revised consensus recommendations of the International Club of Ascites. J Hepatol 2015;62(4):968–74.
45. Wong F, et al. New consensus definition of acute kidney injury accurately predicts 30-day mortality in patients with cirrhosis and infection. Gastroenterology 2013; 145(6):1280–8.
46. Wong F, et al. A cut-off serum creatinine value of 1.5 mg/dL for AKI–to be or not to be. J Hepatol 2015;62(3):741–3.

47. Wong F, et al. Acute kidney injury in cirrhosis: baseline serum creatinine predicts patient outcomes. Am J Gastroenterol 2017;112(7):1103–10.
48. Martin-Llahi M, et al. Prognostic importance of the cause of renal failure in patients with cirrhosis. Gastroenterology 2011;140(2):488–96.
49. Godfrey EL, et al. The decreasing predictive power of MELD in an era of changing etiology of liver disease. Am J Transplant 2019;19(12):3299–307.
50. Singh V, et al. Noradrenaline vs. terlipressin in the treatment of hepatorenal syndrome: a randomized study. J Hepatol 2012;56(6):1293–8.
51. Israelsen M, et al. Terlipressin versus other vasoactive drugs for hepatorenal syndrome. Cochrane Database Syst Rev 2017;(9):CD011532.
52. Allegretti AS, et al. Prognosis of patients with cirrhosis and AKI who initiate RRT. Clin J Am Soc Nephrol 2018;13(1):16–25.
53. Seymour CW, et al. Time to treatment and mortality during mandated emergency care for sepsis. N Engl J Med 2017;376(23):2235–44.
54. Bajaj JS, et al. Nosocomial infections are frequent and negatively impact outcomes in hospitalized patients with cirrhosis. Am J Gastroenterol 2019;114(7):1091–100.
55. Gw T, Sh A, Vd D. Chemical, clinical and immunologic studies on the produce of human plasma fractionation. The use of salt-poor concentrated human serum albumin solution in the treatment of hepatic cirrhosis. J Clin Invest 1946;25:304–23.
56. Garcia-Martinez R, et al. Albumin: pathophysiologic basis of its role in the treatment of cirrhosis and its complications. Hepatology 2013;58(5):1836–46.
57. Caraceni P, et al. Long-term albumin administration in decompensated cirrhosis (ANSWER): an open-label randomised trial. Lancet 2018;391(10138):2417–29.
58. Fernandez J, et al. Effects of albumin treatment on systemic and portal hemodynamics and systemic inflammation in patients with decompensated cirrhosis. Gastroenterology 2019;157(1):149–62.
59. Guevara M, et al. Albumin for bacterial infections other than spontaneous bacterial peritonitis in cirrhosis. A randomized, controlled study. J Hepatol 2012;57(4):759–65.
60. Bajaj JS, et al. The impact of albumin use on resolution of hyponatremia in hospitalized patients with cirrhosis. Am J Gastroenterol 2018;113(9):1339.
61. Arora V, et al. Paracentesis-induced circulatory dysfunction with modest-volume paracentesis is partly ameliorated by albumin infusion in ACLF. Hepatology 2020. [Epub ahead of print].
62. Piano S, et al. Including relative adrenal insufficiency in definition and classification of acute-on-chronic liver failure. Clin Gastroenterol Hepatol 2020. [Epub ahead of print].
63. Levesque E, et al. Impact of acute-on-chronic liver failure on 90-day mortality following a first liver transplantation. Liver Int 2017;37(5):684–93.
64. Hernaez R, et al. Prevalence and short-term mortality of acute-on-chronic liver failure: a national cohort study from the USA. J Hepatol 2019;70(4):639–47.
65. Bahirwani R, et al. Factors that predict short-term intensive care unit mortality in patients with cirrhosis. Clin Gastroenterol Hepatol 2013;11(9):1194–200.
66. Artru F, et al. Liver transplantation in the most severely ill cirrhotic patients: a multicenter study in acute-on-chronic liver failure grade 3. J Hepatol 2017;67(4):708–15.
67. Gustot T, et al. Clinical course of acute-on-chronic liver failure syndrome and effects on prognosis. Hepatology 2015;62(1):243–52.

68. O'Leary JG, et al. Outcomes after listing for liver transplant in patients with acute-on-chronic liver failure: the Multicenter North American Consortium for the study of end-stage liver disease experience. Liver Transpl 2019;25(4):571–9.

69. Huebener P, et al. Stabilisation of acute-on-chronic liver failure patients before liver transplantation predicts post-transplant survival. Aliment Pharmacol Ther 2018;47(11):1502–10.

Printed and bound by CPI Group (UK) Ltd, Croydon, CR0 4YY

03/10/2024

01040407-0005